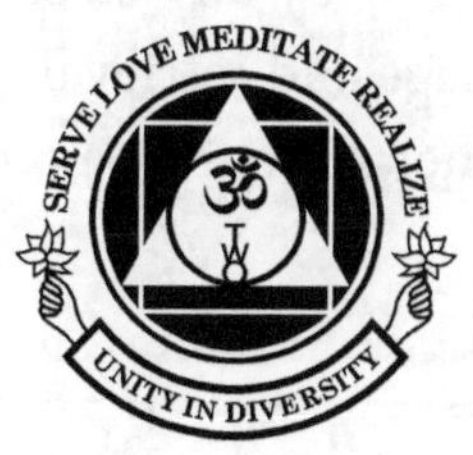


YOGA AND VEDANTA METHODS FOR HOLISTIC HEALTH

# YOGA SADHANA for *Self* healing

*Text and compilation by*
Swami Sitaramananda

SIVANANDA YOGA VEDANTA CENTER

First Edition: 2025

ISBN: 978-1-6086-9292-7
Library of Congress Control Number: 2025936603

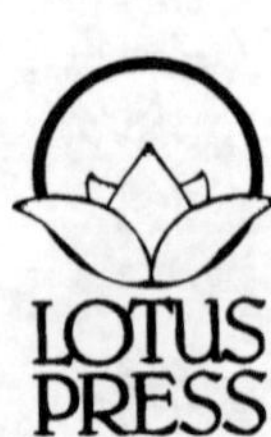


Published by:
**Lotus Press**
P.O. Box 325
Twin Lakes, WI 53181
www.lotuspress.com | lotuspress@lotuspress.com
Ph: (262) 889-8561

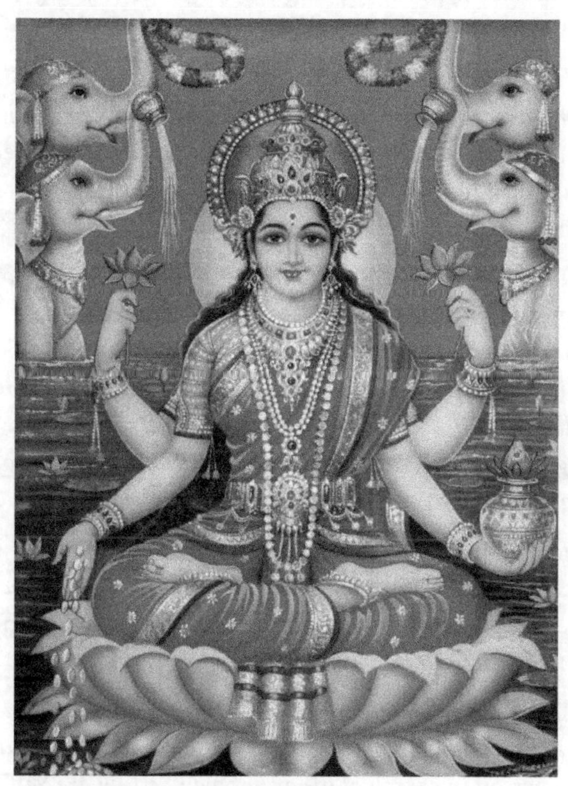

*In service of the seekers after Truth and Bliss and students of Yoga and Vedanta*

# Preface

*The Sivananda teaching is a traditional Yogic teaching coming through a lineage of Yoga Masters, including Swami Sivananda and Swami Vishnudevananda.*

*Master Sivananda's approach to Yoga, the synthesis of Yoga, is well-rounded and practical, written in almost 300 books.*

*Swami Vishnudevananda, founder of the International Sivananda Yoga Vedanta Centers, taught students in both the East and West, giving innumerable lectures and writing two bestselling books:* The Complete Illustrated Book of Yoga *and* Meditation and Mantras. *His teachings are practical, humorous, and well-suited to modern life.*

*In this book, you will learn the essentials, the basic aspects of this profound spiritual, mental and physical self-healing. Later on, if you want to know more, you will have to dive deeper—for example, learn to heal yourself while teaching Yoga asanas and holistic lifestyle in the Sivananda Yoga Teachers Training Course and after, take the deeper, 800-hour Sivananda Yoga Health Education Training course to become a Yoga Health Educator and instrument in the process of empowerment of people to heal themselves and to be free from suffering.*

*There are many books on Self-healing and Self-realization, as well as a host of materials on the process of healing. This book, however, attempts to addresses a deeper spiritual and Vedantic approach to health and healing, in a practical way, from the viewpoint of conscious training of the practitioner.*

*It is about Yoga's specific way of seeing Health and about the process of Self-healing, the journey home to completeness of being. It is about the process of awakening for a person in search of his or her own Self-aware Self, more known as the process of Self-Realization.*

*There are many Vedic and Vedantic scriptures or teachings by spiritual teachers available today. However, I obtained this knowledge from my specific lineage of spiritual knowledge stemming from Adi Sankaracharya (8th century AD) and many books and writings of my Master Swami Sivananda, as taught and infused with the shakti of devotion by my teacher Swami Vishnudevananda.*

*The knowledge from this book was passed on through the traditional system of Gurukula wherein the students are immersed in Yoga life under the daily guidance of his/her teacher. All in all, in the context of the Sivananda Yoga Vedanta Centers,*

*I have imbibed the knowledge and passed it on to thousands of students through 40 years of learning, practice, teaching and serving. This book is a result of my own Self-healing journey and my teaching on Health Education and on Self-healing.*

*This Yoga journey is the application of the Yoga of Synthesis as taught by Swami Sivananda (1887-1963) and Swami Vishnudevananda (1927-1993).*

*The teachings came to me through countless stories of students who came to the ashram for Self-healing. I learned with each student, with each story. They are the many faces of the same suffering humanity with its core issues in the quest of Happiness and Peace.*

*May this book pave the way to Health, Peace and Happiness for countless more students to come and save them time and tribulations on the journey.*

*May we all attain Peace and Harmony*

*Loka samasta sukhino bhavantu*

*Swami Sitaramananda*
*Grass Valley, CA*
*November 1, 2023*

# *Table of Contents*

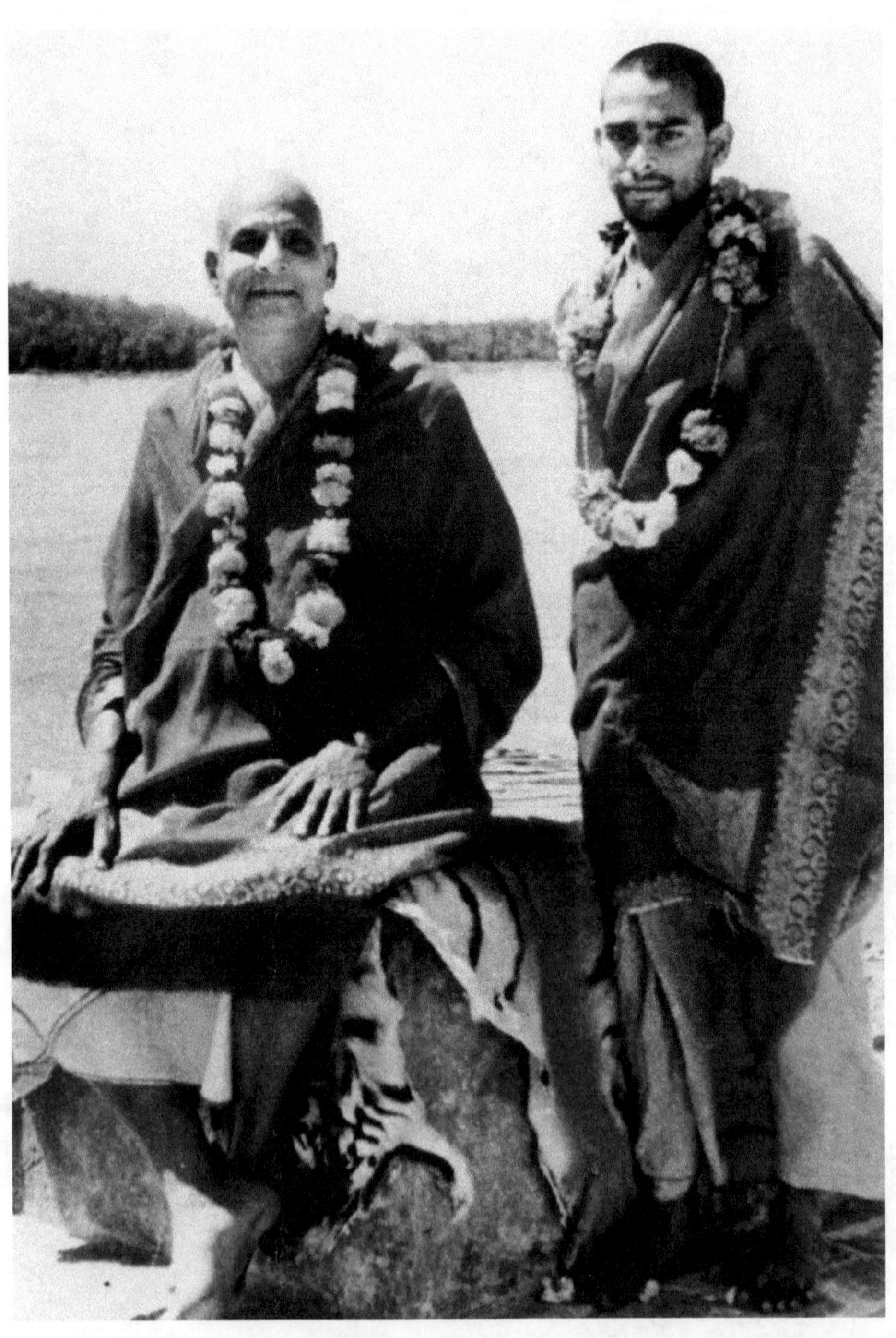

SWAMI SIVANANDA AND SWAMI VISHNUDEVANANDA,
RISHIKESH, HIMALAYAS

CHAPTER 1

# The Deeper Path of Holistic Health: Knowing the Self

***"Serve, Love, Give, Purify, Meditate, Realize."***

– *SWAMI SIVANANDA*

## 1. HOLISTIC HEALTH

*Yoga Vasishta,* one of the great classical Yoga texts, describes the causation of disease as the essential disease of being caught in the birth and rebirth cycle. This *vyadhi* (disease) doesn't cease until *Atma-Jnana,* Knowledge of the Self, is attained. Knowing the Self is the most powerful, deepest, truly lasting way of Self-healing.

Yogic health is very different from the common idea of "health." The word *"yoga"* means completeness, wholeness, union of body, mind and spirit. Self-healing is not the same as getting help from a doctor, nurse, or therapist. In the process of Self-Healing, you are your own healer. Through the process of self-training, or sadhana, you elevate and heal yourself and you naturally become a healer of others.

Self-healing is to become whole, perfect, and complete. Self-healing is equated to "Self-Realization." It means you realize the perfection of yourself and you are completely healed.

Since the COVID-19 crisis in the world, people have become very concerned about their health. But they have the misconception that health is only physical health. Yoga health and yoga Self-healing includes physical, mental, and spiritual healing. Yoga is the original mind-body medicine to maintain a state of *sukha sthanam,* well-being of body-mind-spirit.

This book is about *Yoga chikitsa* (Yoga healing practices) which are not just physical Yoga therapy using only asanas for the health and fitness of the physical body. *Yoga chikitsa* is the Yogic use of yoga practices for prevention and alleviating of mental and physical conditions integrating many levels of healing. *Yoga chikitsa* includes Yogic techniques stemming from the classical 4 paths of Yoga: *Hatha Yoga* and *Raja Yoga* (path of control of mind, breath and body), *Bhakti Yoga* (path of transformation of emotions), *Karma Yoga* (path of selfless action), and *Jnana Yoga* (path of self-enquiry).

## 2. CAUSES OF DISEASE

As mentioned, according to *Yoga Vashishta*, the essential manifestation of disease is the disease of rebirth. This refers to our primordial ignorance. This highest teaching states that we reincarnate on earth to pay our karmic debt and we need to live life wisely to avoid creating new karmic debts. New karmic debts will cause rebirth, a new life to learn our difficult lessons. We live in karmic ignorance, not knowing the meaning of our life. We learn from each birth and eventually realize our True Nature as immortal spirit, free from birth and death, free from karma and rebirth.

The primary manifestation of disease, once reborn in the body and mind, is the vasanas (the thoughts, the mental tendencies) in the mind. When the vasanas are strong and the ego is out of control, diseases manifest.

We struggle in life when we believe ourselves to be body and mind interacting in this world. We feel that we are imperfect, and yet, we feel that we are perfect. We know that we are ignorant, but at the same time, we feel inside we have all knowledge. The ego switches back and forth, sometimes identifying with our lack of knowledge, feeling that we are small and incomplete, and at other times, feeling we know everything. The ego holds fast to an attitude of, *"Don't tell me, I won't learn from anybody."*

Self-healing means to recognize that we are perfect by nature, however, we are struggling. We must face ourselves with compassion to see through our illusions, our habits, and mental tendencies, to discover this truth about ourselves. An attitude of compassion towards our own struggles and the struggles of others is necessary in the process of self-healing. Everyone is at different levels in their heart-of-heart struggles, even though some may appear to be knowledgeable, powerful and successful. The truth is, they do not realize their True Nature and the True Nature of the world clearly.

The secondary manifestation of disease is when it affects the physical body. At that time, conventional medicine and prevalent healing modalities are to be applied to alleviate the issues.

## 3. WHO IS THE SELF? WHO AM I?

When we say the *"Self"*, we talk about our essential nature. Our essential nature is obscured by our false ideas of identity. Therefore, self-enquiry or asking yourself the question *"Who Am I?"* is necessary for Self-healing. Self-healing means being aware of the true Self, to understand and to come closer to the realization of the true Self. The Self is your own Consciousness. It is the experience of Peace that surpasses all understanding. It is experienced when you function out of your healthy transcendental space. Self-knowledge is the most essential knowledge because it is about your true Self. It is about your life.

If you don't have a sense of your true Self, you cannot make decisions. If you don't know who you are, you will be lost in illusions and worldly things and suffer more. You need to know yourself to heal from suffering. Suffering can be physical, mental or emotional, and also spiritual, when you don't know why you are here and you feel that you are in darkness.

You cannot begin healing if you don't know what you are seeking. What is to be healed?

What are the steps to have a better sense of Self? What are the steps to control the mind and to have calmness of mind? What are the steps for meditation and for Self-enquiry?

## 4. CALMING THE MIND TO KNOW THE SELF

When the mind is agitated, restless or fearful, it is always looking for something external. It is like a drunken monkey—running and jumping around. The mind will run like a wild horse, refusing to be reined in. When the mind is not calm, it is hiding your Self. When it is out of control, constantly agitated, you cannot know yourself, you cannot realize your Self, you cannot be peaceful, you cannot be happy.

Yoga science teaches you many techniques to calm the mind and, the moment the thought waves subside, you will find yourself. You will find peace and happiness. In the *Yoga Sutras* of Patanjali, this state of yoga is defined as *"Yogas chitta vritti nirodhah"*—Yoga is that state where the thought waves of the mind are subdued.

In calming the mind, we must explore the connection between the breath, the prana (life force) and your mind. If you want to calm your mind, you need to calm your breath. If you know how to work with your breath through pranayama, you can slowly bring your breath to a regulated rhythm. You calm your breath to an imperceptible movement. This means to the point of silence of the mind.

If you learn to work with your breath, your mind will become more focused. You will experience your peaceful, contented self, then and there, in that moment. The mind that is very calm is like a lake without waves, which acts like a clear, clean mirror in which you can see a true reflection of your Self.

## 5. THE PROCESS OF FINDING SELF ACCORDING TO VEDANTA PHILOSOPHY

The Vedantic process is to remove the wrong thinking about yourself. According to Vedanta, an ancient spiritual philosophy, the nature of the Self is *Sat-Chit-Ananda*, meaning Truth-Consciousness-Bliss. That is the nature of the *atman,* or the Self, according to Vedanta philosophy. The teachings in the Sivananda lineage stem from the teachings of the great sage and philosopher Adi Shankaracharya of the eighth century CE, who taught Advaita Vedanta philosophy, the philosophy of unity of consciousness. This philosophy expresses the non-dual nature of Reality or Brahman. Non-duality implies that there is One truth and only One, that the individual *atman* and the Universal Brahman are One.

Adi Shankaracharya created ten classical lineages of monastic Yogis. The Sivananda lineage belongs to one of these ten lineages. The teaching espoused in this book comes from this classical source, coupled with personal and practical knowledge acquired through observing a multitude of practitioners, both East and West.

### The Vedantic process: hearing/thinking/realization

Knowledge of the immortal *atman*, your own essential Self, begins with learning about the nature of the Self through scriptures and enlightened teachers. In Vedanta (and the Sivananda lineage), there is a three-step process in this journey: Shravana (listening), Manana (thinking) and Nididhyasana (meditation). Listen to the teachings of the Upanishads and other key scriptures of Vedanta, think deeply about the teachings and then you come to know the *atman* through deep meditation. When one goes through these three steps, awakening of Consciousness and Self-Realization follow. This is our approach. We hear about the Self from the teachers and then we contemplate. In the following chapters, you will learn ways to think about the Self. You must contemplate, reflect and meditate and then you realize the Truth within yourself.

The True Nature of the *atman* is *Sat-Chit-Ananda*, Truth-Consciousness-Bliss. The *atman* is the core of being. The *atman* is your Self. The *atman* is the "I" thought.

You think "I" all day long and you talk about "I": *"I like this," "I don't like this," "I am in a relationship with this person," "I love this person," "I go here, I go there."* But you don't understand who this "I" is.

You are here now, on this earth, in this human body, and you have a certain idea of "who I am". That idea of "who I am" started when you were born. When you were a baby, you already tried to understand the limits of your body and *"Who am I?"* From a young age, you are defined by your gender, your family, your nationality, your religion, your status in society. You have been receiving these ideas about yourself since birth—they are very much related to the body, mind, environment and what people say about you. Then, whatever your external condition, you think this is who I am. The teachings of Vedanta suggest that you need to rethink and question all these ideas of "I."

However, you cannot rethink about *"Who am I"* from your current state of mind. You need to have a technique. Why? Because you need to remove all the preconditioning that has been on your mind for a very long time. That is why the process starts with listening to the teachers. "Hearing" means listening to the teachings about the truth from enlightened teachers that have known themselves and from the scriptures. These are two sources of authority: the lineage of teachers and the scriptures.

In a lineage, knowledge is passed from teacher to student, passing on the same consciousness, the same knowledge, for thousands of years. The teaching is passed, not just through words but, through living the teachings and through experience. The teacher passes the spark of knowledge.

The teachings are also confirmed by the Vedic Scriptures. These ancient scriptures are thousands of years old. They confirm the teachings of the masters of all times. You need to hear these teachings. How long will you practice hearing the teachings? If you attend a one-week course, you'll hear them for only one week. Some will hear them for one month. Some will hear them for ten years, and some for twenty years. Anyway, you will need to hear the teachings for a long time.

I heard from my own teacher while sitting at his feet. Why do you need to sit at the feet of the teacher? What does hearing have to do with the feet? This is all the language of respect from the spiritual traditions of India.

You are not on equal footing with your teacher. If you think you are, then the teacher's opinion is given the same weight as your own and you select the one you like best. You will not go to the essence of the teachings if you do not have the utmost respect towards the lineage of the teaching, towards the truth. You have to sit for a long time to absorb that knowledge, hearing the truth. The teacher will not ask your opinion nor what you think about this. The teacher will ask if you understand what is taught. And you will reply *"Oh, it's not really correct."* You will need to listen more, until you really understand. By hearing from the scriptures and the teachers, new ideas come into the darkness of our mind. When we believe something for a very long time, we are blind to our errors of perception. We carry a lot of wrong thinking in our minds and perpetuate the suffering for ourselves.

Self-healing means understanding these mistakes of thinking and realizing that they were superimposed upon the truth. Then the search of the essential truth needs to go first. It's like in Sivananda asana practice, we do the headstand first and standing poses at the end of the practice session. Standing on the feet implies that you are already balanced through the whole practice—your feet are on the ground, on this earth, and you are composed and harmonized with everything else around, and at the same time not losing your balance. With the headstand coming first, it implies that consciousness needs to be considered first. Blood flows down to the brain and everything is awakened. As you go through the asana sequence, you eventually find yourself. You find that harmony, that inner power, that inner quiet who you are. With that inner power, balance and strength, you are ready to interact with the world.

When we say "I" in Vedanta philosophy, we talk about the *atman*. The *atman* is the Self. This is the beginning of the teaching. The Self is the *atman*. When you are seeking the *atman*, in fact, you are seeking the truth about yourself. When you use the word "I"—*"I like this," "I like that," "I do this," "I do that," "I go here," "I go there"*—in reality, you are truly talking about the unchanging, immovable *atman*. The *atman* is your true, eternal, enlightened Self. It is the all-conscious, all-blissful, all-knowledgeable Self. The root of the Self, the root of the "I" is your own true Self, it is the most important thing.

When you don't have the sense of Self, it is as if something has overtaken you; you have been kidnapped. If the sense of Self is not there, you lose your balance, you are not experiencing your life, you are not conscious, nor are you able to digest your experiences. You are like a robot. The robot speaks and moves, but the "I" is missing or the "I" is mixed up with the emotions, with the worries, with the memories. That is why you are confused. You don't know who you are. You feel weak. Your mind is not calm. You are not aware of your surroundings. You are not aware of everything that has happened to you. You cannot recognize the thoughts that confused you. You suffer.

This is why it is necessary to calm the mind and to feel the Self. You have to realize that you are capable of recognizing the projected thoughts that confuse you. You have to learn to calm your mind and witness all the underlying, disturbing thoughts which are the source of your anxiety. When the mind is active, it is always projecting a distorted reality. It has preconceived ideas of this and that. However, it is only a projection. It comes from your mind and it projects a twisted reality. You cannot stay still. The mind cannot stay still. Like a turbulent lake, it cannot reflect your true Self. That's why we have so many imaginations, so many desires, so many emotions and so many fears and anxieties. When you project an idea of yourself externally, you will run after it, because you want to know what it is, but it's not the truth of who you are. When you project these ideas outside, you are compelled to go out and experience it, thinking it will bring back your peace. When you mistake this experience for happiness, you want to explore externally to find peace and happiness. Consequently, you are continually running and projecting.

The technique of yoga and Vedanta is to find yourself, to calm the mind down, to be the witness of all the thoughts in your mind that are disturbing, to recognize the source of your anxiety. This is the journey of Self-healing that we are talking about. When the mind is active, it is always projecting different ideas, different thoughts. It keeps you very busy, but it hides the truth within. You can have an ordinary mind or you can have the super mind of a computer. It is still the mind; it is a projection. It projects a twisted reality and doesn't help you to reflect on the nature of your own true Self.

Shankaracharya explained the phenomenon in three sentences. The first statement is *"Brahman is real."* Second,

*"The universe is a projection, an appearance, an illusion." What is the universe? The universe of names and forms. And the third statement is "The individual soul is in reality atman, and atman and Brahman—the Absolute Truth—are one."* This is his summary of the teaching about the Self. Roughly translated, it says that, in reality, you think you are this separate self, but actually your essence and the essence of the universe are one. In reality, you are *Sat-chit-ananda Atman*, Existence Absolute, Knowledge Absolute, and Bliss Absolute.

You live in this world of names and forms and you think it is very central to your existence. Philosophically, we say that the universe is unreal, because the names and forms we experience are constantly changing. Nowadays, we use a new kind of telescope and we discover more distant galaxies. All the planets and all the galaxies are still philosophically considered to be the "universe of names and forms." We experience the universe through our mind and senses. However, Vedanta philosophy declares that the world as you see it, the world that you live in, is, in fact, only an appearance. It is not absolutely real and is not true, because it is constantly changing. We need to remember the substratum of consciousness, that is the unchanging truth on which these different scenarios are playing. Similarly, different movies and fictions are being projected on a movie screen without which there is no movie.

The oak tree I see out the window is beautiful. It is more than 100 years old. It is protected, because it has been classified as historical. It looks like it will stay forever. But it is only temporary. Nothing is forever in this universe of names and forms. It changes. It changes constantly. If you can name it, it is part of the universe. If you can see it, it is part of this illusory universe. When I first learned about artificial intelligence and something called a chatbot, I asked, *"What is that? What are they talking about?"* Then I realized it is automated to generate words and data. Words? Data? Millions, billions, trillions of words generated very, very, quickly. But they're still just words, names and forms.

Sankaracharya said the universe of names and forms is unreal. Now you understand that everything, including our body, our mind, our environment, and everything that we are attached to are just appearances. It all comes and goes; it will not last forever. The problem is we mistake what we perceive for reality.

We perceive everything with our mind, and our mind has preconceived ideas about everything. We have our memories; we have our characters. We have what we think is our knowledge; we perceive through our mind; and we make a mistake. This is the fundamental mistake, according to Advaita Vedanta. We take what is an appearance projected by our mind, the universe of names and forms, to be the truth.

We take our bodies for our real selves. This nice yoga hall in the early morning sunshine, the grass, every blade of grass is shining; and our thirty smiling faces are sitting in this hall and listening to Swami Sita; and this is our reality. The teachings say, "No." This is what you think it is, but there are not just thirty people. You can technically demonstrate this illusion. If you put a radio here and turn it on, you can receive all kinds of information, all kinds of voices and music. This body and mind cannot receive this information. You have the computer trying to catch lots of information but, still, you think this is the reality, but it is not. It is a projected reality that comes from the mind.

## 6. THE STORY OF MISTAKING THE ROPE FOR A SNAKE

A fundamental story of Vedanta philosophy illustrates how we mistake projection for reality. The story of "the snake and the rope" is about mistaken identity and perception.

In the dark, as you walk home, you see a snake in front of your door. You are very frightened. You jump, you run, and almost have a heart attack. You call somebody who is not afraid of snakes to help you. The person comes with a flashlight and shines it on the snake. Under the light, you realize that the snake is just a rope. The snake, which caused fear, disappears and the truth of the rope is revealed. You breathe a sigh of relief and joy!

You have mistaken the rope to be a snake. Your mind has played a trick on you. When you look at the rope and see the snake, you superimpose an idea of the snake that is already in your mind upon what you see. The fear associated with the idea of encountering a snake is already there in your mind, and it is now associated with the reality of the rope. You react to the perception emotionally and take action to deal with the snake. What makes you restless or fearful is a mistake in seeing. You are projecting what is in your mind, the perceived snake, on top of reality, the rope.

Because we do not perceive ourselves and the universe truly for what they are, we do not perceive the truth of the Self and the truth of the universe correctly. It is projected by our mind according to what we have ingested in the past; and it stays in our mind. We project it out in order to realize our mistake, to realize the truth. But, instead of seeing the truth, we react to the projection. We have all kinds of emotional reactions, physiological reactions because we are frightened of the danger created by the snake. We fear for our very survival and we run away. Only when light comes, when knowledge dawns, can we take a long deep breath and realize our mistake.

When knowledge of Truth allows you to see the error of perception, you'll gain your strength. You'll gain your power. You'll gain your intelligence. You'll see yourself properly. And you say, *"Oh, it was too bad, it was a mistake. When I was running, I fell in a ditch. I was having a heart attack. Next time, I need to see properly."* You say this because the imprint in your mind is deep from the past. You know it and yet you see the snake again the next day when you go home—and you get scared again. But this time you have a little bit of memory of yesterday, *"I just saw it correctly; it is just a piece of rope."* You are stronger. You aren't as frightened as the first time. You dare to glance at it, but then the fear returns and you run away again. The third time, you become even stronger. You dare to look at it. Your heart is still pounding, but you look at it. You realize you don't need anybody to come with a flashlight to help you. You look at it and confirm again that it is just a rope. There is nothing to be afraid of.

What does the story mean? What we perceive to be ourselves and what we perceive to be reality is actually a projection. It is not the truth. Many ills and difficulties come out of our false perceptions of the truth, of reality, and of ourselves. Self-healing is returning to the Truth. You can stop the fear, stop the anxiety, stop the projections, stop all the conflicts that are created when you see something that is not real. In our ignorance, in the dark, we misperceive. When the light comes, we see correctly.

Darkness represents our spiritual ignorance (avidya). Light represents our Self-knowledge. Fear represents suffering due to ignorance. Realization under the light represents a moment of awakening to our True Nature. Similarly, in our ignorance, in our darkness, we project our habitual preconceived idea of what constitutes happiness (the snake) and then we act on it in order for us to find it. We chase it frantically. But when we wake up from our illusion, when the wisdom insight dawns in the light of Self-Knowledge, we realize the truth that happiness is already there (the rope). It is our True Nature and cannot come and go.

This story of mistaking a rope for a snake teaches us that we need to always remember that life as we know it is a projection of our mind. We need to stay calm and not fall for the same mistakes in seeing. Self-healing means you need to realize it yourself. No doctor, no psychiatrist, nobody can see what you see, feel what you feel. You need to cleanse yourself of these wrong impressions which tend to repeat themselves.

When something is repeated, it becomes real. A fleeting thought can be powerful. When it is repeated, repeated, repeated, it materializes. It becomes real. You live in that world with that thought. You believe it to be real. You can repeat something wrong again and again. It becomes solid, and then you believe it to be true. That's the problem. We superimpose the wrong impressions on our True Nature, which is eternally-existent as peace and bliss. But we don't see the peace and bliss, we see this-and-that projected from our mind.

Why do we keep re-expressing the same experience, the same suffering? We're experiencing the same situation again—seeing the snake and getting scared by it—in order for us to become stronger and stronger; and to have more awareness of the underlying eternal perfect Self that is entirely distinct from what you perceive to be true. You say, *"Okay, next time I will pay attention. I'll be more aware. I won't make the same mistake. I won't let my mind fool me."* Well, the next time comes and you make the same mistake. Again, you project whatever is in your mind—your fear, your obsession, your trauma, your memory—upon reality. You see things according to what your mind tells you and create more trouble and suffering—until you recognize your mistake. Light coming means knowledge coming, and you recognize there was no snake; there was no victim; there was no danger; there was no threat. *"I was afraid for nothing. I remain who I am—Sat-Chit-Ananda Atman, strong and free."*

The snake is in your mind, in your imagination. The impressions in your subconscious mind are what create fear and attraction.

This story shows that you have to watch what is in your mind, so you will not be fooled by it. Learn how to purify your mind, learn how to keep your mind calm, so this mistake of losing yourself will no longer happen.

Here are a few examples of common mistakes and illusions: People work very hard to change themselves and their natural appearance. They wish to be more beautiful, in order to attract a romantic partner. They work very hard to get what they think will give them happiness. Their life becomes very busy, going to beauty shops, going to the gym and shopping for clothing and jewelry, in order to be more adorned and attractive, all this in search of happiness.

Or you work very hard, for example, in your job to get a promotion. You have to compete with other people; you try to build your skills. You are very active and very busy devoting all of your precious time and energy to this. You think if you get the promotion, then you'll be somebody special—and then you'll be happy. You accept this and, consequently, have no time for yoga and meditation. Our projection is always telling us what we need to do to get happiness.

But then when you get what you thought you wanted, you find that you're still not happy. You get the partner you wanted and the perfect wedding, but after some time, you're not happy. Or you get the promotion, your dream job with a signigicant raise, more prestige, and soon afterwards you are not happy. Why?

This thing that you think will make you happy is an object. It is outside of you and that which is outside of you can never complete you or make you happy. This external thing is not you. You are looking in entirely the wrong place. Happiness comes from the Self which is found only through an internal search. Your Self cannot be something external, but quite the opposite. Instead of getting busy and running, you need to keep yourself quiet and be still. Look within instead of running outside. Learning the different yoga techniques will help you to become calm.

You need to have certainty that the Self is a source of happiness, and a source of healing. When you are unhappy, recognize that mentally you are not healthy. Learn to sit and quiet and calm your mind. Breathe calmly and it calms your mind.

Do pranayama and your mind becomes clear. At that time, you feel that you don't need this external thing anymore and then you don't run anymore.

**The idea of subject/object**

Subject is you, the consciousness, the Self, the true I. Object is something external to the Self, impermanent, and always changing. I can say, *"This is my hand,"* but it is still an object. I say *"my hand,"* because it is something very close to me. I say: *"my heart," "my nose," "my hair"*... but it is still *"mine"*; *"my table," "my house," "my car," "my property"* is still *"mine."* It is still an object. We talk about objects. We don't talk about the subject. The subject is "I" and something that is"mine" is an object. We always have that split: subject/object. I am here and that thing is there. And then we live in the illusion. That thing is separate from me. I run after it, in order to make it belong to me, I want to possess that thing. The more I possess it, the more I feel good, convinced it is not separate from me. But, whatever you possess changes. The house changes, the car changes, the relationship changes; and you come back to the same illusion again, the illusion of missing something, of incompleteness, of being let down.

## 7. THE FALSE SELF, THE EGO

When you find the "I," the source of the "I," you find your own Self. In reality, the "I"-thought is your own Self. It's not the ego. It is not your false self. It is the *atman*. When you're running in the outside world, in fact you're seeking the Self, but you mistakenly think that it is our ego's desire. The idea of the ego is the idea of the false self. In Vedanta, it is the self-asserting principle, that means, you identify yourself with the characteristics of the body and mind and assert yourself to be that.

It is *avidya* or ignorance, which is the root cause of the ego idea. When you identify with the thoughts in your mind, you will be very restless as there are lots of waves in the mind. At that time, you are already thinking, "I am so and so, I am big, I am small, I am male, I am female, I am rich, I am poor." The "I" is connected to some idea, and then you feel you have to make that idea bigger, stronger. *"I am rich,"* so you want to be richer. "*I am female,*" so you have to be more female; *"I am intelligent,"* so you have to be more intelligent, because the "I" is attached to some condition and you want that to be real. So, you have to work on the idea of cultivating "more", but you go in the wrong direction, which brings suffering. You are in need of healing, which means getting back to your True Nature.

Avidya manifests in many ways. Always the "I am" is linked to something, this creates problems. You identify with your culture— *"I am Vietnamese, I am Chinese,*

*I am French, I am American"—or your age—"I am thirty years old", "I am sixty."* You say, *"I am Mr. So -and-So"* and compare yourself with other people, *"I am better than you, I am worse than you."* If you feel incomplete, you tend to compare yourself in terms of your relationships, *"I am your wife, I am your husband, I am your teacher, I am your student, I am your Mother, I am your friend."*

Self-healing means gradually learning new ways of thinking and adopting techniques to free yourself from all those wrong notions of who you are. There is a lot of attachment in your mind. You are very attached to that identity. You are not just having this thought once. You keep repeating this assertion of the false self and interpreting everything that happens in your life accordingly. Whatever happens, you have the excuse, "*Oh, it's because I'm not intelligent*" or "*Oh, it is because I'm female.*"

## 8. CLEANING OUT THE HABIT OF WRONG-THINKING

You become very attached to your deeply-buried patterns of wrong-thinking, the samskaras. You build walls to imprison yourself as you keep repeating these ideas in your mind. You have begun to see things according to these wrong thought tendencies. When these become aggravated and the ego becomes out of control identifying itself with the tendencies, disease will happen.

A very common example of wrong-thinking is: *"I am what people think about me."* With this assertion, not only do I think of myself wrongly, but I end up being what people think about me! But who are these people and what exactly are they thinking? The truth is you don't know. People's opinions about you are never really true, never really who you are anyway, because people see you through their own eyes. Can you imagine how serious this mistake is, and the harmful illusion and the delusion? You imagine yourself as seen through the illusory perception of others, which is impossible to really know—and then make decisions and live according to these illusions. This is a source of great confusion, pain and suffering.

Instead of loving yourself, you check to see if other people love you. You try to please them. Only through their eyes do you love yourself. But then, other people and society change their opinions about themselves and others constantly. Can you imagine the entanglement? By repeating the idea of false ego, false self, you suffer so much. You look for yourself, in a mirage, a kind of illusion, appearance. That is the mistake. That's why you're always restless, you're always unhappy.

When you try to find yourself through others, you miss the beauty of the Self that is already there, unchanged. It has been there all the while—quiet and peaceful inside.

You can heal all these emotions. You can heal this mind. You can heal this habit of wrong-thinking and when you do, it affects your whole body. You can heal all diseases in your body. Correct your thinking. Focus on the unchanging, the peace inside, and thus, Self-heal.

*INSPIRED STORY*

**Healing from grief and sorrow**

*At four years old, I was hospitalized with pneumonia. I always had a weakness in my lungs. Lungs are related to the emotion of grief. I asked myself why a four-year-old would have grief? What kind of grief? Throughout my upbringing and adulthood, I noticed grief as an important underlying feeling and realized that it came with my attachment to the idea of a just world—a world with no pain, no loss, and no sorrow. I have worked on releasing attachment for a very, very long time. If I meditate on my mindset, I can see the theme of many lifetimes trying to understand and alleviate sorrows. During this lifetime, if I witnessed individual or collective suffering, I was stirred to action; I spent twenty years of my life doing social and community work.*

*After more than 40 years of turning inwards and going to the root cause of suffering, I found that spiritual ignorance is the root cause of all ills, and that an external world without spirit is an illusion.*

*In 2023, after three years of the whole world being deeply immersed in COVID, and miraculously I did not get it, I realize that I have healed from my karmic disease of grief and sorrow. (COVID, as you know, is a disease involving the respiratory system.) This discovery gave me tremendous joy—as if I had passed an exam. I have finally overcome the negative feelings that I had, coming into this life, this karma of grief, of attachment, of sorrow for the whole world, a mental disease inherited through countless lifetimes.*

*Now I understand the cause of suffering, the cause of attachment, the illusion of objects, the illusion of attachment, and what detachment means. I feel that I have healed myself from this particular karma. And I am very happy about this. It's the completion of life, 70 years of life struggle to sort out the cause of personal and human misery.*

Swami Sita

**A doctor's view about health care vs. disease care**

Addressed to trainees in the Sivananda Yoga Health Educator Training (SYHET)

*The health sector has two functions: health care and disease care. The healthcare industry today is mainly focused on patient care. The health care part has mostly been abandoned due to too much work. It is the students in this [SYHET] course who do that job, taking care of their own health and other people's health. Health care is critical. If there is health, there is no disease. Sickness indicates poor health. The healthcare industry is doing its best to take care of the sick. Then we need to do the rest, to take care of health. Healthcare is the unsung hero. Doctors taking care of the sick are heroes known by everyone. And even, while doing that, we make a lot of money with diseases.*

*But we live this life not to make money. We live for fun and health. Be healthy and heal yourself. It is a compassionate and wise approach. If I make people happy, I'm happy. You are taking this course and you are going to do a very meaningful job in your life, that is health care. Increased health means increased quality of life. Living without quality of life is a disease, a pain. Having good health ensures quality of life and prevents disease recurrence.*

*True health care requires firstly time, secondly determination, and thirdly an open heart. Only a person with a good heart can become a healthcare provider or healthcare educator. I hope that after this course you will continue to practice and improve your knowledge, in your way.*

Dr. Quan Van Hung

**Self-healing is the purification of self and healing of others**

*In these two years of the SYHET course, I have learned a lot. The knowledge and love have touched my heart. It is a journey of self-healing. When I started the Sivananda Yoga Health Educator Training, I didn't expect this much. I was arrogant.*

*After two years, I have become much humbler. I always suffered when I did a practicum with my students. When they suffered, it became also my suffering; I suffered a lot. But I learned from Swami Sita that we need to be conscious, detached, and compassionate. We need to be rooted in the Self, in our True Nature. We cannot be drowned in the suffering of the world. Now I try to practice Sadhana and come back to myself.*

*I'm very grateful to be part of this course.*

*Thank you very much.*

N.

**QUESTIONS**

1. *What is Self-healing according to classical yoga?*
2. *What is holistic health?*
3. *Spiritual ignorance is the first disease according to classical text. The second cause of disease is aggravation of the vasanas and aggravation of ego. Please comment based on your personal experience.*

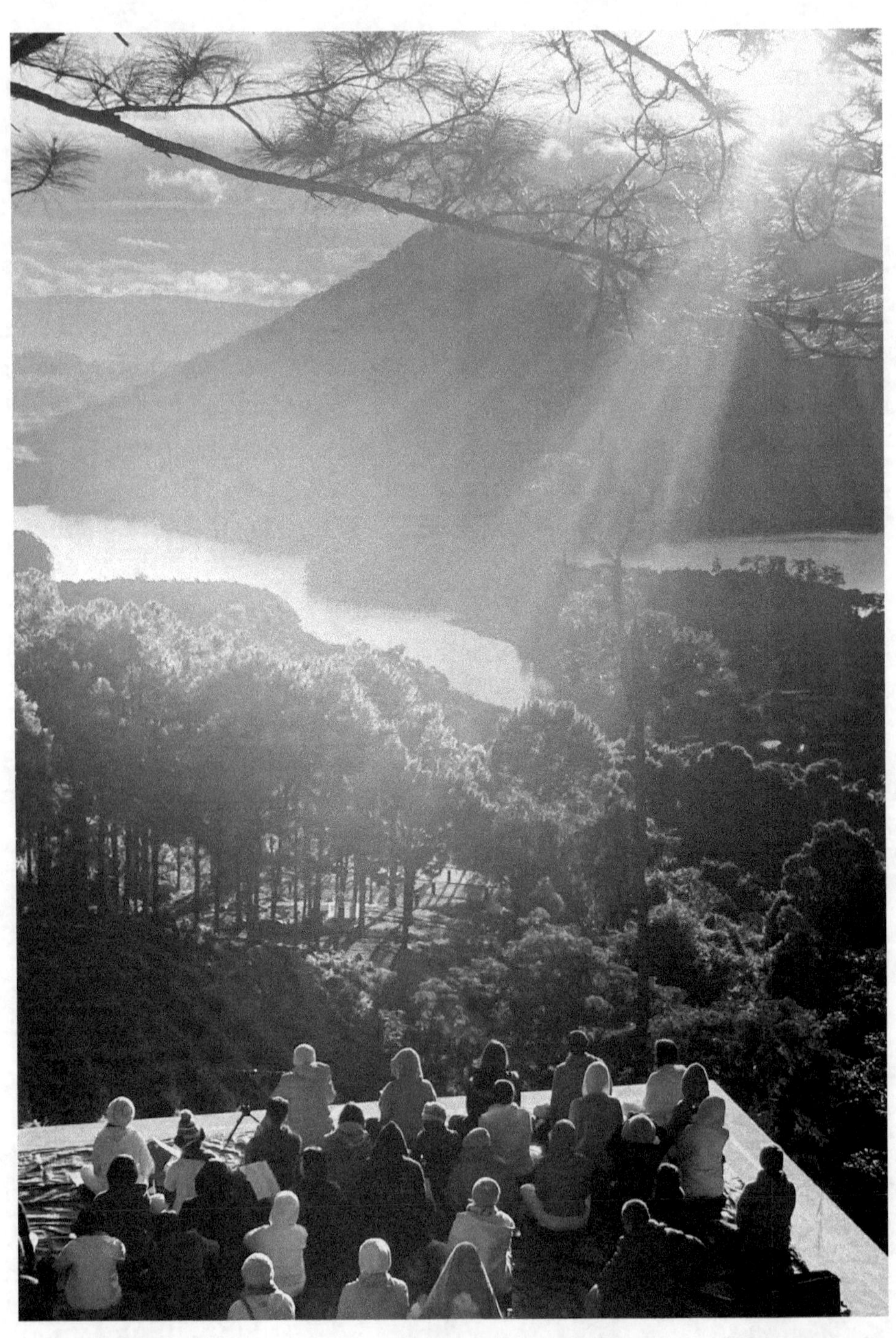

GROUP OF MEDITATION IN ASHRAM, DALAT, VIETNAM

CHAPTER 2

# Understanding the 3 Qualities of Nature (3 Gunas) and Knowing the Way Out of Suffering

*"Yield not to Tamas and Rajas, stick to Sattva."*

– SWAMI SIVANANDA

Our journey of Self-healing is a journey from darkness to light, from ignorance to knowledge. It is a journey of purification.

Yoga philosophy talks about three qualities of nature: Tamas, Rajas and Sattva. Tamas and Rajas come from ignorance and Sattva comes from knowledge. Tamas and Rajas are binding, Sattva is leading to knowledge, balance and freedom from suffering. In this chapter, we examine how these qualities work in our consciousness.

## 1. SELF-HEALING IS PURIFICATION AND RETURNING TO YOUR SAT-CHIT-ANANDA NATURE

The process of what we call holistic healing is not just healing of the physical body and the mental body, but it is seeing ourselves and others under a different light, the light of the *atman*. It is a return to our True Nature as Spirit. The *atman* is compared to the radiant Sun, giving light and life to all around. Self-healing is allowing your consciousness to be enlightened, to understand the body and mind as your instruments, and to no longer see them as your Self. You come to recognize that you are the driver of the body-mind vehicle; the vehicle is not driving you. If you think the body and the mind are your Self, you will be restless, and experience a lot of limitation and suffering. The Yogic and Vedantic approach to Self-healing is based on the subtle understanding of a philosophical, consciousness-based interpretation of reality, a reality in which the whole person, the Self, occupies the central role and, as it were, governs the body and mind from within. From this perspective, we can understand the concept of three vehicles or bodies, the concept of the three levels of health and the concept of five veils of consciousness.

Vedantic scriptures and enlightened teachers describe the Self, the *atman*, as being complete, perfect *Sat-Chit-Ananda* nature.

- **Sat:** The Self, the *atman*, is Existence Absolute. It has never been born and never dies. This means that your True Self is beyond the body and mind and is eternal. As you come closer to the realization of your immortality, you move away from the fear of death and the fear of not being seen. Self-healing is understanding the context of your soul's greater journey, a journey beyond this limited life, and seeing the mistakes you have made in the whole perspective of your soul life.
- **Chit:** The Self, the *atman*, is Knowledge Absolute. The Pure Consciousness that is your True Self is beyond the intellect and the intelligence. This means that your knowledge and your understanding comes from a source that is beyond the intellect and the mind. If you remember this, all knowledge will come to you as the Self is pure underlying Consciousness and True Intelligence itself.

  You are knowing because your True Nature is all knowledge. There is nothing hidden from you, because you are one with everything. You are unlimited in your knowledge. The identification with the body and mind makes us feel limited, creates feelings of low self-esteem, pride and competition. The remembrance of the *atman* brings us peace as we know we are not missing something and that we are at the core of everything and essentially we are in everybody.
- **Ananda:** The Self, the *atman*, is Bliss Absolute. Bliss Absolute means permanent bliss in all conditions. This means that whether you get what you want, or you don't get what you want, wherever you live, whoever you live with, whatever you do, whether good things happen or bad things happen, you are Bliss Absolute.

This teaching cannot be applied literally. There is a process of purification and tuning inward which will allow you to understand the complex, subtle philosophy correctly. For instance, if you have an accident and as a result you break your leg and you need to have your leg amputated, it is difficult to say, "*I am Bliss Absolute*" while you are in the hospital and they are removing your leg. However, at that time, remembering your True Nature as *atman* transcending the body will give you much solace and strength.

This subtle philosophy, when applied correctly, gives you a different perspective on life and your experiences in life. There is a whole process of retraining your mind, re-training your intellect, so you understand the subtle aspect of things. In learning this wisdom path, you need to learn patience, not jump to conclusions too quickly and you need to trust the process.

## 2. PURIFICATION OF THE BODY AND MIND AS INSTRUMENTS

Purification means living a conscious lifestyle to make the body-mind-spirit function healthily, optimally and harmoniously. We experience the three vehicles of ourselves (three bodies) when we go through three states of consciousness daily.

- **The gross physical body** is the vehicle we use in the awakening state of consciousness. The physical body is an aggregate of the five gross elements of nature: earth, water, fire, air and space. Heaviness of the body comes from earth and water. Fire creates heat in the body. There is a lot of air and space in the body.
- **The astral body (mental/emotional)** is the vehicle we use when we are functioning out of our subtle mind and subtle energies in the dream state. It is called our inner instrument and is composed of subtle energies and our mind.
- **The causal body (seed body)** is the vehicle we use when we experience life at the core level which is similar to what we experience in the deep sleep state. From the seed comes the tree. From the karmic seeds come the body and mind. All the characteristics of the seed will be manifested in the tree. The seed here is the seed of karma.

As the three bodies are, in fact, consciousness operating on a gross or subtle level, purification of the instruments means to make them strong and function optimally so that they can reveal the True Nature of the Self (the *atman*), the underlying consciousness distinct from the instruments.

Purification of the physical body means keeping the body and its organs functioning optimally through healthy and moderate lifestyle. Purification of the astral body means rendering our energy, our mind and our emotions pure and balanced. Purification of the causal body means understanding the cause of our suffering and mistaken thinking and no longer repeating the same incorrect understanding of the Self.

**Detachment as the result of purification**

Purification leads to self-awareness and self-healing. To know that we are not the body is to be detached from it, no longer identifying ourself with it. Purification of the prana or energy means having abundant and inexhaustible energy and yet not identifying with our energy. Purification of the mind and emotions leads to calmness, peace, and pure love. We no longer identify with our mind and our emotions. The mind is no longer occupied with momentary ups and downs, confused, attached and deluded. It can, instead, reflect the beauty of our True Self. Purification of the intellect leads to the capacity of self inquiry and self awareness that reveals the Truth about the blissful and self-delighting nature of our Soul. When the intellect is purified, we no longer identify with the limited imperfect ego self, but with the eternal, powerful and knowledgeable *atman*.

## 3. THE PROCESS OF TRANSCENDING THE FIVE VEILS TO REALIZE PURE CONSCIOUSNESS

The Self, the *atman*, is always present and yet we do not see it. We believe ourselves to be something else. We experience the *atman* as veiled. In the same manner as we fail to see the true nature of the rope because we perceive it to be a dangerous snake, we fail to perceive the True Nature of *atman*—our pure, all fulfilled consciousness—because we project different ideas of our limited beliefs of ourselves upon the *atman*. We identify with a distorted vision of ourselves and react as though this is the true Self.

Failure to see the Self correctly is due to our veiled vision. Thinning out and removing the veils is the way to liberation and Self-realization. Light is shining brightly from within us but we are unable to see it, because thick layers of dust are covering the light bulbs.

There are five veils that are covering our consciousness, our awareness, or the idea of who I am. The essence of Self-healing is to be able to see through the five veils. If we see through the five veils, we see ourself, and ourself is perfect, always perfect. We don't need anything from outside. We just need to see through the veils. How can we do this?

To see through the veils we have to inquire, meaning to think correctly about ourself, to open our eyes and see through our illusion of self due to our belief of separation. The veils are the false beliefs about ourself, believing ourself to be the body, the prana, the mind and emotions and the separate ego self. However, consciousness is one, but due to the identification with the body and mind, we think that there is separation between individuals. In the same manner, the space inside an empty cup seems to be separated from the space outside of the cup, but it is an illusion due to the presence of the separating factor which is the cup. We can't really remove the veils, but we can make them thinner and more transparent through Yoga, meditation, purification practices and Self-inquiry.

In the analogy of the cup and space, when the walls of the cup are thick and dark, the separation appears to be more real as we can't see through the veils. When the cup is replaced by a clear glass, with thinner, lighter, transparent walls, we can see clearly through the walls of the glass what is behind them. The veils are still there, the separation is still there, but we have an idea of unity as we can see through the veils. Similarly, because of our identification with our body and our mind, we feel separated from each other. The more we identify with the body and mind, the more we feel separated. This identification with the body and the mind becomes the veil that hides the truth from us. It becomes the separation factor between ourself and others.

That which separates us from our peace are the veils over our consciousness.

Awakening and beginning on the path of Self-healing starts with the realization of our illusions and the sincere search for Truth. We must want to see behind the veil. We must want to get out of the condition of being ignorant, blind and in the dark. We must strive to move away from wrong beliefs about ourself. We must start to look within and question ourself for the first time. This is how our journey of Self-healing begins to unfold.

## 4. SEEING THE FIVE VEILS OF CONSCIOUSNESS (THE PANCHA KOSHAS) AS THEY ARE

The veils are the different ways of understanding ourselves, when our Satchidananda consciousness becomes perceived as the physical gross body, the subtle mind, emotions, intellect and ego. Understanding the veils leads us to the conscious practice of detachment from the veils and the conscious practice of identifying with pure consciousness.

- **Veil 1: Annamaya Kosha, the food sheath**

  The food sheath corresponds to the physical body and is made of the five gross elements: earth, water, fire, air and ether. The physical body has different functions: birth, growth, change, decay and death. What we eat becomes our physical body. Eating sattvic food will lead us to a sattvic state of mind. If the food is tamasic, dead or impure, our body will become heavy and our consciousness will become tamasic and dark. The separation we experience will become thick, leading to more suffering. If the food is tamasic and rajasic, for example alcohol and drugs, it makes us excited and then gives us a hangover, brain fog, isolation and feelings of guilt. A lack of self-worth follows. If we eat and drink the type of food that is more pure, or more Sattvic, our body and mind become more sattvic.

Identification with the physical body can be thicker or thinner, depending on the individual. A person involved in competitive physical sports, in muscle-building, or a person involved in beauty contests or in cosmetic surgery would be more attached to the annamaya kosha with greater identification to the physical body.

Purifying this sheath involves proper diet and asana practice, working on the body, taking care of the body and detaching from the body at the same time.

- **Veil 2: Pranamaya Kosha, the pranic sheath or vital energy layer**

  Yoga philosophy pays much attention to the subtle body layer, which is subtler than the gross physical body.

  Different energies are operating to allow us to be alive and to act in life —to breathe, eat, drink, digest, feel heat and cold, procreate and act in life. Vital energies or prana also govern the mind, the emotions and the senses. Without enough prana, the mind is stressed, the emotions and senses are dull. With too much prana unchanneled, the mind is restless, jumpy and scattered. Blockages of prana create disease.

  Purification of this sheath by Pranayama gives energy to the body and mind, opens blockages of energy, and channels and balances energies.

  We need to purify the prana so that we can see ourselves as the source of all prana. Our life continues after the prana departs from the physical body. We need to ask the question "Who am I?" so we don't identify ourselves with our koshas and, thus, we remain who we are.

- **Veil 3: Manomaya Kosha, the mental sheath**

  The mind, the senses and the emotions of the mental sheath create a thick layer that can easily make us forget our True Nature and cause us to identify with the mental, emotional and sensual perceptions of the external world. We experience this physical world through the five senses and the mind which perceives the subtle, non-physical aspect of the five gross elements. These five subtle elements are each associated with one of the five senses: earth to smell, water to taste, fire to sight, air to touch and ether to hearing. The mind interprets the information provided by the senses based on past experiences and preconceived notions in our subconscious mind (lower mind). We identify with our lower emotions: anger, fear, greed, hatred, envy, jealousy and lust and thus are trapped in the tamasic and rajasic sensual world (of the five senses).

We lose ourselves in this sheath because we identify with the senses, mind, memories and habits. The more we identify ourselves with these mental impressions, the more we need to purify. When our identification with the mental sheath is thick, we are engulfed by tamas, we live only in the past, we are in the dark and we are unable to think and discern what is good for us. When we lose ourselves in our desires, and the mind is excited and jumpy, our mind is rajasic. We need to render the mind sattvic, clear and calm so we can perceive our Self.

Purification of the manomaya kosha involves:

- clearing the subconscious of tamasic and rajasic patterns and imprints;
- installing sattvic habits and positive thinking and feeling;
- remaining in the present in order to control the resurgence of subconscious impressions;
- consciously focusing on positive thoughts and emotions, such as mantras;
- sublimation of tamasic and rajasic emotions through devotion and chanting;
- keeping the mind calm and observing ethics (yamas and niyamas).

- **Veil 4: Vijnanamaya Kosha, the intellectual sheath**

The next veil in our subtle body is called vijnanamaya kosha, the intellectual sheath, which gives us the sense of ourselves, either the ego self or the awareness of our true Self. We need to sharpen our intellect in order to discriminate between real and unreal, truth and illusion, in our perception of ourselves and others. Our self-knowledge and self-awareness will improve when the discriminative intellect is sharpened. This self-awareness allows us to navigate ourselves, make correct decisions and evolve. Humans are more evolved than animals and are equipped with these capacities of self-transformation, self-knowledge, self-awareness. This is a very precious gift, but we are not using these faculties as much as we might.

Most of the time we function from our instinctive lower nature, animal-like. We eat, sleep, procreate, and die without using our higher intellectual faculty. The purpose of Self-healing is a significantly different process, requiring you to see through the veils, to see the truth and the light. This Truth and light behind the veils are pure consciousness, your own Self, the *atman*. It is the source of knowledge and healing. You are already equipped with this intellect that enables you to see your Self.

As we have made clear here, the ego is not your Self. It is an idea of yourself that is related to the body and mind. It comes from the self-assertion principle. You need the ego, the idea of your separate self, related to your body and mind, in order for you to learn your lessons and to be free. The ego is, in fact, not the Self. The ego is only a tool. It is not your Self, it is a tool to make you think and realize your mistaken identification so that you can transform yourself, so you can find yourself.

The ego idea is something you need to purify. If my ego is very big, I identify with whatever I think I am—my body and my mind. My ego can also project an idea of myself very strongly and make me behave in various ways.

There is the tamasic ego, the rajasic ego and the sattvic ego.

The sattvic intellect sees the Self more clearly and does not create conflicts and problems. A sattvic ego means a detached ego. I still feel that I am separate from you, I still feel that I am this body, this personality, this role, but, at the same time, it's not really important. I can see you, I don't just assert myself, I don't identify with my differences from you. With a pure, sattvic mind, I identify myself in oneness with you, recognizing our sameness. I see myself as the same essence as you. I have a more expanded idea of myself, not just the selfish idea of myself. This is the sattvic ego we are striving for in this life.

Thus the vijnanamaya kosha, or the veil of intellect, can be thick or thin, and it can be purified.

- **Veil 5: Anandamaya Kosha, the bliss sheath**

  The last of the five sheaths is called the anandamaya kosha, the bliss sheath which operates in your deep sleep and when you are happy. It relates to your core self that is happy at all times. You access it when you do a good action and you feel very satisfied. Or, when you desire something and you get the object of desire, your mind stops for a moment and you feel very happy. In this moment, you access the anandamaya kosha, the blissful sheath, the blissful Self that is within yourself. But it doesn't last long, because you don't stay there. You need to go beyond it to find the bliss that is absolute.

## 5. HOW TO PURIFY THE VEILS

The *atman* is the only reality, the only Truth, but we identify with one or another of these sheaths because we are veiled. Some people will see more of their body, constantly thinking of their physical body (for example, athletes). Some people think of their prana more (for example, healers). Some people think of their mind and emotions all the time (for example, a person in love). A scholar will identify with his intellect, a meditator with his blissful sheath. There are five veils, which means there are five ways the idea of the *atman* can be obscured. Consciousness is attached to this or that idea of the self. Eventually, all the different veils get thinned out, so that consciousness shines in its pristine glory.

**How to purify the veils to see the *atman***

- How do you purify the gross physical body? Through asanas and proper diet.

  Asanas make your body fit and allow the prana to flow to all organs and systems of the body. That's why asanas can heal, because they open the blockages in the flow of prana. Let's say you sit in a slumped posture and constantly feel pain in your back. If you sit straight, the energy can flow and you lose awareness of your spine, because it is perfectly aligned. So, when you do asanas, you purify the body because there is no blockage of the energy and all the different systems of the body are enhanced and working in harmony; the structure is well-aligned. You do not think of your physical body when it's healthy; it's no longer an obstacle. It's as if you want to go somewhere but the car doesn't work. You are constantly fixing the car. You cannot get in the car and go where you want. You want to be physically healthy so that you're preoccupied by the body. That's called purification of the body.

The second practice of purification of the physical sheath is proper diet. If we eat sattvic food, our mind becomes sattvic, and consciousness about ourself becomes clear. The sattvic lifestyle gives more chance to see the true Self. Natural, plant-based food is considered to be sattvic.

- Pranayama purifies the pranic sheath. You work with the prana so that it flows, so that you have an abundance of prana, so the prana that's in the universe is serving you, and you can recharge yourself with prana. The organs of action are in the pranamaya sheath. When you have a lot of prana, you can do a lot of things, and it helps you to live this life meaningfully, to think clearly, and to realize your Self. You need a lot of prana to think, make decisions, see, love, live, understand. So you need to do pranayama. We will talk more about prana and pranayama in later chapters.

- The third veil is the mental veil, which includes emotions, senses, thoughts and all the impressions/samskaras in your mind, impressions from the past that stay in your mind. This undigested material remains in the mind and obstructs the flow of energy. Undigested thoughts and emotions are information and experiences that are repeated in the mind, even though they are not understood or are wrong.

  When we have too many emotions, we react strongly even to minor events. The intellect is drowned in the emotions. It is difficult to balance and regulate the emotions and we become driven by them. Sublimation of emotions by the practice of devotion or Bhakti Yoga is needed *(see Chapter 11)*.

  How do you transcend the third veil, the mental veil? Through the guidelines of conduct, the Yamas, the Niyamas, Bhakti Yoga and Karma Yoga (selfless service). You purify yourself through pure love, through serving somebody as your own self. That also helps your heart to open, to get the rajasic emotions out of your system and bring about pure love. When the heart is open and you feel pure love, you can see through the mental veil.

- How do you see through the intellect and the ego? How do you make the intellect and the ego become more clear? You need to study the scriptures, because the scriptures will tell you correctly who you are. This knowledge then guides your thinking so you are not subject to the ego. When you ask yourself the question *"Who am I?"*, it is called vichara, the practice of right inquiry, you are attempting to transcend these false ideas. For example, we question "*Who am I? Am I this body?*" Let's say there is a pimple on your face and a feeling of inadequacy arises, the questions "*Who am I? Am I this face? Am I this skin? Am I this body?*" will eventually bring about the answer: "*I can think I look ugly, but I am the same. I am not my body.*" In the same manner, we can ask "*Am I this size? Am I this appearance? Am I this man? Am I this woman?*" in order to disidentify with age, gender, race, false identity, false idea of reality. Reality becomes fragmented, split in genders, races, age groups. However, when you are in awe looking at the sunrise, for example, you and the sunrise are one. The person merging with the beauty of sunrise is pure consciousness, neither young nor old, neither black nor yellow, rich nor poor, male nor female.

- You can do inquiry with all five koshas, the five veils. "*Am I my prana?*" "*Am I this veil?*" "*Am I this angry mind?*" "*Am I this intellect?*" "*The anger is in my mind, I observe the anger in my mind, but I'm not angry, I'm not lost in the anger.*"
- How do you transcend the fifth veil? Through meditation. You transcend the fourth veil of intellect by the study of scriptures and the right inquiry of "Who am I?" and through meditation, because when you meditate you go beyond the intellect. Then you transcend the fifth veil through Samadhi, which is the highest state of meditation, when you completely become one.
- Rejecting the false self and affirming the true self are two facets of the same process. Self-inquiry leads to the rejection of the false self: "*I am not this body, I am not this energy, I am not this mind, I am not this emotion, I am not this wrong thinking, I am not this temporary bliss that comes because I get something that I like.*" *Self-enquiry also leads to the affirmation of the true Self:* "*I am the immortal Self, I am Satchitananda, I am the pure Consciousness.*"
- So slowly, slowly, by doing this exercise of self-inquiry we transcend the veils. You can make ten thousand mistakes about yourself, ten thousand times you may think wrongly about yourself, but you also have ten thousand or a hundred thousand opportunities to think about yourself correctly.

## 6. THE THREE GUNAS AND THE WAY OUT OF SUFFERING

The three gunas are a key concept in Yogic psychology and essential to a Yogic understanding of the mind. The three gunas are the three qualities of nature, or attributes of the mind, which help to guide us on the Self-healing path heading towards peace of mind and attaining freedom from pain and suffering.

The three gunas are sattva, rajas and tamas. First, we need to understand these qualities and recognize them in our own mind. With awareness of the gunas, we can learn to work with them as one of the main Yogic tools in healing the mind. Second, we need to wake up the inertia of tamas, calm down the passion of rajas and third, nurture the purity of sattva. This is the way out. This is the beginning of Self-healing.

These three qualities of nature are working together at all times:

> **Tamas** guna is the quality of inertia, darkness and ignorance. Its action is pulling down and veiling.
>
> **Rajas** guna is the quality of action, passion and egoism. Its action is going outward and projecting.
>
> **Sattva** guna is the quality of purity, knowledge and balance. Its action is going inward and upward, revealing our True Nature.

**How tamas works:**

- The veiling in our consciousness makes us strongly identify with our vehicles, our external separate ego-self-body-mind.
- When the veil is too thick, we see our own physical desires only and fails to see the feelings and soul of another. A tamasic person can't help another tamasic person. A prisoner cannot liberate another prisoner.
- Tamas creates the feeling of being in the dark—desperate, depressed, stuck, lazy, inert, pulled down, sick, fearful and anxious.
- A tamasic mind is constantly living in the past and feeling that nothing can change, that we cannot move. Everything appears to be heavy and solid. Tamasic minds brood over the past and complain without doing anything to alleviate their situation.
- A tamasic mind has the attitude of a victim, indulging in addictions and self-destructive behaviors, incapable of detaching or being objective. It cannot exercise reason and cannot see the big picture.
- A tamasic mind feels lonely, isolated, separate.
- Tamas causes a sense of denial of ourselves and of others' goodness. It creates fear and delusion, the disregarding of consequences of actions, maintaining numbness, a freezing stress response, resisting change and a sneaking, hiding behavior, not being aware nor sincere.

- The frequent thought in the tamasic mind is *"I do not care."* Carelessness is applied to our daily life, but also in behavior towards others. It makes us incapable of empathizing and feeling others' pain. A tamasic mind thinks *"You are hurt by my actions and I am fine because you are very different from me. I see you and me very differently."* The veils over the eyes are thick, the separation is very great, and the isolation or the limitations of oneself are very big.
- The tamasic worldview is very limited. It is oftentimes mixed with a rajasic world view, bringing fragmentation, suffering, abuse, war, troubles and conflict, because it believes that we are only this body and mind, very separate from everyone and everything else in the world. From that place of isolation, a person with a tamasic mind has a lot of tension and stress, resulting in many ailments and disease due to fear and anxiety.

**How rajas works:**

- Rajas is action, movement, passion. Rajas fails to see unity and harmony, but is motivated by egoism and selfish motives.
- Tamas denies, rajas projects.
- Tamas fails to see, rajas sees only what the ego sees.
- Rajas brings about desires and, thereby, restlessness in the pursuit of desires.
- Rajas creates competition. Comparison with others is based in ignorance and separation. The mind projects things like "*This person is taller than me, this person seems more intelligent than me, and I feel small because it seems that I'm poorer than her.*" etc... There is constantly a vision of myself in comparison with others who are different than me, because I identify myself to be very separate and different.
- Rajas wants to see ourselves better and bigger. It creates stress and tension due to selfish greed, insatiable desires and over-exertion. *"I am the richest man in the world," "I am the most powerful person."* Rajas can breed the opposite as well, which drives thoughts like *"I am the most unlovable person," "I am the most pitiful person."*
- Rajas exaggerates and leads to extremes.
- While tamas is completely dark, rajas has some knowledge, but it is selective knowledge. It is like "I'm seeing you only because we do something together," but I don't care about other people.

- Tamas and rajas work together. Because of ignorance of reality, our sight is veiled by tamas and rajas. In the analogy of snake and rope, because of our ignorance of the true nature of the snake, we run and react in fright. Disease and conflict are due to tamas and rajas.
- Tamas and rajas are friends, often found linked together. Nowadays our society is tamasic and rajasic, unwise and upside down. Out of ignorance of the Truth of the Self, wealth, name, fame, status and external beauty are projected as the goal of life, at the expense of the common good and common sense. Our consumer society and pleasure-seeking tendencies are due to the gunas tamas and rajas, the energy of darkness and ignorance and the energy of projection. One is denying, unable to see the Truth and the other is seeing, but seeing it incorrectly.
- Family division, community split, racial division, gender division, political and national division, all sorts of division, animal abuse, irresponsible actions creating environmental damage, mass shooting, are all coming from tamas and rajas.
- Tamas and rajas make you do lot of actions in order to get the happiness and improve your life according to your own criteria.
- Tamas and rajas perpetuate suffering due to our vision of the same self-created view and its constant repetition. We cannot solve problems created by our tamasic and rajasic minds with the same mind. Only when we change consciousness will the problems resolve themselves.
- Most people are subject to rajas. Busy-ness is due to rajas. People are very engrossed in being busy with their lives and find no time to stop to think and feel. They have a very strong idea of who they are and they project this idea until it is all they see. The ways in which they try to make their lives better are motivated by rajas.

**How sattva works:**

- Sattva is revealing. Sattva is harmonizing and calming. Sattva is understanding and wisdom. Sattva comes from a sattvic lifestyle: proper exercise (asanas); proper breathing (pranayama), proper relaxation (savasana), proper diet (vegetarian) and positive thinking and meditation.
- Yoga asanas—when performed correctly without strenuous exertion or competition, but with the balance of effort and relaxation and with inner focus, awareness and relaxation—wake up tamas, calm down rajas and transform the mind to sattva.

- Pranayama purifies and balances the vital energies and leads us to go inward towards truth instead of outward with cravings for the objects of the senses.
- Proper relaxation in nature allows meditation and self-awareness. It is not stimulation of the senses nor indulgence in tamasic and rajasic dramas or games.
- The sattvic vegetarian diet is based on respect, moderation and understanding of nutrition and health. Sattvic food uplifts the mind and consciousness. We feel free when we are able to see the big picture.
- Positive thinking gives us opportunities to see things differently and to turn unfavorable circumstances into favorable ones. Meditation helps us to calm and transcend the mind.
- Sattva enlightens. Sattva reveals the underlying unity. Sattva allows a beneficial collective view, collective good, collective endeavor. The walls of the cup separating the inside and outside are still there but the cup now is made of crystal glass, transparent and revealing. We are able to see through to the other side. The upadhis, identification with our body and mind, are still there, the separation is still there, but we are able to see through to our unity and our commonness.
- Philanthropy, humanitarian actions, selfless actions and charitable actions are possible in sattva.
- Sattva balances tamas and rajas. Tamas wakes up and rajas calms down in sattva.
- The movement of sattva is turning inwards and upwards.
- All Yogic practices calm down the mind and promote sattva.
- Sattva allows peace and lasting happiness.
- Sattva gives hope. Sattva brings Light. Sattva makes a person virtuous.
- Sattva awakens intelligence and clear thinking.
- Tamas complains, rajas points fingers, and sattva teaches.
- Sattva allows connection with the consciousness of Self. All conscious decisions and motivations are sattvic by nature.
- In the previous example of the wall of a glass which separates the space inside and outside, or the individual person identifying with the body and mind, thinking him/herself to be a separate entity, sattva means the walls of the glass are now transparent. The person is able to connect with Self by detaching from body and mind and see themselves as part of a whole.

- If your mind is enlightened by the light of Self-knowledge, if your intellect is clear and unselfish, if you are conscious in your actions for the benefit of others, then what you see in your mind and the reality are almost the same.
- The result of this vision of oneness is that you will make less mistakes, bringing fewer karmic consequences and sufferings. You will feel more expanded, more peaceful, more calm, more connected, more wise. Your vision is pure, because the veil is pure. You see the Truth with less distortion. It takes going beyond the three gunas to completely embody Truth. The ego has to be completely transcended.
- In the sattvic mind, I understand that if I hurt you, I am actually hurting myself. Whatever I do to you, actually is being done to me. If I help you, I help myself.
- If you understand this, then you will see the path toward Self-healing. It is a path towards thinning the veils of our consciousness. It is not finding the solutions outside of ourselves. Instead, it is relieving our suffering through the awakening to our selfishness and through the revelation that we are already fulfilled and complete within ourselves. The path of Self-healing brings fewer ideas of happiness outside of ourselves and more peace and happiness from within, less delusion and restlessness, more connection and knowledge. Less "I" selfishness and more "we" consensus. More questioning and less laziness. More acceptance and less selfish ideas of right and wrong. More peace and light.
- This journey of purification starts from within and will set us free. Free from what? It will set us free from present and future suffering stemming from our distorted view.
- Purification means turning around and cleaning our glasses (mind) to correctly see our Self and reality.
- All Yoga practices lead to purification or transformation of consciousness from gross to subtle, from tamas to sattva, from hatred and conflicts to love.

In summary, the body is a vehicle and you are not the vehicle. The approach is to see things as vehicles and as veils of consciousness. The first vehicle is the physical body, made of five elements, that goes through the cycle of birth, growth, change, decay and death. So when the body dies, when the body gets old, don't be surprised. Its nature is to be born, to grow, to change, to decay and to die. But you continue as the astral body continues. You're not dead when the physical body is dead. The astral body is the second vehicle. It has the five organs of action, five senses, five kinds of prana, the mind, the intellect, subconscious mind and the ego. (Five organs of action: you do actions with your mouth, hands, feet, anus and genitals. Five organs of knowledge: you see, hear, smell, taste and touch things. Your inner instruments are like the engine of your car—you have the mind, the intellect, subconscious and the ego, that's how you think. So two people who are twins have the same physical body, but the way they think is different, because the inner instruments are different. Deeper still, you have the causal body, the seed body, seed of your karma.

## *INSPIRED STORY*

### Holistic healing

*H, a 42-year-old woman, has been working for a bank for 17 years. She is married with four children and is her family's main income source. She currently lives with her husband's parents and has little connection with her in-laws. She is close with her biological parents and regularly takes care of their meals and nutrition, as well as her siblings. She always prioritizes the well-being of her immediate family members and considers it her joy, often neglecting her own needs. She spends 60 minutes commuting to work daily and has limited friends or people to share her thoughts with. She rarely takes time to relax, exercises little, and goes on family vacations 2-3 times a year.*

*She was diagnosed with stage 2 breast cancer and turned to Yoga and Ayurveda as a healing method. After surgery and completing half of the prescribed chemotherapy, she took a leave of absence from work to participate in a panchakarma Ayurvedic detox treatment for three weeks in India and a month-long Yoga Teacher Training Course (TTC) followed by an additional two months in the ashram living a classical Yoga lifestyle. This includes practicing the five points of Yoga in daily life. Upon her return four months later, all cancer indicators had completely disappeared, and her history of hepatitis B also was gone.*

*She found a new job closer to home, experienced less stress, dedicated time to practicing Yoga and meditation, and took walks in nature daily. She found joy in self-care and improved her overall health. She registered to study to become a Sivananda Yoga Health Educator. Her initial cancer was attributed to her strong attachment to her family and lack of self-awareness. When taught the Yoga lifestyle, she learned to detach herself from others and prioritize self-care, leading to a physical and mental recovery. It has now been fiveyears since her illness, and she continues to maintain a Yoga lifestyle without any metastasis complications.*

**QUESTIONS**

1. *Describe the three bodies which are vehicles of the soul. What do you want to achieve when seeing the body and mind as vehicles?*
2. *Describe the five koshas. How do you purify each of the koshas?*
3. *Describe the three gunas, or qualities, tamas, rajas, sattva. Describe the process of purification moving from tamas to rajas to sattva. Give an example from your own experience.*

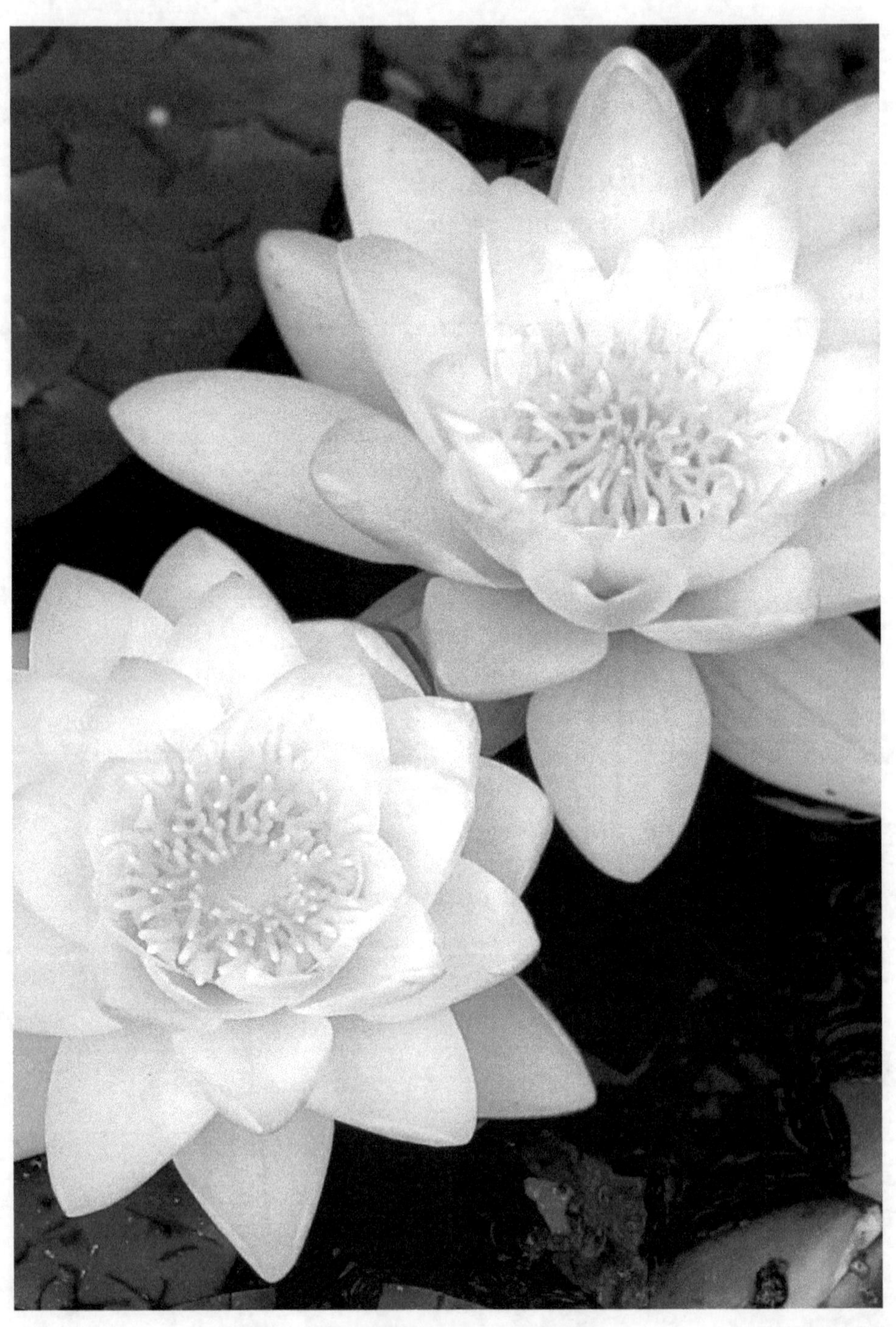

LOTUS OUT OF MUD

CHAPTER 3

# Resilience in Life Struggles - Conflicts & Stress

***"Yoga leads us from ignorance to wisdom, from weakness to strength, from disharmony to harmony, from hatred to love, from want to fullness, from limitation to infinity, from diversity to unity, from imperfection to perfection."***

*– SWAMI SIVANANDA*

In a world of conflicts and stress and in the constant inner battle between the past impressions *(samskaras)* and the newly-acquired positive thoughts, the Yoga practitioner needs to develop resilience, the capacity of inner strength and endurance and the capacity to tame and harness the mind and emotions, staying in balance amidst conflicts deriving from both internal and external factors. Resilience is the ability to bounce back from the trials and tribulations of life and keep going onward. It comes from seeing life clearly and accepting that life is changing. Resilience is key to positive mental health as well as to spiritual health.

Let's examine life and its inherent struggles and understand the five causes of stress and how Yoga is the unique way offered to all to face life challenges.

## 1. THREE TYPES OF SUFFERING ACCORDING TO BHAGAVAD GITA

A scripture of yoga, the Bhagavad Gita, describes three main causes of suffering, three types of affliction.

- **Adhyatmika** refers to afflictions of the body. The body is thirsty, hungry and sick. It is a very complex network. The nine different systems of the body are intricate and the body needs to maintain homeostasis to keep the entire system healthy. The nine body systems are: 1) musculoskeletal system, 2) respiratory system, 3) cardiovascular system, 4) nervous system, 5) digestive system, 6) endocrine system, 7) urogenital reproductive system, 8) immune system, and 9) lymphatic system.

Swami Sivananda, who was a medical doctor, said, *"Physical health is when the body organs function optimally under the intelligent control of the mind."* He said about health: *"Every human being is the author of his own health or disease. Disease is the result of disobedience to the immutable laws of health that govern life. The laws of health are the laws of nature. In the vast universe, only man breaks and violates rules and laws. He willfully disregards the laws of health, leads a life of dissipation and then wonders why he suffers from disease and disharmony."*

Upon graduation, many medical students take a modern version of the Hippocratic Oath from 1964, vowing, among other things: "*I will prevent disease whenever I can, for prevention is preferable to cure.*"

The sciences of anatomy and physiology teach us that the body systems need to maintain homeostasis—a state of balance among all body systems needed for the body to survive and function well. We need to learn the sciences of the body. We need to understand its anatomy, physiology, pathology and dietetic needs in order to use our vehicles properly.

- The second cause of suffering is called **adhibhautika**, which means the afflictions caused by beings around you. You are born in a certain family and you go through life interacting with people around you. These are the people you are connected with, people you are working with or people you live with. When you drive in traffic, you will also be affected by the people driving around you. We need to examine the relationships we have with new, clear eyes and know how to deal with them.
- The third cause of suffering is called **adhidaivika**, which means the suffering caused by the forces of heaven or by the divine forces. These forces include natural disasters like cyclones, hurricanes, floods, drought, excessive rain, excessive heat. Recently, there were many earthquakes; a big earthquake in Turkey killed 47,000 people and the earth kept shaking. This created a lot of fear, a lot of trauma, a lot of suffering. People get angry, but it was from a divine cause.

Facing the three types of suffering, we have to learn to build up our resilience, so that we can be strong to meet our challenges.

## 2. TRUE MEANING OF LIFE: A SCHOOL WHERE WE LEARN TO DRIVE OUR VEHICLE

Swami Sivananda said, "Life is a school in which every sorrow, every pain, every heart-break brings a precious lesson. Life on earth is the means for Self-perfection. The world is your best teacher. There is a lesson in everything. The world is the best training ground for developing various divine virtues, such as mercy, forgiveness, tolerance, universal love, courage, patience and strong will."

**Life is a struggle**

Swami Sivananda said, *"If you cease to struggle, you cease to live."* The more we understand the battle of life, the more we are able to use our tools, our equipment correctly to support our journey. Why is life so difficult on earth? How can we win the battle and come out on the other side?

Yoga equips us with all the tools needed to lead our lives successfully. Yogic discipline is a necessary path to explain, inspire, and support this life struggle. The Yoga teachers understand the struggle of life and help us with Yoga discipline with compassion. When we do not understand the need to practice Yoga and Yoga discipline, we think we can win life's battle by ourselves without sadhana.

**Life is a conscious stream**

Life is meant to be lived consciously, even as it constantly changes, like a river. If you stand at one place and watch a river flow, you are always watching different water. It looks like the same water, but it just keeps flowing past without stopping for a moment. Life is like this conscious stream. We have to accept that our life is constantly changing. With acceptance of constant change, we will not be fearful or anxious, trying to stop the natural progression of life. We need to remember that life is a stream of consciousness. This means we are constantly evolving, from being unconscious to being more and more aware.

Embrace the flow of life and recognize the divine intelligence and presence in every movement of life.

**Life is a journey**

But you need to know from where to where so that you can interpret the struggles of life. You have gone through different experiences in this life, but also in past lives. According to the theory of karma and reincarnation, there are past lives, and there will be future lives. There will be future experiences in order for you to purge yourself from impurities. This life is only a chapter in the book of your life. You have come to this life with weaknesses and strengths, but remember that both weaknesses and strengths can lead you to pain when there is no awareness. It is awareness that is most important to see what is happening and to find our lessons so we can learn from them. We are in no way a victim of what is happening in our lives: This is understood if we are conscious of our path.

**Life has a direction, life is progress**

Even though it keeps moving, life has a direction. From outward to inward and downward to upward. We are constantly evolving, like a river that is turbulent or smooth-flowing and may take many twists and turns, ceaselessly, moving until it merges with the ocean. And when it merges with the ocean, it becomes peaceful. It dissolves into it, blends into it and becomes one with it. Before that, it was restless. Even in those stretches of life when we feel we are stagnating, we are still progressing. Changing and struggling means learning. The more the struggle, the more the triumph. Learn resilience and understand the meaning of life in order to derive courage. Come to accept struggle, but with less stress and strain. Aim to learn the lessons faster, without having to repeat the class. Train yourself to bounce back. Pick yourself up again and carry on.

We have all made mistakes. The blemishes and dirt are on our glasses, but while looking through them we perceive what is around us to be blemished and dirty. It is our vision and how we see things that is tainted. We need to clean and purify our way of seeing things while remembering our pure consciousness. We are the source of Light; we are Light itself. When we purify our vision, we will not see the imperfection outside anymore. The sooner we can do that, the sooner we will become peaceful. Why wait?

**Life is a journey from impurity to purity**

According to the theory of yoga, there are three kinds of impurities:

- First is impurity that comes from egoism, which means the wrong idea of self. Practice selflessness in order to thin out the ego. When we have pain, when we struggle, when we have stress, we have to know it comes from our egoism.
- Second is impurity that comes from the restless and jumping nature of the mind that is always projecting different ideas, stories and scenarios. Calm that mind down to realize the beauty and fulfillment behind the projected desires.
- Third is impurity that comes from the veiling nature of the mind. We believe we are the body, *"I am a man, I am a woman,"* and we believe ourselves to be the mind, *"I am sad, I am angry."* This third kind of impurity creates

false identification and is more difficult to manage. Do self-inquiry and meditate in order to be more self-aware and awaken to your True Nature. Ask the question *"Who am I?"* Refute the appearances and find the Self.

Impurities are like dust lurking under a seemingly clean carpet. You say, *"Oh, the carpet is clean."* But if you start cleaning, you will see all kinds of dust. Along the way you might get discouraged from the spiritual path, you might throw down your vacuum cleaner and your broom and walk away. The carpet is too dirty. The reality is you never really looked within; you thought you were perfect. When you start to see your imperfections, you realize there are many and you blame Yoga for giving you these problems.

*"When I came to the ashram, I thought I would be walking three feet above the ground and talking to the butterflies. I thought that yoga would give me an easy, wonderful life. But soon I realized this is a romantic idea."*

It takes time and patience to cleanse the impurities. Facing ourselves and realizing our illusions and imperfections is already great progress. Swami Sivananda said that in the beginning of Yoga life, you will feel ups and downs; but you will progress in great strides once you train yourself in new habits.

Life is a journey of learning how to be free from these three kinds of impurities.

**Life is a journey from hatred to cosmic love**

We have a lot of hatred in our hearts, lots of liking and disliking. We might not say these inner feelings of discontent and contempt out loud, but they are always there. When we become adults, we learn not to say, *"I hate this, I hate that"* so often. We learn to hide our feelings.

On our journey, we may love plants, pets, animals, our kith and kin, but it is difficult to have unconditional love for people we do not know. When we are able to do that, we expand our heart and we feel bigger, lighter, freer. Life gives us a lot of challenges in order for us to open our hearts and overcome our emotional challenges in relationships.

**Our story is a reflection of what is happening within**

You must come to recognize the inner journey.

When we tell our story, we always tell the story of what is happening externally - *"I lived in this country; I moved there; I did this job; now I started this business,"* and so on. However, we neglect to explore and understand what's happening inside, and it is the inner journey that is most important to recognize. The same lesson will keep repeating whether you are here or there, with this husband or wife or this or that job. The same karmic lesson keeps happening until we learn it, and the first step is to honor our inner journey.

Examples of these lessons might include being more tolerant, loving, and content; not being perfectionistic and hypercritical. You might hate yourself and other people for not being perfect. Recognize that you are projecting the idea of perfection externally, which leads to being overly critical, judgmental, or extreme.

Whatever is happening, the core lesson is that *"true perfection is within"* and *"everything outside is relative."* The journey inward and upward helps us become less critical and more tolerant, having less expectations of things going our way. The more we are aware of the inner landscape, the more we'll be able to find the tools and resources to help ourselves progress. We don't have to spend so much energy, so much effort, in uselessly blaming, in stress and disease.

**Life is a journey from death to immortality**

There is a connection between improper ways of living, destruction of our instrument faster than necessary, and disease and death. Going from death to immortality is not about this physical process. It is about the soul's journey to liberation. Going from death to immortality means eventually understanding all our lessons and not making more mistakes. We become complete and fulfilled and that journey, that cycle of life and death will automatically cease, because we have attained the full knowledge of ourselves.

**Life is a journey from imperfection to perfection**

Know that everyone is progressing towards Self-healing. Everyone is moving from imperfection to perfection. Have compassion when you see people struggle. Hold space for them. Keep the highest vision of them. They might not see themselves this way, but you will.

**Life is a journey from slavery to freedom**

There is false freedom and true freedom. False freedom comes from external conditions, to travel where we like, to eat what we like, think what we like, talk as we like. True freedom, which is the boundless, limitless freedom of the soul, needs to come from inner self-discipline.

**Life is a journey from diversity to unity**

In this phase of the journey, we start to see less external differences between ourselves, cultures, languages, religious beliefs, characters, gender, and color. A vision that sees people and things as different and separate creates the unnecessary struggles we endure. With the attachment to our own way of seeing, we get into war, crime, and all kinds of crazy, unnecessary conflict. Growth is to recognize and appreciate our diversity, and at the same time see the oneness that is always there. This is what we call "unity in diversity." Waves of the ocean might look different, but they are simply part of the same ocean.

**Life is a journey from ignorance to wisdom**

Academic study is not wisdom. Intellectual study is not wisdom. Erudition will not set us free from repeating mistakes. Wisdom makes us feel fulfilled and free. The more we are able to understand that we do not know, the more we have a chance to know. All crises we go through in life are there to teach us to become wise.

**Life is a journey from pain to eternal bliss**

Life is full of pain—physical, mental and emotional. Doctors and psychiatrists administer to pain and symptoms through external measures. The Self-healing journey goes to the root causes of pain and heals from a source deep within. The path of Self-healing understands the connection between different levels of pain by understanding the connection between the three bodies and the five sheaths. Spiritual ignorance and the egoism thereof is seen as the root cause of suffering. Self-healing starts from within through Self-awakening. Remembering the Self, the painless, diseaseless *atman* allows us to be detached from pain and to remember peace and bliss.

**Life is a journey from weakness to infinite strength**

Pain, suffering, and disease are opportunities to gain strength. We always think that our suffering comes from some external source, but actually it comes from our own weaknesses. Life is a journey to become stronger. Weaknesses and strengths can be seen in our mental tendencies and can be remedied by yoga practices catering to the individual. We need to be very patient when working on our weaknesses. Eventually everything will balance out.

**Life is service and sacrifice**

Life is service. Understand the relationship between you and others around you. They are your own Self. If you work for others, if you love others unconditionally and serve them, you actually elevate yourself.

There is a story of a disciple and a teacher going through the different compartments of hell. They come to one place and see people suffering greatly, because all the people in the room have fused elbows. Their elbows cannot bend, so they cannot eat food, pick things up, or scratch their head. They are very frustrated and angry. Then the disciple and the teacher go to another compartment where they see people are very happy, despite having the same problem. All the elbows are fused and yet people are very happy. Why? Because they feed and scratch each other.

We need to help each other. We need to serve each other because it serves ourselves. It makes us happy. Life is service and sacrifice. Our life is a quest for our lost inheritance. Our destination is our perfection. The central goal of life is the realization of our oneness with the source from which we came.

Realization can come in many forms:

> *"Oh my God, I did not understand that. I did not understand that when I harm somebody, I harm myself, and when I forgive others, I forgive myself... When I abuse animals, I suffer from the flood, the virus, the fire. Those things are happening to me. I did not see the connection!"*

There is a connection in everything. We need to come to the conscious realization of our oneness. The opportunity to understand it is now. Dive deep within and find the way to realize it. We cannot transform something outside so we must transform ourselves. The more we try to change something outside, the more we are powerless. As we equip ourselves with the right attitude and practices, we improve our well-being and immune systems and the well-being of the planet.

One lady, who tends to complain, testified about her Self-healing journey:

*"Oh, I realize that I am not alone. My life is not that bad really. Look at this other person's life. They struggle much harder than I do. They have no food to eat. They are starving and I am complaining that my preferred food is not being served."*

**The central goal of life is to come into the conscious realization of our oneness with God.** Life has no meaning as a separate life. That's why you need to see the connection between yourself and others. Be compassionate and serve others so that you can be free yourself. There is a Buddhist prayer that "we can be free when everybody is free." You don't ask for yourself to be freed and then disregard other people. So, the Buddhist prayer is, *"I will be free when everyone else is free."* This is beautiful! It is beautiful because, in that prayer, you recognize the oneness.

**Life on earth is a school to learn to see spirit in matter**

Boldly face all the difficulties and tribulations of this earthly life, be a person of courage, and know that life is a school. Live a simple life in an unassuming manner. Serve, love, give, purify, meditate and realize. See life as one, as a whole. See the unity of life. Smile with a flower and the green grass. Smile with everybody and everything that you meet.

## 3. LIFE AND STRESS

We need to understand what stress is, and the relationship between stress and disease so we become aware of how we heal ourselves.

It's like when we have a good vehicle, but we don't know how to drive. If we drive in the wrong manner, accelerating and pushing on the brake at the same time, what happens? We damage the vehicle. Not going anywhere, we create stress and tension for ourselves and maybe even crash the car.

We cannot be free from stress. Let's say a person buys a yacht and sails on the ocean alone for years. He doesn't have to deal with people and he doesn't have to deal with work, but he does have to deal with storms, cyclones, and his own loneliness. It will never really work. Escape is not the way. It is better that we endeavor to understand what stress is, and what life is. Sometimes when we are very stressed, we conclude, "It's me, I'm being cursed; it's me that has a problem." In actuality, it's everybody's general condition.

### Stress and anxiety stop the flow of life force

If we don't follow the flow of life, we will stop the flow of prana, or life force, and that's when we come into stress. We expend prana, our life resource, uselessly when trying to do things that are impossible or not worthwhile. When we don't know how to connect with nature, or how to connect with the source of prana within us, we become very anxious.

With anxiety, we become rigid. Anxiety comes from fear. When we are fearful, we become paralyzed and rigid. The more we become rigid, fearful, less accommodating and less flexible, the more the flow of life is obstructed. The things we fear become more serious. We aggravate our problem and it escalates.

The alternative is to face the challenge, become strong. Avoid creating unnecessary problems by your negative reactions. Think of it as a positive opportunity.

Anxiety is quite rampant these days. When feeling apprehensive about the future, the best remedy is to bring the mind back to the present with the Yogic techniques of asana, pranayama, relaxation and meditation. Yoga helps to alleviate anxiety in this world of uncertainty. If everyone develops their faculty of self-control and learns to live in the present, the world will be a peaceful place.

From stress comes disease. Medical research estimates as much as 90 percent of illness and disease is stress-related. Stress can interfere with your physical functioning and bodily processes. High blood pressure, cardiovascular disease, and heart disease have been linked to stress factors.

**COMMON SIGNS OF STRESS**
**(from American Institute of Stress)**

| General | Nervous System | Psychological |
|---|---|---|
| • Lost efficiency at work<br>• Allergies<br>• Addictions<br>• Dizziness<br>• Vertigo<br>• Fatigue<br>• Eyes irritation/ redness<br>• Insomnia/ nightmare disturb dreams<br>• Nose bleeding<br>• Rash and skin irritation<br>• Anemia<br>• Infection<br>• Swollen lymph gland | • Frequent headaches<br>• Tense yawn<br>• Difficulty talking<br>• Tuttering<br>• Stammering<br>• Hands and lips trembling<br>• Cannot share and communicate<br>• Tremors<br>• Panic attack<br>• Difficulty concentrating<br>• Cannot learn new information<br>• Difficulty making decisions<br>• Crying for no reason<br>• Minor accidents<br>• Obsessive compulsive behavior<br>• Ringing sound in the ears | • Anxiety<br>• Depression<br>• Memory lost<br>• Mood swing<br>• Addictions<br>• Overwhelmed<br>• Forgetful<br>• Confused<br>• Difficulty Concentrating<br>• Anger/hostility<br>• Irritability<br>• Edginess<br>• Loss of balance<br>• Suicidal thoughts<br>• Lonliness<br>• Worthlessness<br>• Social Withdrawl<br>• Isolating |

| Digestive System | Cardiovascular System | Muscular Skeletal System |
|---|---|---|
| • Heart burn<br>• Stomach pain<br>• Nausea<br>• Excess belching<br>• Dry mouth<br>• Problem swallowing<br>• Flatulence<br>• Constipation<br>• Diarrhea<br>• Increase/Decrease in appetite | • Rapid heart beat<br>• Cardiovascular problem<br>• Heart attack<br>• Stroke<br>• Coronary problem | • Neck aches<br>• Back ache<br>• Muscle spasms<br>• Tapping Feet |

| Respiratory System | Immune System | Endocrine System |
|---|---|---|
| • Coughing<br>• Sneezing<br>• Difficulty breathing<br>• Frequent sighs | • Frquent colds<br>• Frequent infections<br>• Constant fatigue | • Diabetes<br>• Thyroid problem<br>• Urinal/ reproductive problem<br>• Frequent urination<br>• Infertility<br>• Cold hands and feet |

Classical yoga teachers understand the deep relationship between Yoga and stress relief as they go to the root cause of stress. Seek out these yoga teachers or other experienced and wise people to get support in dealing with these psychological and philosophical causes of stress.

If you don't address the real inner problem and instead blame external circumstances, stress will become chronic and aggravate disease. The body and mind cannot sustain stress for long. When we are able to tune back within, get in touch with the inner ruler, correctly understand what life is, we will regain our inner power, become resilient—less afraid and much more healthy and peaceful.

## 4. THREE RESPONSES TO STRESS

There are three stress responses, depending on personality type:

**Fight** - You're always agitated and fighting against a perceived threat. With this response, you'll tend toward health problems like high blood pressure, heart attack, and cardiovascular problems. An example of the fight response: if you have stress at work, you will work harder.

**Flight** - You run away from stressors, anything that causes you discomfort. You run away and don't face your problems. For example, if you have stress in work or relationships, you will frequently change jobs or romantic partners.

**Freeze** - You are conflicted between fighting and running; you don't know what to do. You respond in fear and freeze. You want to live, you want to feel, you want to love, you want to experience life but, at the same time, you are paralyzed and cannot act. The freeze response prevents us from acting, talking, feeling, basically from living our lives.

Any of these responses is ultimately damaging to the body and mind. In response, many people die at an early age. For example, many famous actors and actresses, who live intensely with a lot of emotional ups and downs, feel the need to take prescription medicine or street drugs to calm their stress, to calm their anxiety or to help them sleep. They are chronically anxious and on edge. They go through life pressuring themselves to appear to be perfect—and then die early. The underlying cause of almost all premature deaths is stress-related. The human body is a vehicle like a car, with a certain expected life span. Proper use of the vehicle maximizes the life expectancy. Learning to live a more stress-free life is essential for longevity and well-being.

Swami Sivananda said that the secret to being healthy is to live in moderation. In our fast-paced society, it is best to take time, slow down, relax, and lead a simple life. Understand the goal of life. The answer lies within and not externally. Taking extended spiritual retreats and supporting ashrams and yoga retreats are alternative personal and collective solutions. We don't need to take on one more project, or take on more work. Relax! We don't need more information in our mind, more busy-ness. We need to be still, develop stress resilience, learn to discriminate and detach in order to wisely manage our strengths and weaknesses and progress in Self-healing.

The physical and mental pains in life are there for a reason, to show us something. Don't run away from the challenge.

*Imagine you are driving a car and the flashing red "check engine" light comes on. You get very annoyed, because you just want to get to your destination. So, you take a hammer from the glove compartment and smash the indicator. No more flashing light!!! But is everything okay?*

Like the check engine light, pain shows up in life as a warning. We have to wake up; we have to try to maneuver so that we don't crash. Sometimes it's too late in the process and we cannot avoid crashing. But ideally, as much as possible, as soon as possible, recognize the pain, face it and try to go to the root cause.

**Self-healing is learning to manage stress, pains and weakness.** It's very comforting to know that pain itself will lead us to freedom from pain. Weakness will lead to strength. If you feel you're weak in something, you become strong. How? When you have a weakness, you think about it all the time. And by thinking about it, you will become stronger. Conversely, sometimes you feel you are strong and maybe take it for granted, then you fall down. In the arrogance of thinking you are so good or so strong, you become blind to your weaknesses and they arise again to bring an opportunity for your learning.

But if you know that you have a weakness, you will become stronger and stronger. Since you are aware of it and you think of it all the time, you work on it. You make progress. Also, realize that you are not alone. All your struggles are not just unique to you. This is already a very big step.

**Self-healing is the path of wisdom, recognizing our human condition, and not taking things personally.** It is universal. If you only think personally, you will constantly repeat to yourself and everyone around you, *"I suffer from this," "I like this," "My life is this," "I suffer."* When you think in this way, you are trapped by one very big problem—it is called egoism.

Egoism is the root cause of all your problems. You need to get out of this trap of egoism and see it as the universal condition. You might be a little different from others, but the differences are very small. Many people suffer like you. The problem is universal and it is not yours personally. You can detach from it and become objective in your view of situations and feelings. It becomes less self-involved. When you understand the problem is general then the problem is alleviated because you are not investing all your energy in all-consuming self-pity.

Stress is subjective and emotional. It can be dealt with by classical Yoga. Stress, in reality, is independent of external conditions. A stressor may not create much stress for one person, but may create terrible stress for someone else. Stress is subjective. Because it is subjective, you can change the way you look at things.

Example: Two people lose their job. One person cries and becomes anxious and feels like it is the end of the world. The other person has a different outlook and says *"Yeah, great. Now there is an opportunity for me to be creative, and do something else."*

## 5. FIVE CAUSES OF STRESS AND HOW CLASSICAL YOGA HELPS

1. **The first cause of stress is lack of prana.** If you don't have adequate prana, you cannot deal with the situations of your life and the situations become aggravated. Yoga's unique specialty is to help increase, conserve, balance, channel and purify prana *(see Chapter 5 on prana)*

2. **The second cause of stress is negative emotions.** Negative emotions come from the struggle of life we have been discussing. This struggle brings anger, frustration, fear, anxiety, hatred, greed, desire, envy, jealousy and lust. These emotions can accumulate and become habitual, creating recurring stress responses. Classical Yoga teaches the uplifting methods of devotion, positive thinking, and meditation.

3. **The third cause of stress is lack of adaptability.** The changing nature of life requires us to be flexible and adaptable. We have difficulty because of our attachments, because of our ego. Classical Yoga methods help us detach from our ego and expectations and learn to cope and adapt.

   Yoga teaches you to be flexible. That's why you exercise your body in Yoga - forward, backward, sideways, twisting, and upside down! *"Flexible spine, flexible mind."*

   Yoga teaches you to drop the expectation that things should follow your preferred way, but try to adjust yourself so you have less stress. In the time of the global pandemic, the biggest lesson that everyone learned was flexibility, as the very manner in which we lived changed. While we used to frequent coffee shops and restaurants, go to parties, and relax, socialize with friends, we were urged to adjust to living indoors all day with the same few people. We had to adapt to an altered way of living and changed relationships with people in our lives.

4. **The number four cause of stress is our existential anxiety.** Existential anxiety is simply the stress of being alive and the struggle to understand what it's all about. Unanswered existential questions make us uneasy. The existential questions are the big questions: "*Why am I here on this earth? What is the purpose of my life? Where am I going? Why are things the way they are? Who am I? What is life? What is death?*" Spiritual wisdom and yoga philosophy about the Self and the not-Self, the truth and the illusion, help to answer a lot of these questions and help to alleviate our existential stress.
5. **The fifth cause of stress is karma.** As a cause of your stress, karma is the most difficult to address. Everyone is stressed to some extent because of unresolved karma: family karma, personal karma, relationship karma. Classical Yoga scriptures teach many methods of renewing our attitudes that will free us from past karma and from repeating karma. Through a very deep understanding of karma, we can learn to accept it, and learn how to deal with it. So go to the source of your karmic struggles and stress.

**Yogic methods to decrease stress:**

- Learn basic Yogic skills to increase prana.
- Learn basic skills for how to be adaptable.
- Learn to increase your faith to prevent anxiety.
- Learn to see your attachment, because attachment creates anxiety and fear.
- Learn to affirm courage and inner strength to face challenges in life.
- Remind yourself time and time again to live in the present. Experience the power of the present, and don't let your mind go too far into the future or be too attached to past experiences. "*Present is superior to the past,*" according to Swami Sivananda.
- Build the habit of being calm under all conditions.
- Learn to relax in your own power of being. Improve your body awareness and your breath awareness. Learn to work with your breath especially.
- Adopt a positive attitude toward life. Increase your sense of gratitude so you are not anxious when you don't get what you want. Become thankful for what you already have and be content.

- Learn to let go of desires and adopt the attitude of contentment. Create a sense of security and emotional relaxation. Remember that anxiety and stress are a part of life. Learn to calm yourself down, to soothe yourself, to love yourself, to feel secure within yourself.
- There is a power of sustenance within you, called *ojas* according to ayurveda. We need to replenish *ojas* in our system all the time as *ojas* gives contentment and joy. Depleted *ojas* creates exhaustion and discontentment. Learn to improve your *ojas*, the energy of contentment, endurance, and sustenance. This can be done through nutritious diet, positive thinking and devotion. *Ojas* gives you security and stability and counteracts anxiety.
- Practice remembering the Self, being detached from things that are not true about yourself and others. Know how to positively affirm yourself instead of doubting all the time.
- Learn to use your subconscious mind.

**A story about acceptance**

*A woman is crying because her son died and she can't accept it. She goes from place to place to find all the teachers and all the monks and says to them, "I want my son back, I don't accept this!" She comes to a Swami and says the same.*

*The Swami responds, "Okay, I will give your son back if you take this bowl and go to different houses and ask for a few mustard seeds. When you fill up the bowl, I'll give you your son back. But the condition is you can only take mustard seeds from houses in which no one has died." The woman agrees. She goes and visits many houses. At every door, in every encounter at each home, there is someone who has died. She continues and goes here and there and everywhere.*

*At long last, she has been to all of the houses and isn't able to fill up the bowl. She returns to the Swami who sent her on this mission and concedes, "I return the bowl. I accept. I don't want my son back anymore. I now understand death is a universal phenomenon."*

## 6. CULTIVATE THE THREE LEVELS OF FAITH FOR SELF-HEALING

To counteract stress and anxiety, we need to develop positive thinking and faith. **The three levels of faith for self-healing are faith in yourself, faith in the practice and faith in the teacher.**

**You must have faith in yourself** and believe you can change and heal. Without faith towards your Self, you cannot self-heal. You might try, but then, not believing in yourself, you give up.

**You have to have faith in the practices.** The Yogic practices for Self-healing are thousands of years old and have been proven to be highly effective. You have to believe and have faith that they will work to be motivated to show up and practice every day. If you don't have faith in pranayama, asana, prayer and meditation, you won't do the practice. You must have faith to carry you through the more difficult days. Even if you don't feel well, or you feel stressed or agitated, with faith, you will sit down to meditate, do asana, do pranayama… and you will soon feel better. Your faith in the practices will keep you committed to doing them day after day. Trust the process.

**Faith in the spiritual teacher and in the Supreme Being.** The spiritual teacher has tread the path before you. He /she has encountered the same trials and tribulations on the path and will be able to support you as you go through yours. He/she has the enlightened vision that will inspire you.

Beyond having faith in yourself, the practice, and the teacher, you have to have faith in the Supreme Being. You need to believe that everything is actually good, that you can be helped, supported and nurtured. You have not been abandoned. You are not alone. The universe is helping you and upholding you. Have faith in that.

Have faith and trust in Mother Nature. Mother Nature is all of creation and it is also your own body. Have connection to, and faith in, Mother Nature that gave us life. It's amazing how everything is being taken care of!

For example, Mother Nature gave us the liver. This organ helps us detoxify and reduce our stress and anger. The liver can renew itself. It works very hard every day to keep us healthy and alive. We need to think about the liver and be thankful for the liver.

Think about your heart. The heart is working all the time. Think about the brain. Think about the lungs, think about the marvel of the skin. Think of the eyelids. You put weight on the eyelids and the relaxation response comes. There are a lot of things that Mother Nature has given you in order to help you. Just trust in Mother Nature and learn.

When you feel stressed, go out in the sun for 10 minutes. Just by the sun's nature, the sun will take all of the stress and give you energy right away. Similarly, fresh air will take your stress away and refresh you. Go out and breathe in air, fresh air. You might be stressed and thinking what to do to help yourself. Breathe! Breathe! Fresh air responds, "I'm fresh air. I'm here. I'm helping you. I'm helping you." You breathe and your stress dissipates.

In a time of stress or distress, when you don't know what to do, go hug a tree. "*Tree, please help me. I'm so stressed,*" you implore. You touch the tree, you hug the tree. "*You have been here for 100 years. I'd like to be like you. Please give me stability like yours.*" You hug the tree and your stress melts away.

There are so many things you can do in a forest; it's a bath of prana. Birds are singing, leaves are fluttering. Your thoughts also become lighter and lighter. Mother Nature surrounds and supports you.

**Things to avoid (obstacles to Self-healing):**

- Negative company
- Negative spaces
- Avoid watching too much negative news or stories that you cannot digest
- Negative habits of smoking, drinking alcohol, using drugs of all sorts
- Wasting your energy and draining your prana
- Rigidity and lack of adaptability
- A sedentary life, and anything extreme
- Too much moving around, too much shopping, too much desire.
- Comparison with others for more name, fame, power, success
- Denial and isolation

When you're stressed, you don't know you are stressed. Or, when you are stressed you have been conditioned to think that it is weak to be stressed or to admit it, so you deny it. Accept that stress is part of life and give yourself compassion. Ask for help.

There's one lady, she said: *"I have stomach pain, I have a headache..." I tried to console her, "Ok, ok." I touched her hand with my hands... Her hand was cold and wet, she said her stomach was cramping and she had a bad headache... I said, "You're stressed. Calm down, breathe slowly." She had all the symptoms and yet she kept saying: "I'm not stressed. I'm not stressed."*

## *INSPIRED STORY*

**How Yoga helped me physically, mentally, and spiritually through difficult times**

*I was in a severe auto accident in a remote area of Mexico. I was on the bed in the back of an RV and was flung against a wall when it flipped. I was knocked temporarily unconscious, my right hip was over on top of the left, and my right shoulder was ripped up. A vehicle showed up with a woman who was a nurse and yoga teacher. She called an ambulance and helped me get into a stable position and breathe through the spasms. She was my first "angel" in the chaos of the accident.*

*I had no pain relief and was transported to a clinic down a dirt road—a painful, bumpy ride! I imagined Jesus holding my one hand and Krishna holding the other to help me through the pain. I did long, slow breathing and visualized swimming away from the lower part of my body when the pain was extra-intense. Sixteen hours from the time of the accident, I received some drugs for pain relief. The doctors were amazed that I didn't go into total shock. I credit it to my belief that God (in many forms) was with me, plus my breathing exercises and visualizations.*

*The journey of rehabilitation was long and intense, from being bed-ridden to slowly learning to walk again. However, I continued with my very limited version of the sun salutation in the morning, visualizing my body doing the full motions. I also modified my breathing and meditation practice to sitting in my recliner, because I couldn't sit on the floor or sit straight up for very long. I credit the visualization and keeping a regular sadhana (spiritual practice) to my healing.*

*All during this time I felt SO grateful. The idea of cultivating gratitude went from a concept in my head that I learned through yoga into a deep-seated feeling in my heart. I become a changed person after this encounter with karma and grace!*

R.

**QUESTIONS**

1. *Life is a struggle, but at same time, it is a school for Self-healing and Self-knowledge. Stress is inevitable. Give a short discourse on how understanding the meaning of life helps to decrease stress.*
2. *What are five causes of stress?*
3. *What are your five preferred Yogic methods to decrease stress?*

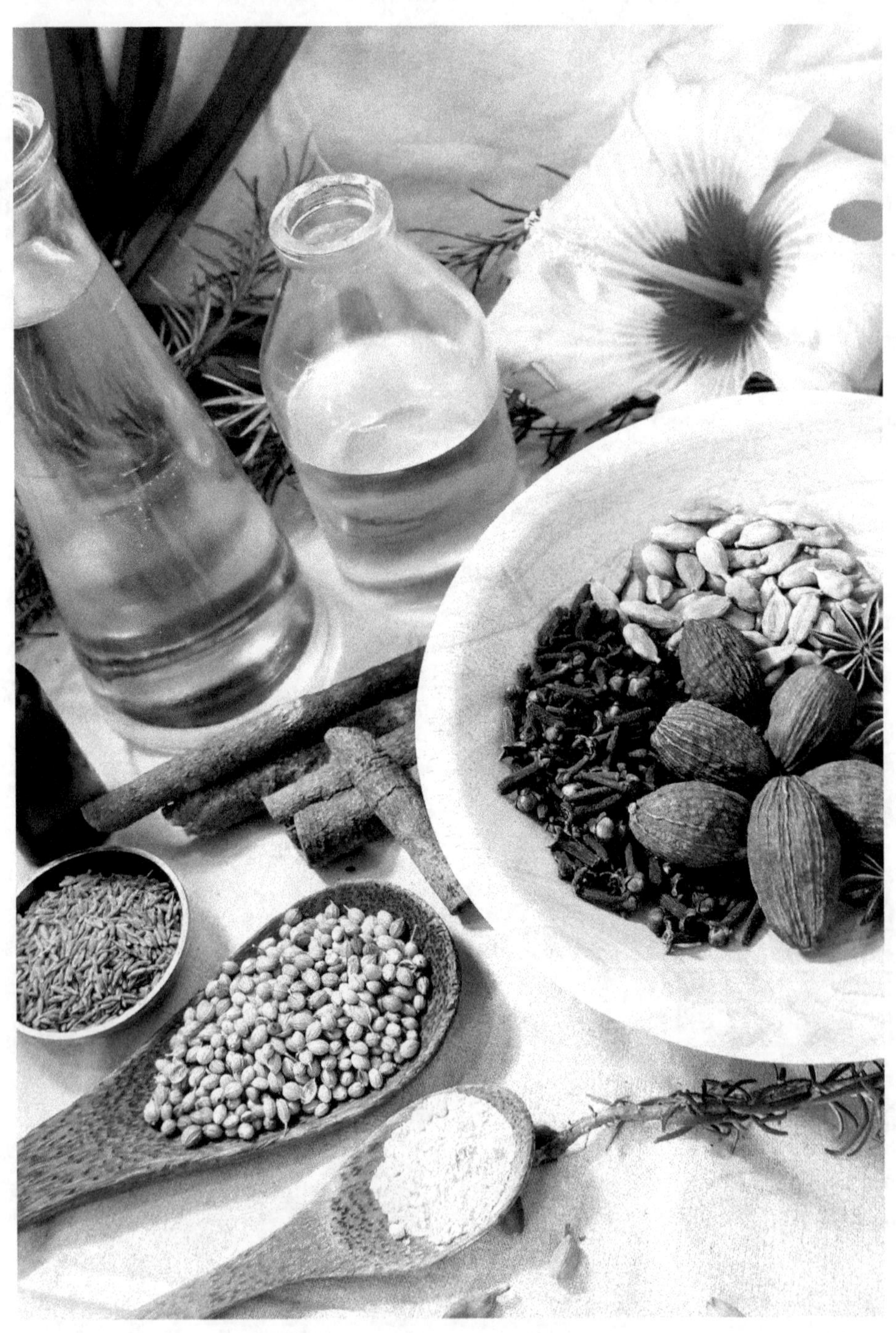

AYURVEDIC OILS AND HERBS

CHAPTER 4

# The Yoga and Ayurveda Way of Life

***"Yoga is a life of self discipline built upon the tenets of simple living and high thinking. If you follow these five points, which compose a true holistic approach to our whole system of body, mind and soul, you will gain strength and balance in this demanding stressful world. Obstacles become stepping stones to success, and life is a school for the development of character and compassion and the Realization of the Divine all-pervading Self"***

– *SWAMI VISHNU-DEVANANDA in The Complete Illustrated Book of Yoga*

## THE GOAL OF LIFE

The aim of life is to advance as far as possible on the path of Self-healing and Self-realization until the body-mind vehicle ages and is no longer able to actively pursue the demands of the spiritual path. In order to go on, we must conserve our strength and health as much as possible, diminish stress and strain, and provide proper nutrition for optimal function of both body and mind. Meant to be practiced together, the Vedic sciences of Yoga and Ayurveda both propose the wisdom of observing a daily routine. Ayurvedic principles support the health of the yoga practitioner as he/she embarks on the spiritual path to find the deeper truths of this life.

## 1. WHAT IS AYURVEDA?

Ayurveda is the ancient medical tradition of India and one of the oldest systems of medicine in the world. Its origins have been traced back more than five thousand years. It is recognized as the root of many systems of healing throughout Asia and the West. Based on the theory of the five elements—earth, water, fire, air and ether—Ayurveda is the science of how to live in accordance with nature. The more you tune to nature, the healthier you are. In modern times, we live a life that is far from nature, alienated from nature and we suffer the consequences.

**Three causes of disease, according to Ayurveda**

1. Ayurveda and Yoga both state that the prime cause of disease is *avidya* (forgetting our True Nature as Spirit) and that remembrance of who we are constitutes health. Everything we do throughout the day is an attempt to remember who we are. Therefore, spend less time in Tamas or forgetfulness, less time in Rajas or false ideas, and more time in Sattva—a balanced, calm, peaceful state in which you remember who you are.
2. Misuse of the senses and intellect: This misuse causes identification with objects rather than the Self. Seeking temporary sensual pleasure rather than permanent peace of mind, we fall into unhealthy lifestyles.
3. Time and use of the body: While aging is inevitable, living out of alignment with time, the seasons, and natural rhythms causes the body to age and decay more rapidly.

To recover health, you must remember your True Nature as Spirit, nourish Sattva in all daily activities, be wise in your lifestyle choices, be regulated in diet, sleep and live in accordance with nature.

**Ayurvedic Constitution**

In order to pursue our individual goals and realizations in life, each person is given a unique constitution at birth. With the ebb and flow of life, it can evolve and be modified into a less balanced version of the self. Ayurveda says health is achieved when you come back to your original constitution, as much as possible, by incorporating healthy dietary and lifestyle practices in daily life.

The body is an external manifestation of the subtle mind. The physical constitution also represents the psychological and mental constitution. Ayurveda classifies all the different types of physical bodies and minds into three types (or *doshas*) depending on the constitutional elements: Vata, Pitta and Kapha.

**Vata** is made up of the elements air (movement) and ether (space). Vata provides movement and has the characteristics of dryness, subtleness, and lightness. Vata governs movement, expression, blood circulation, breathing, transmission in nerves and sensation, and elimination of waste. When balanced, all of these functions occur without symptom or distress; when imbalanced, the dosha is seen in the presenting symptoms. The seat of Vata is in the colon, so imbalances there may be the first indicator of Vata dosha imbalance.

**Pitta** is made up of the elements fire (transformation) and water (fluidity). Pitta governs transformation—digestive and metabolic actions in the body—and has the characteristics of heat, sharpness, and oiliness. Pitta governs digestion, fuels the digestive fire (*agni*), produces blood, colors the skin, provides self-confidence, intelligence and sight. When balanced, these functions occur without excess heat, but when Pitta dosha is imbalanced, its heat may be seen in the symptomatic expression in these or other bodily processes. The main seat of pitta is in the stomach and small intestine, where its imbalance may first be seen.

**Kapha** is made up of the elements earth (mass) and water (fluidity). Kapha is the dosha of sustenance and has the characteristics of stability, heaviness, and moistness. Kapha provides density to tissues, moisture to food in the stomach and to all the mucous membranes, provides strength and cooling to the heart and the sensory organs, stabilizes and lubricates the joints, and provides taste. Kapha gives the body substance, strength, cohesion, lubrication, cooling and immunity. When balanced, the body has adequate fluidity and stability in its organs and tissues; when imbalanced, the heaviness of Kapha may create sluggishness and stagnation in the body. The main seat of Kapha is in the stomach and the chest; imbalances in Kapha dosha may reveal themselves in this region first.

A person's constitution is reflective of the relationship of the three doshas to each other. This is the relative presence of each of these three doshas, since everyone has all three in some amount. A person's constitution can be dominantly Vata, mixing with Pitta and Kapha to a lesser degree; predominantly Pitta mixing Vata and Kapha to a lesser degree; or Kapha with a mixture of Pitta and Vata. (For a glimpse into your own constitution, see the assessment questionnaire in *Practical Ayurveda*, Sivananda Yoga Vedanta Center, 2018).

The birth constitution is assigned according to your allotted karma for this life. You have a body type that comes with certain physical structural qualities and functional tendencies. You also have a certain mental type that determines the qualities and tendencies of the mind. When you make choices based on the doshic tendencies, you create doshic imbalance that is seen as symptoms or disease. As you live and go through different life circumstances, your body constitution and your mental constitution might change because of the dietary and lifestyle choices you make. Ayurvedic practitioners like to regain the original constitution as much as possible— to return to a state that existed before the unconscious indulging of the doshic tendencies. The original constitution is called Prakruti, and the present constitution that has changed and become imbalanced is called Vikruti.

To know your constitutional tendencies is to be empowered with the knowledge needed to create balance in your life.

**Vata Dosha**

The Vata dosha's elements are air and ether, giving it the qualities of lightness and mobility, or being capable of moving.

- A balanced Vata mind is creative, joyful, a fast learner, fast thinking and is a spiritual person.
- An imbalanced Vata mind is anxious, scattered, restless, learns quickly and forgets quickly and has a poor memory.
- A balanced Vata body has fast metabolism and is usually thin, light and tall.
- An imbalanced Vata body has dry skin, irregular digestion, is malnourished and is prone to constipation, and is hyperactive and restless.

**How to pacify Vata**

Vata imbalances create the problems of anxiety, restlessness and lack of stability in both body and mind. It is difficult to control the Vata mind. Vata-natured people might be inspired and insightful, but lack endurance and forbearance to sustain their inspiration. Symptoms of Vata imbalance can be ungroundedness, lack of concentration, constipation, anxiety and overall dryness. Vata is irregular, mobile, light, dry, cool, fine, quick and rough. To pacify Vata, do practices that are regular, stable, heavy, oily, heating, viscous, slow and smooth.

**Diet:** Eat grounding food that is warm, soupy, with more grains and fats and fewer processed or convenience foods. Hydrate more. Sip hot drinks frequently. Minimize pungent, bitter, astringent, dry, crunchy, cold and raw food. For best results, favor eating foods with sour, salty or sweet tastes.

**Lifestyle:** A Vata person needs to balance themselves by rest and routine. They don't like routine, but they need routine. They need to do slow and calming activities, because they are typically very fast, and this creates exhaustion. Avoid stimulants, overexertion and sensory overload as these will lead to depletion. Daily hot oil massage (abhyanga) is the best remedy for problems of Vata imbalance.

**Yoga Practice:** Vata is suited for the paths of Bhakti Yoga and Jnana Yoga; these cultivate more of the qualities of Kapha and Pitta dosha, which will balance the Vata. However, it is good for them to practice Hatha Yoga to balance and slow down the Vata dosha as well. Restorative and gentle yoga practices are beneficial and create greater stability.

**Pitta Dosha**

The Pitta dosha's elements are fire and water, giving it the qualities of hot, oily, and transforming.

- A balanced pitta mind is focused, intelligent, able to solve problems very quickly.
- An imbalanced pitta mind is aggressive, overly critical, judgmental, demanding and expresses anger.
- A balanced Pitta body has strong digestion and medium build with well-built musculature.
- An imbalanced Pitta body has excess heat that presents as inflammation, heartburn, rashes, acne, hypertension.

**How to pacify Pitta**

Pitta-natured people's tendency is toward intensity in their emotions and activities. They will benefit from moderation in work and personal life.

**Diet:** Eat food that is cooling, heavy, and drying. Eat more vegetables and greens than a Vata diet. Limit the oily, sharp, and overly-spiced foods and minimize sour, salty, pungent tasting foods. Favor the sweet, bitter and astringent tastes.

**Lifestyle:** The Pitta person does well with moderate exercise, cool baths, swimming, walks in the woods or in the shade, and listening to calming music. They also need to favor rest and stable routines. They do well to avoid excess exposure to sun and any activity that could overheat the body and mind. They should drink plenty of water and avoid stimulants, overworking, stress, and overly competitive activity.

**Yoga Practice:** All four paths of yoga are beneficial when pacifying Pitta dosha. The rigors of Raja Yoga support control of the Pitta mind, body and breath and Jnana Yoga stimulates and directs the Pitta mind; these two paths of yoga are their preference, while the other paths help them to address other Pitta challenges. Karma Yoga is helpful to channel their energy and help them to release their focus on the ego, and Bhakti Yoga will help them to relax and calm down and cultivate their compassion while opening their hearts.

**Kapha Dosha**

The Kapha dosha's elements are earth and water, creating the qualities of coolness, moistness and heaviness.

- A balanced Kapha mind is calm, loving, nurturing and patient.
- An imbalanced Kapha mind is attached, lazy, greedy and depressed.

- A balanced Kapha body is strong, in general, with good immunity and power of endurance.
- An imbalanced Kapha body is lethargic, has excess fat, slow digestion and congestion.

**How to pacify Kapha**

Kapha's tendency is towards conservation of energy leading to a sedentary life-style and an over-commitment to habits and routines that may exacerbate the Kapha qualities of heaviness, sluggishness and immobility. They will benefit from an active lifestyle and fostering an openness to change.

**Diet:** Kapha dosha should eat foods that are light, warm and spicy and minimize heavy foods, excess oils and cold food. They do well to limit sweet, sour, and salty foods, focusing more on pungent, bitter and astringent tastes found primarily in vegetables, greens, and legumes.

**Lifestyle:** Kapha needs to exercise. Waking early and stretching first thing in the morning helps them to feel lighter during the day. They need to favor spontaneity, change their habits, do new activities that stimulate them, go outside and engage with nature. They should avoid excess sleep, inactivity, sedentary lifestyle, darkness and over-attachment to the same habits.

**Yoga Practice:** Kapha nature is naturally devotional and loyal to their teacher and their system of learning and practice. They are steady on their chosen spiritual path. However, they might be stuck in their ways and routines and need to combine their approach to mobilize energy. Bhakti Yoga is their preferred practice, however, they need to make an effort to do Karma Yoga to detach from their sense of doership, Hatha Yoga to move the body and invigorate the prana, and Jnana Yoga to encourage detachment and to lighten both body and mind. They tend to be content and attached to their emotions and actions, and do not easily detach. Practicing inquiry into the nature of the Self and not-Self is highly beneficial.

## 2. THE THREE GUNAS AND THE DOSHAS

The three gunas combine with the doshas to form our unique way of perception and interaction.

**A Sattvic Vata** person is creative, joyful, and learns fast. They can be very inspirational and spiritual people. Tamasic or Rajasic Vata becomes scattered, restless, and therefore, cannot connect to themselves. They become anxious and worried and doubtful and lack self-confidence.

**A Sattvic Pitta** will be a good leader and good thinker with the power of discrimination and with the courage to reject what is untrue in the pursuit of Truth. They make decisions quickly, are focused, intelligent, and have great power of comprehension. Tamasic or Rajasic Pitta can lead people in the wrong direction and can be divisive, abusive, angry, aggressive, intolerant, and overly judgmental.

**A Sattvic Kapha** person can be calm, content, and present. They are loving, nurturing and stable, and you can trust them.

**Therefore, nurturing Sattva in all doshas is the path of Self-healing**

Pain and suffering come from Tamasic or Rajasic Vata, Pitta or Kapha. If the person is tamasic or rajasic, they become lazy, lethargic, depressed, indulgent, incapable of making decisions, and very attached.

Knowing your constitution, you know your strengths and weaknesses. You can nurture sattva through Yogic sadhana, moving from tamas to rajas to sattva.

Yogis on the path of Self-healing seek to eliminate tamas. It is imperative to work against tamas in all aspects, as it brings you down through the thick veils of ignorance and denial. Avoid procrastination, laziness, inertia, darkness, ignorance, self-hatred, and self-doubt. Be self-disciplined and understanding.

Rajas is also detrimental to the Self-healing path. Rajas is activity, movement, passion, desire, always projecting, seeking external happiness. Rajas projects happiness outside. We run after the projected pleasures of the senses and the imaginative emotional rajasic mind. Rajas creates pain through egoism, passion and expectation, suffering from disappointments and anger from desires unfulfilled and the pain of loss. Rajas suffers from fragmentation and does not allow you to see the whole picture, the union and harmony of nature. Rajas exaggerates differences, favors extremes, the liking and disliking tendencies of the mind. Instead of peace of mind, a rajasic person has pieces of mind.

The rajasic and tamasic states of mind occur when we unconsciously follow the longings of the dosha for sensory experience to mirror the dosha. For example, fiery uncontrolled Pitta is prone to aggression and strong feelings: frustration, anger, and radical ups and downs. Combined with tamas, the veils are thick, the separation is great and Truth is illusory. Tamasic-Rajasic Pitta without control can lead to criminal activities, because you want something intensely. You believe it to be true and just. Because you are tamasic, you don't care about other people's feelings. You act out of tunnel vision, creating a lot of pain to yourself and others.

## 3. STRESS AND THE DOSHAS

Dosha imbalances bring about stress and stress brings about imbalance.

Vata responds to stress with escapism.

Pitta responds to stress with fighting, criticism, perfectionism and overwork.

Kapha responds to stress with freezing.

**Sattva** brings stress resilience due to its capacity to remain balanced and detached in changing conditions. The sattvic person accepts their karma, possesses the capacity to adapt, adjust and accommodate, and is able to connect to his/her inner wisdom and surrender to God's will.

**Rajas** brings frustration, stress, negative emotions, inability to adapt, hyperactivity, conflict and overreaction.

**Tamas** creates attachment and darkness, fear and worry. It activates stress patterns that aggravate and strengthen existing negative karmic tendencies.

### The Yogic and Ayurvedic lifestyle

Yogis utilize Ayurvedic practices and knowledge to maintain the health of body and mind to support their sadhana. Rather than following cultural trends, family influences or even their preferences, Yogis take into account their constitution, adapt to the season and time of day, adhere to ethical guidelines to maintain mental and physical purity, and cultivate self-discipline.

## 4. FIVE POINTS OF YOGA: LIFESTYLE MEDICINE

Swami Vishnudevananda synthesized the ancient wisdom of Yoga into five basic principles, which can be easily incorporated into your own pattern of living, to provide a long, healthy and happy life.

Swami Vishnudevananda compared the physical body to a vehicle. For a car to function smoothly and efficiently, it needs a lubrication system, a battery, a cooling system, proper fuel, and a responsible driver behind the wheel.

**The Five Points of Yoga** are the recipe to live a holistic, balanced life by integrating:

1. Proper Exercise (Asana)
2. Proper Breathing (Pranayama)
3. Proper Relaxation (Savasana)

4. Proper Diet (Vegetarian)
5. Positive Thinking and Meditation (Vedanta and Dhyana)

**Proper Exercise** acts as a lubricating system for the joints, muscles, ligaments, tendons, and other parts of the body by increasing circulation and flexibility. The fundamental difference between Yogic exercise and ordinary physical exercise is that physical exercise emphasizes violent movements of the muscles, while Yogic exercise promotes slow and conscious movements of the body, thus avoiding the build-up of lactic acid in the muscle fibers which causes fatigue. The main purpose of exercise is to increase circulation and the intake of oxygen. This can be achieved by simple movements of the spine and various joints of the body, with deep breathing, and without violent movement of the muscles.

Yogic exercise is called yoga asana. Asana means steady pose. Asanas done correctly influence and positively energize all systems of the body: the circulatory system, the muscular and skeletal systems, the endocrine system, the respiratory system, the digestive system, and most importantly, the nervous system. In terms of muscles, Yogic exercises not only strengthen the muscles, but also stretch them. There is a great emphasis on the flexibility and the youth of the spine. Swami Vishnudevananda said: "Flexible spine, flexible mind."

**Proper Breathing** aids the body in connecting to its battery, the solar plexus, where tremendous potential energy is stored. The Yogi taps into this energy by specific yoga breathing techniques (pranayama). This energy is used for physical and mental rejuvenation.

Yoga emphasizes breathing correctly (the Yogic full breath using the diaphragm). We substantially increase the intake of oxygen through deep inhalation and release the toxins appropriately through our deep exhalation. Yoga teaches us to be constantly aware of our breathing patterns and to breathe consciously in our daily life. Specific breathing techniques (pranayama) are devised to further purify the nadis (energy channels), balance the breath and the energy in our system, and to store and channel the subtle energy (prana) for higher purposes.

The word Hatha is composed of the syllables 'Ha' and 'Tha', which mean sun and moon, respectively. This refers to the balance between the prana vayu (the positive vital air) and apana vayu (the negative vital air). Prana (vital air) in the body of the individual is a part of the universal breath. Regulation of the harmonized breath helps the Yogi to regulate and steady the mind. Pranayama needs to be practiced by all serious Yoga practitioners. Advanced practices should only be done by those already leading a pure lifestyle, and it is recommended that they are done under the supervision of a teacher in a pure environment, like an ashram.

**Proper Relaxation** techniques, such as Savasana, cool the system down like the radiator of a car. When the body and mind are constantly overworked, their efficiency diminishes. Relaxation is nature's way of recharging the prana. The state of our mind and body are intimately linked. If your muscles are relaxed, then your mind will be relaxed. If the mind is anxious, then the body suffers, too.

There are three levels of relaxation: physical, mental and spiritual. There are also three levels of tension or stress: physical stress, mental stress and spiritual stress.

Physical stress comes from poor eating habits, sedentary living, repetitive movements of the body, and poor posture. Modern life, especially in big cities, is full of stress as modern work and living conditions are full of unabating pressure and devoid of prana and relaxation.

Mental and emotional stress comes from a hectic lifestyle, highly demanding jobs, distractions of the mind, low vitality due to lack of prana, and negative emotions such as anger, hatred, jealousy, fear, and anxiety.

Spiritual stress comes from existential anxieties and living with questions without answers, such as, *"What are life and death?", "What is love?", "What is the nature of our connection with God?", "Is there a God?", "Why is there unrighteousness?", "How can I find stability in an ever-changing world?", "Why is there suffering?" and "Why can't we achieve enduring peace?"*

**The solution is to achieve the three levels of relaxation:**

**Physical relaxation** is achieved through the systematic practice of conscious relaxation (Savasana) and correct posture (Asana).

**Mental relaxation** is gained by correct breathing, concentrating the mind and positive thinking. A distracted mind is always anxious. A mind concentrated on a positive object is more relaxed and recharged.

**Spiritual relaxation** is a deeper type of relaxation, when we become content, a detached witness of the body and mind. Swami Vishnudevananda taught that being free from identification with the physical body, the mind, and ego-consciousness is the only way to reach a state of complete relaxation.

**Proper Diet** gives proper fuel for the body and mind without creating toxins and digestive problems. Optimum utilization of food, air, water and sunlight is essential. There is medical evidence that a balanced vegetarian diet is extremely healthy and provides everything the body needs. The Yogic vegetarian diet is sattvic (pure), and helps to calm the mind and reveal the spirit, as well as nourish the body.

The body needs food for two purposes: as fuel to supply energy and as raw material to repair the tissues of the body. For repairing and building tissue, the body needs: 1) protein; 2) carbohydrates; 3) fats; and 4) minerals. These elements are found in larger proportions in vegetable tissue than in animal tissue. Nuts, peas, beans, soybean products like tofu, and milk contain protein. Wheat, oats, rice and other grains are mainly carbohydrates. All protein foods and vegetable oils provide fats, and the main supply of organic minerals and vitamins comes from fruit and vegetables.

A vegetarian diet is a natural diet, fresh and wholesome, full of fiber and alkaline in nature, energy-producing, and easy to absorb and to eliminate. To maintain a sattvic diet, free from rajasic and tamasic influences, avoid stimulants and depressants such as caffeine, alcohol, cigarettes, drugs of all kinds, overly-spicy food, onions, garlic, overcooked food, old food, frozen food, canned food, sodas and processed foods, as well as all meat. Yogis advocate "ahimsa", the principle of non-violence, non-injury and respect for life. Everything our body and mind needs for growth can be provided from the vegetable kingdom. By not eating animal flesh, we nourish ourselves in a natural and healthy way.

Changing to a vegetarian diet can be gradual and life-transforming. It consists not only of deciding to stop eating meat, but also learning a new way of life, by being conscious of how you nourish yourself. It includes being aware of not only what you eat, but also how you eat. Yogis promote taking time to cook and eat consciously in a regular manner, with appropriate intervals between meals to allow the digestive fire to activate and digest the food. Blessing meals is also encouraged to sanctify the act of eating and to offer thanks to the Creator. Proper diet includes periodic fasting as well, to give a break to the digestive system, purify body and mind, and to make the mind more perceptive, sattvic and more conducive to concentration, contemplation and meditation.

**Positive Thinking and Meditation** puts us in control. The intellect is purified. The lower, instinctive nature is under the control of the clear and concentrated mind. Just as the driver of a car manages to bring themselves to their destination without accidents and setbacks, so the Yogi learns to manage his/her mind and emotions to stay positive at all times. Positive thoughts are energizing and facilitate growth, while negative thoughts are draining and inhibit growth. Only with a positive outlook about ourselves can we maintain a meditative life, which will ultimately lead to intuitive knowledge and inner strength.

## 5. THE TRIANGLE OF LIFE

The Yogi sees life as a triangle; the physical body undergoes birth, growth, change, decay and death. The growth period reaches a plateau at about the age of 18 to 20 years. In the first years of life, the 'youthful period', the rate of cell rejuvenation (anabolic) exceeds the rate of cell decay (catabolic). In the average person, the body maintains these processes in equilibrium from the age of 20 until around 35. Then the decaying, or catabolic process, begins to take precedence, and the body starts its decline. This process later results in 'old age' with its accompanying ills and despair. However, Yogis say that we were not born merely to be subject to pain and suffering, disease and death. There is a far greater purpose to life. But the spiritual investigation of life's purpose requires a keen intellect and a strong will; these are the products of a healthy body and mind. For this reason, the ancient sages developed an integral system to ward off or retard the decaying or catabolic process, and to keep the physical and mental faculties strong.

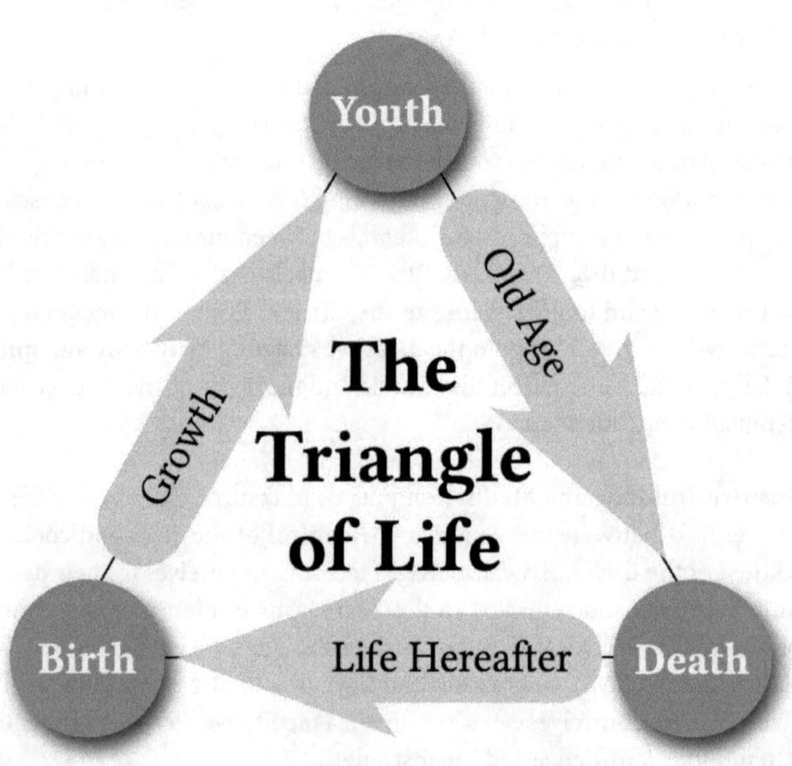

## 6. ASANA ROUTINE: WHAT IS PROPER EXERCISE?

Asanas help to stretch and balance the entire body, increasing flexibility of the spine, strengthening bones and stimulating the circulatory and immune systems.

Asanas move the prana, help to focus and calm the mind and reduce stress.

Yoga exercises are slow and conscious movements which integrate relaxation before and after the practice session and in-between the postures, thus improving awareness.

Yogic exercises have psychological and emotional effects. For example, Fish posture expands the chest and improves self-confidence and fearlessness. Yogic exercises increase sattva and induce the mind to turn inwards. Yoga helps with detachment (or less attachment) to the physical body and can bring awareness of what is beyond the body and mind through the final deep relaxation.

Yogic exercises affect not only the physical body but also the astral body (the energetic body and the mind).

**The twelve basic asanas**

Asana means steady posture. It implies that the practitioner holds a posture with attention and concentration.

The Sivananda system has twelve basic postures and begins with practice of sun salutations, which give you the full benefit of the practice session. There are 84,000 yoga postures in total. Swami Vishnudevananda summarized all the postures into this sequence; many variations can be added. The basic twelve postures are pictured on the next page.

**General guidance:**

- When you practice asanas, dedicate your action at the beginning of the session with a prayer such as Dhyana Slokas. You may conclude the session with the Maha Myritunjaya mantra or other prayer. These sacred prayers help to generate the right mental attitude of turning inward, and prevent you from practicing asana like other forms of exercise.

  Chant OM three times in the beginning to be in harmony with the universe. Upon conclusion of your practice, repeat the dedication prayer to the teacher who has given you this knowledge.

- We need to care about how the asanas are performed to receive the full physical, energetic and spiritual benefits. Sun salutation can be accompanied with mantras as prayers to the sun, honoring the sun as the source of light, energy and health.

- Sun salutations are part of the warming-up sequence, mobilizing all the muscles and joints in preparation for the postures. The sun represents vitality and health. Salutations to the sun with awareness are important for health and well-being.
- Note the order of the twelve-asana sequence. It begins with the headstand and ends with standing postures, turning the energy first inwards with focus on the head and brain (and consciousness) in an inverted position and moving the energy downwards in subsequent postures.
- The logic of the sequence is energetic, putting energy on consciousness, centering the person first, then moving outwards with balancing and standing poses to conclude the sequence.

**Benefits of the practice of asanas:**

- balances your doshas
- improves the structure of the body
- facilitates the movement of prana; circulates the prana helping to avoid blockages
- promotes sattva by removing tamasic and rajasic thoughts in the mind
- helps regulate emotions
- improves Self-awareness by slowing down
- balances energies
- facilitates detachment from identification with the body/mind vehicle
- calms and energizes the mind; turning inward, allowing for inner connection. This is achieved through relaxation before, after and in between the postures, and by exclusive concentration on the body and the breath, moving the prana.

- Observe the three phases of the asana: entering the posture, holding the posture, and coming out of the posture. Come into the posture step-by-step, then hold the posture, relax the breath, and concentrate on a specific energy center. The posture needs to be comfortable to avoid creating more tension that would block the flow of prana. Stay calm and positive in the posture and breathe. In case of any physical limitation, still aim to stretch gently. Visualize the asana mentally, allowing for the flow of prana and a relaxed attitude.

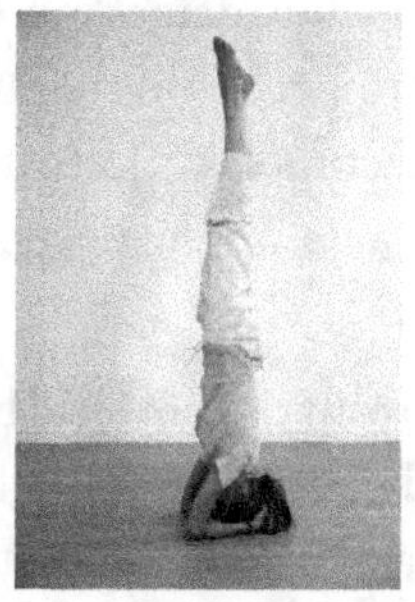
1. Headstand

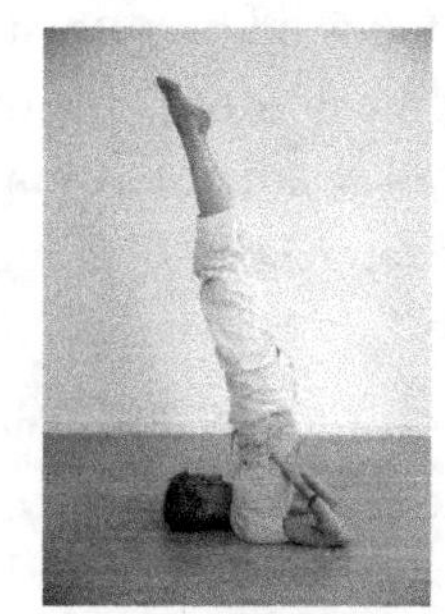
2. Shoulderstand

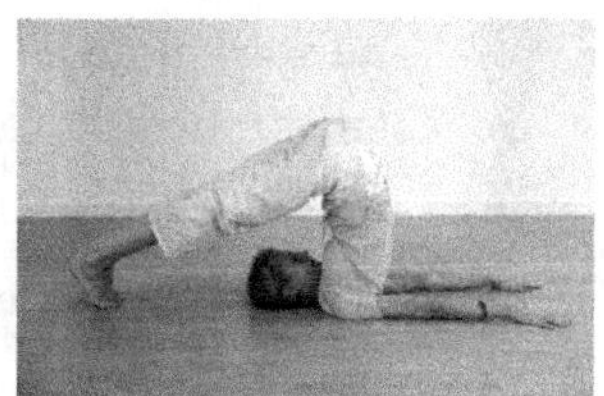
3. Plough

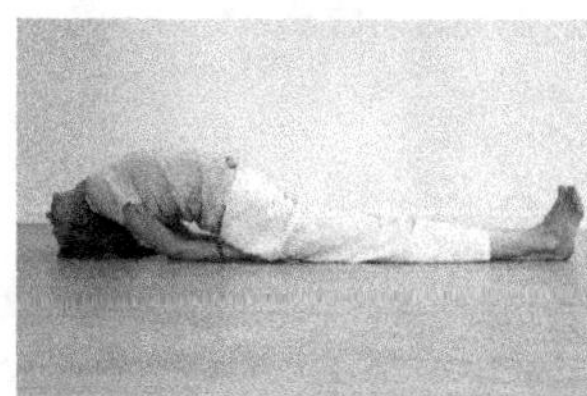
4. Fish

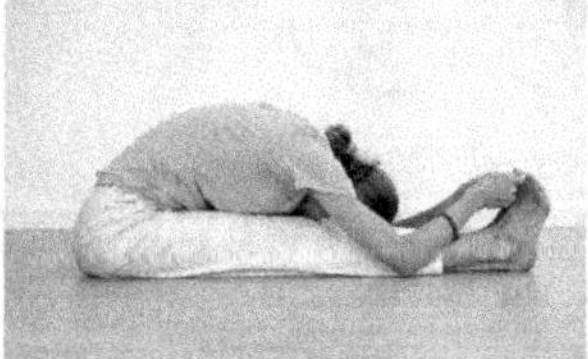
5. Forward Bend

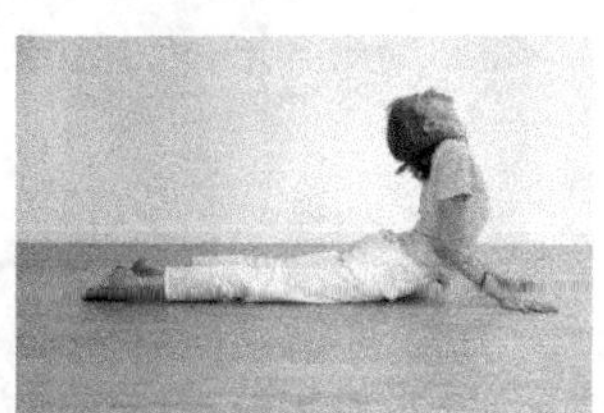
6. Cobra

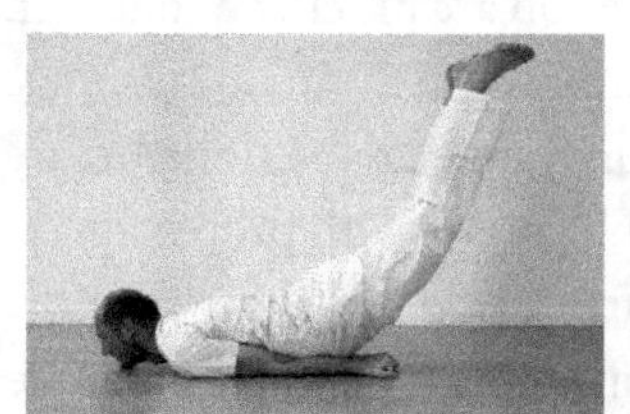
7. Locust

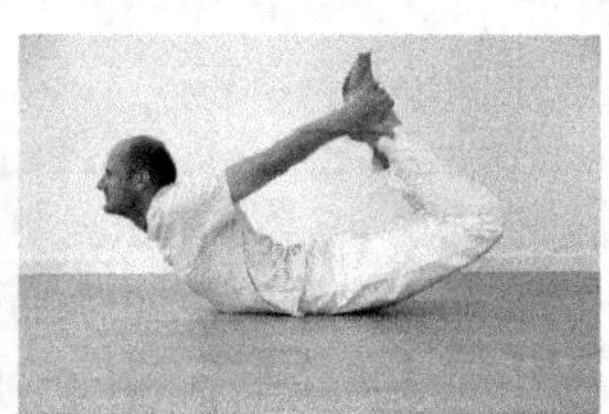
8. Bow

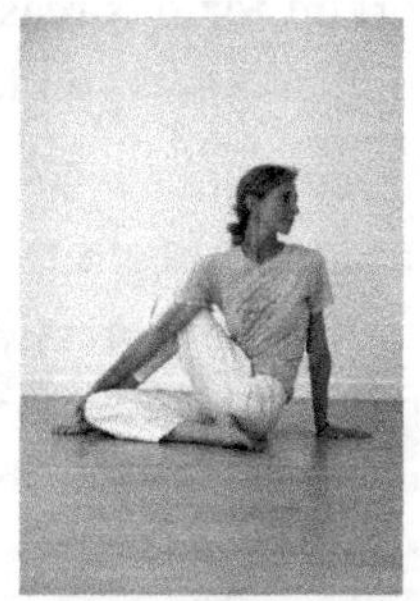
9. Spinal Twist

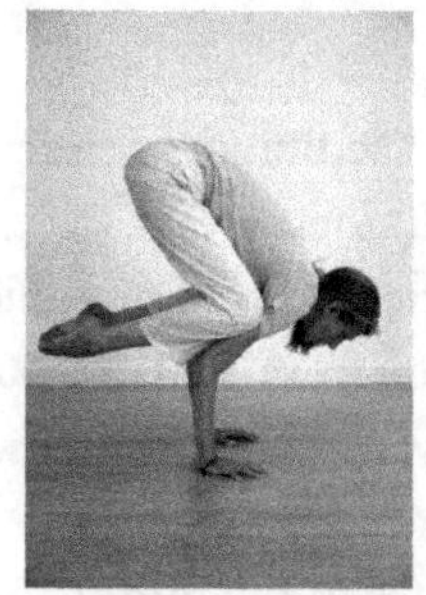
10. Crow

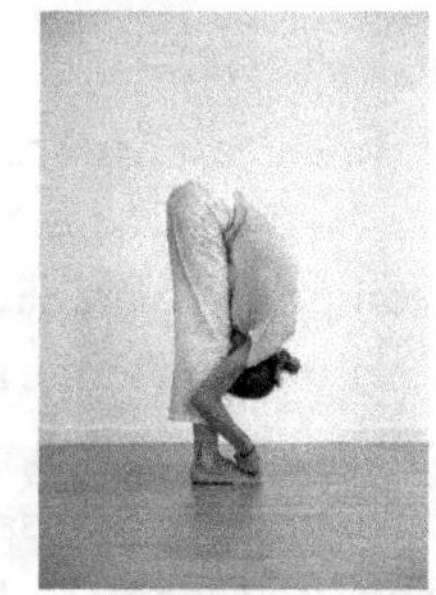
11. Standing Forward Bend

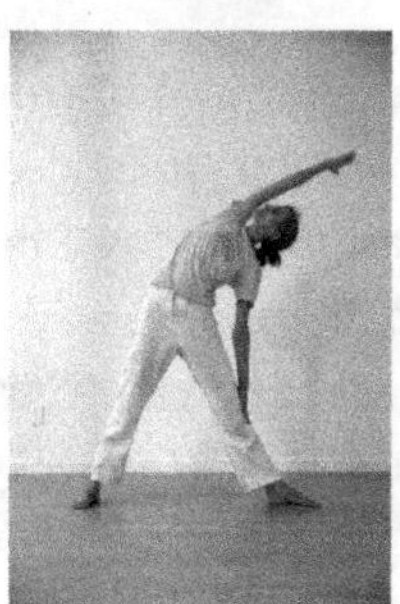
12. Triangle

- The longer savasana relaxation at the end is necessary for you to receive the benefits of the practice. This is done after the successive tensing and relaxing of all the muscles, followed by auto-suggestion, thus detaching from the body and sweeping the flow of prana from feet to head. This complete relaxation clears away all residual tension and attachments. Body, mind and spirit plunge into deep relaxation almost equivalent to the deep sleep state or meditative state.

  The main benefit of savasana is the detachment from the physical body. As you let go of identification with the physical body, you feel very light, as you function now with your subtle energy body. Many healing insights occur during savasana. The sun salutations and the twelve-posture sequence all lead to that final experience of deep relaxation that recharges and brings you back to yourself.

## 6. YOGIC AND AYURVEDIC DAILY ROUTINE

Ayurveda promotes waking up in the early morning. This is the nurturing time to become strong in body and mind to prepare for the day. The morning routine is important for this reason. The afternoon routine is for recovery. A routine in the evening prepares you for sleep.

In the Sivananda system, asanas, pranayama and meditation are practiced together. For example, begin the day with meditation for a minimum of 20 to 30 minutes. Follow with the practice of asanas and pranayama. Pranayama can be done before or after asana. Pranayama can take 15 or 20 minutes, then asana with proper relaxation which can take about 60 minutes for twelve postures. For the evening routine, repeat the same, but you can do a lighter asana and pranayama session. This can be followed by 30 minutes of meditation to close the evening.

**Frequency and timing of practice**

Asana can be practiced twice daily or at least once every day. Meditation is practiced at least once a day. Pranayama can be practiced every day. It doesn't take long, just 15 to 20 minutes a session. You can practice pranayama twice a day, if possible, in the morning with your morning routine, and in the afternoon, from 4:00 to 6:00pm. For those who are very active, are tense, or live in a big city, it is very beneficial to practice pranayama more than once per day. Savasana relaxation can be done with the asanas, but can also be done by itself for 10 to 15 minutes in the middle of the day or afternoon to recharge yourself for the evening. This gives you a picture of the Yogic discipline as a daily routine. This routine needs to be systematic, regular and integrated into daily life. Then it becomes your sadhana (conscious practice) for Self-realization.

**Pillars of health**

According to Ayurveda, there are three important pillars of health: sleep, food and brahmacharya. Time should be reserved to prepare yourself for sleep.

Nowadays, many suffer from lack of sleep, insomnia or difficulty falling or staying asleep. Stress manifests in the form of an inability to rest. When you are not resting or not sleeping well, it affects your health. Having a daily routine can improve your sleep.

You can eat two meals a day—or you can eat three times a day with a light breakfast, heavier lunch and light evening meal. How we take the food, with reverence, is important to support full and healthy digestion of the food. In addition, we may consider how we "feed" all the senses with our sensory intake and make sure that it's of the highest order. Brahmacharya includes sensory and sexual restraint and supports maintaining the sattvic state of body and mind.

**Morning routine**

- Wake up early at brahma muhurta (sunrise) regularly. It is best to have 6-7 hours of sleep in which deep sleep is achieved.
- Practice daily hygiene. Drink warm lemon water first. Wash face and eyes, clean the mouth, teeth and gums and then evacuate the bowels and the bladder in the first hour. Do a little *abhyanga* (self oil massage).
- Clean the nose with a neti pot; drop Nasya oil into the nose.
- Take a bath.
- Use a tongue scraper to remove *ama* from your tongue.
- Meditate.
- Practice asanas and pranayama.
- Eat a light breakfast or skip breakfast if you do intermittent fasting (16 hours in between dinner and lunch). Try to extend the number of hours between meals, so the body has time to digest.
- Prepare for your day.

**Afternoon routine**

- Ayurveda doesn't promote sleeping during the day, but take time to rest and recover.
- In your recovery routine, you can have some simple light asanas or restorative yoga.
- Ayurveda is very clear on the time of day, every hour has some quality such as Vata time, Pitta time or Kapha time. The activity has to follow this rhythm of nature, according to the time of day and the season.
- Your evening meal should be lighter than lunch and taken two hours before your evening meditation session to allow time for digestion and not disturb your meditation.

**Evening routine**

- Meditate at sunset time, generally between 6:00-8:00pm. If you have dinner at 6:00pm, meditation can be at 8:00pm. Meditation helps to calm and cleanse your mind from the activities of the day.
- Take all beverages before sunset. If you drink too close to bedtime, you may wake up in the middle of the night.
- Avoid eating after sunset. Eat at least two hours before you sleep, otherwise you have not digested your food and cannot sleep.
- Switch off your cell phone before you go to sleep. Set a regular time each night that you do this.
- Switch off all the lights in the room to promote the production of melatonin by allowing the body's circadian rhythm to recognize day vs. night.
- Ideally, go to bed around 10:00pm. Sleep the appropriate number of hours according to your age. Children sleep more. Consider your lifestyle, as well. If you do asana, pranayama, meditation, lead a Yogic life and don't have so much stress, you won't need as much sleep. Six hours of sleep per day will be fine. The greater your attention to the cultivation of a sattvic state of mind, the more satisfying your sleep will be.
- Learn to prepare yourself for a deep sleep. Mantra repetition helps to calm the mind and prepare you for good rest. Repeat the mantra *"Om Tryambakam"* for healing. Pray for the protective power of

the universe to bless you with health and peace and liberation in due time.

- Deep sleep is vital for health. It is the closest state to Samadhi, or deep meditation. In deep sleep, the mind does not operate. You cease to identify with the body and mind, with who you are, your relationships, your job. This is where deep healing takes place, recharging you in the pure consciousness of who you are.

## 7. YOGIC AND AYURVEDIC DIETARY DISCIPLINE

- Eat according to your constitution. Choose the appropriate Vata-pacifying diet, Pitta-pacifying diet, or Kapha-pacifying diet.
- Proper diet is a sacred activity; you are feeding your temple. Pray before you eat. Dedicate the action of eating and the food that you eat.
- Abstain from food that causes harm. Transition to a vegetarian diet.
- Eat in a conscious manner at regular times. In the ashram, we eat at 10:00am and 6:00pm. In between, as there is a big interval of time, we may have a light snack and do asana and pranayama. Observe a minimum of three to four hours in between meals.
- Focus on what you eat. Chew well. Abstain from the "eat and run" mentality and fast food. Abstain from worldly conversations and cell phone activity during meals. Do not eat in a moving car as this increases Vata, which means you will not be able to digest and you will become anxious.
- Eat simple food, seasonally available and minimally processed. Swami Sivananda said, "*We do not have to eat what we do not like, but we should not eat all that we like.*" Some people want to eat raw food, but it depends on your constitution. Pitta people can eat raw food, but Vata constitution needs to avoid raw food. Cooked food supports the digestive fire. By being aware of the effect of food on the body, we can cultivate the ability to make wise choices about our foods.

According to Ayurveda, it's important to stoke *agni*, the digestive fire that helps to digest, burn or consume the food. Digestion is considered the key to health. It's the heat of the fire that fuels the metabolic changes, that digests our food. The liver has multiple fires inside that perform metabolic functions. Each of the tissues in the body also has fire. All these fires burn brightly to keep us alive. The main fire to maintain is the digestive fire, the fire in the belly. That's why cooking the food is so important, it helps food digest more easily.

According to Ayurveda, the first symptoms of disease appear as disturbances in the digestive system. If you don't have a strong digestive fire, you cannot digest the food. Cook your food in accordance with the state of your digestive fire.

To determine the state of your digestive fire (*agni*), you may assess your appetite. Ayurveda advises eating only when you are hungry. If you eat too much before you are hungry, it will dampen the fire. After dining, note if there are any digestive symptoms such as gas, bloating of the stomach, or acidity. These are the digestive symptoms to check daily to evaluate the balance and strength of the *agni*. A strong *agni* provides complete digestion that is free from symptoms. An imbalanced and weak *agni* results in digestive distress. Elimination patterns are another indicator of the state of *agni*. If you don't eliminate daily, your stool is not evenly colored, has abnormal color, or is not well formed, something is wrong. You have to consider what you have eaten and what you have done during the day. Why are you so upset or stressed that you cannot digest your food? To summarize, take time to eat with awareness, to digest your food, to eliminate properly and to detoxify. Digestive health is physical, but also strongly influences the mind and emotions.

If you digest well, you won't have *ama*, toxins that come from undigested food. Make food choices and live your life in such a way that you minimize *ama* accumulation.

From time to time, especially at the junction of seasons, Ayurveda advises a period of detoxification, where time is dedicated to a simple and cleansing diet, plenty of rest—without cell phones, talking, or mixing with people—and reduced activity. Allow the body to completely rest, recharge and detoxify. During this time, with the help of an Ayurvedic practitioner, you can work to remove all the accumulated *ama* in the intestines and colon, completely detoxifing all the body systems.

## 8. AMA - AGNI - DETOXIFICATION

***Ama*** indicates the presence of toxins. Symptoms that may indicate *ama* include: exhaustion, fatigue, lack of prana or energy, feeling congested or blocked, feeling groggy in the morning when you wake up, bad moods, laziness and lack of motivation, feeling physically weak without reason, digestive symptoms, excess salivation that you need to spit, lack of taste, weakened immunity, frequent colds and flu. *Ama* comes when your *agni*, or the digestive fire, is disturbed. If your fire is low, you are stressed, eating a lot of food and the food is not digested, you will have *ama*. Poor diet is the main cause of *ama*. Taking food that is too heavy, cold, sugary or deep fried are the main contributors to a buildup of *ama*. Irregular mealtimes, over-eating, sleeping after a meal, high stress, daytime sleeping, lack of exercise, and repressed emotions weaken your *agni* and cause the formation of *ama*. It's very important to get back into balance by removing the *ama*. Learn to be aware of what, when and how you eat in order to regulate your digestive fire and thereby digest food well. Doing exercise helps activate the metabolic activity of the tissues and increases the flow of blood, cleanses the body and all the different tracts: liver, skin, urinary and respiratory tract. Eating a light diet will allow the *agni* to burn up *ama* in the digestive tract.

***Agni***, as mentioned, is the heat of the fire that fuels the metabolic changes. That's why cooking the food lightly helps the fire. If you don't have the fire, you cannot digest the food. Assess your appetite; listen. Often we eat too much before we are hungry and that will dampen the fire. Be aware and take note of any digestive symptoms that you have such as gas, bloating or acidity.

## 9. IMPORTANCE OF OJAS

***Ojas*** is the subtle energy that sustains health and life. The best portion of the digested food becomes your *ojas*, the power of sustenance, the energy of connection, life and love. If you don't eat well, digest well, and live your life well, if you don't sleep well, if you waste your prana on excessive worry or self-destructive thoughts, if you over-indulge in addictive substances, you will deplete your *ojas*. That's when you find yourself discontented, depressed, lacking in love for yourself or other people and become incapable of maintaining a steady practice—and then you become sick.

It's very important to live well and build up your *ojas*. *Ojas* is increased when you have regulation and moderation in your use of sexual energy, when you have good relationships, good devotion and good rest. You accumulate *Ojas* like accumulating money in a bank. When you rest, you put money in the bank. When you use your mind or body, you're taking money out and can go into debt, which means you have depleted your resources. This is called a pranic debt situation leading to pranic bankruptcy and disease. To build *ojas*, you need to have physical rest, mental rest and good food. Don't worry. Doing asanas will build *ojas* and help with your tiredness and exhaustion. Spend time in nature and live according to the flow of the day, the flow of the year and the flow of your life. Do pranayama to create mental balance and mental *ojas*. Eat foods that are *ojas*-building such as cashews, almonds, ghee, dates and avocado. Have an internal use of good oil to protect the cells and also external oil with your daily self-massage to support your nervous and immune systems.

It's a lot to do to keep yourself balanced, sattvic and healthy! Take time to study more about Ayurvedic diet and daily routines and the benefits of Hatha Yoga. Learn how the asanas helps you regain balance both physically and mentally. Employ the science of relaxation and the science of the five points. Practice integrally the five points Yoga life.

May you become a shining Yogi radiating joy and life force to all around!

**QUESTIONS**

1. *Describe the three dosha constitutional and psychological types.*
2. *Explain how to pacify, balance and purify (reduce ama) for each dosha type.*
3. *What are the Five Points of Yoga. Describe the yoga lifestyle.*

*INSPIRED STORY*

**Yoga Life gave me my life**

*Practicing the synthesis of Classical Yoga has opened doors and cleaned the windows of my vision to see and know things about myself and my connection to others in ways I never knew possible, yet somehow felt deep inside that it must be. The four paths of Yoga hold a space for every kind of person. I had the room to grow in my strengths and learn to balance, by strengthening my weaknesses. When I first came to take the Sivananda Yoga Teacher Training Course in October 2014, I had no idea the impact it could and would have on my life. I had never practiced Sivananda Yoga before and had no idea really what it was.*

*After a month of following the same schedule, I was able to observe a big change. The routine of the TTC gave my mind the ease and space to have more time and energy. It is such a powerful phenomenon. I stayed for another three months to soak up and integrate into myself all that I had learned. When I went home after four months of life in the Ashram, it was wonderful to see how my perspective and interactions came with a little more ease. After the initial three months, I extended my stay to three more months and eight life-changing years.*

*I am blessed with compassionate and knowledgeable teachers who have walked their path and can guide me on mine. I have met the most loving and caring people, who have encouraged me to go beyond my ideas of limitation and who have nurtured me to be the best version of myself. This complete transformation of my limited outlook into a more sustainably cheerful, confident, and caring human being, I attribute to the practices I have learned here at the Ashram. I continue to grow. Over the last nine years, it has been so important for me to keep my connection, not just to the Ashram, but to myself. The Ashram and the practices support this inner connection, which increases my capacity for confidence, self-love, contribution, and generosity; I have more energy, joy, strength, health, and Love.*

R.

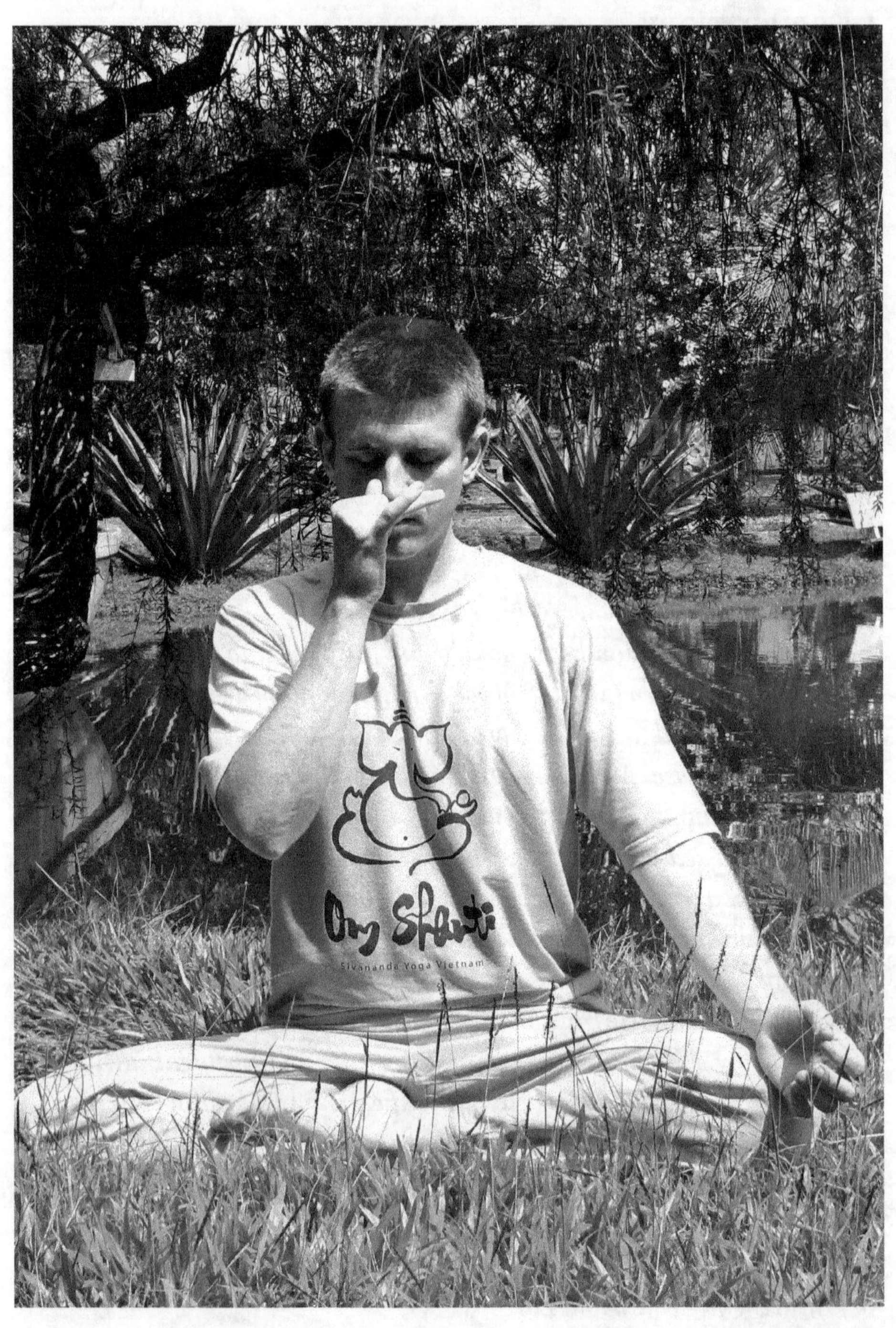


PRANAYAMA – PRACTICE OF CONTROL OF PRANA

## CHAPTER 5

# Increasing & Balancing Prana

***"It is prana that shines in your eyes. It is through the power of prana the ears hear, the eyes see, the skin feels, the tongue tastes, the nose smells, the brain and the intellect do their functions... Prana is force. Prana is magnetism. Prana is electricity. It is prana that pumps the blood from the heart into the arteries or blood vessels."***

– SWAMI SIVANANDA in *Bliss Divine*

### 1. WHAT IS PRANA?

According to Swami Sivananda, prana is universal energy or life force. Prana is vital energy that is everywhere in the universe, that is all-pervading and present in all aspects of life. Prana gives energy to all of our faculties and has many levels of meaning. In its grossest manifestation, prana refers to the breath. Prana can refer to the energy of consciousness itself. Prana also refers to the basis of life. Prana is the animating force that drives the body, the mind, and all expressions of life. So too, the highest kind of spiritual force, the kundalini shakti or serpent power, the awakened inner force that transforms consciousness, is prana. The entire universe is, in fact, a manifestation of prana.

#### Prana and the Physical Body

It is important to understand the connection between prana and the physical body. The pranamaya kosha, part of the astral body, lies beyond the gross annamaya kosha, the physical body. The physical body is made of the essence of the food and is composed of the five elements. The pranamaya kosha is formed by prana. Prana is the animating force that powers the physical body. When the prana departs from the physical body, we call it death. Thus, prana is the link between the astral body and the physical body.

## 2. PRANA MANAGEMENT

Prana is the most important thing for the Yogi to be aware of in daily life. Prana is everywhere in the universe but the Yogi needs to know how to make use of the prana and recharge. It is like checking your pulse. At all times, the Yogi checks in with him/herself and asks: "What is the state of my prana?" You must be aware of your prana and know how to manage it. The Yogi seeks to increase or restore their prana such that they have sufficient prana for all situations. The supply of prana is taken up, or absorbed, through breathing, but also through lifestyle and thoughts. Abundant prana gives strength to the nervous system. Stress arises from not having enough prana in the body, in the mind, or in the consciousness to understand and transcend the problems that we face every day. Stress depletes the supply of prana. Knowing how to recharge prana, to conserve prana and to manage prana will enhance our quality of life, extend our life and achieve Self-healing. If you have a prana deficit, you tend toward disease. It starts with stress, and ends in physical disease. Recent scientific research indicates a strong correlation between mental emotional stress, and the onset of physical disease.

**Five aspects of prana management**

1. Increase prana through the five elements *(see the table)*
2. Conserve prana through the five elements *(see the table)*

We can classify the ways we increase or lose prana according to the five elements: earth, water, fire, air and ether. The absorption of prana or the expenditure of prana is connected to each element and a corresponding sense organ and organ of action.

***Sense organs and the elements***

How you use your five senses determines whether you increase your prana or deplete your prana.

- the nose, or the sense of smell, is connected to Earth;
- the mouth, or the sense of taste, is connected to Water;
- the eyes, or the sense of sight, is connected to Fire;
- the skin, or the sense of touch, is connected to Air;
- the ears, or the sense of hearing, is connected to Ether.

# Prana: Increased, re-charged or spent through the 10 senses

| | | | | | |
|---|---|---|---|---|---|
| ELEMENTS | Earth | Water | Fire | Air | Ether |
| SENSE ORGANS | Nose | Tongue | Eyes | Skin | Ear |
| FUNCTION | Smell | Taste | Sight | Touch | Hearing |
| ORGANS OF ACTION | Anus | Genitals | Feet | Hands | Tongue |
| FUNCTION | Elimination | Reproduction | Moving | Grasping | Speaking |

| | | | | | |
|---|---|---|---|---|---|
| INCREASE PRANA | Nature Smells<br>Aroma Therapy<br>Good Incense<br>Walking Barefoot<br>Gardening | Pure Water<br>Ocean, Rivers<br>Natural Food<br>Sattvic Food<br>Sweet Food<br>Milk/Honey | Sunshine<br>Color Therapy<br>Flowers<br>Plants<br>Smiles | Clean Air<br>Massage<br>Baby Holding<br>Pets<br>Giving | Music<br>Kirtan<br>Stories<br>Sharing<br>Mantras<br>Silence |
| DECREASE PRANA | High-Rise Buildings<br>Smoking<br>Pollutants<br>Chemicals<br>Overeating | Wrong Food<br>Eating Disorders<br>Alcohol<br>Coffee<br>Soda<br>Drugs<br>Sexual Addictions | Wrong Food<br>Eating Disorders<br>Alcohol<br>Coffee<br>Soda<br>Drugs<br>Sexual Addictions | Synthetic Clothing<br>Taking, Shopping<br>Driving a Car<br>Airplanes<br>Air Conditioning | Cell Phone<br>Noise<br>Rock Music<br>Abusive Words<br>Negative Thinking<br>Talk, Gossip |

***Organs of action and the elements***

How you use your organs of action, that is, how you conduct your daily activities determines whether you increase or decrease your prana.

- the anus, or the action of elimination, is connected to Earth;
- the genitals, or the action of procreation, is connected to Water;
- the feet, or the action of moving, is connected to Fire;
- the hands, or the action of grasping, is connected to Air;
- the tongue, or the action of speaking, is connected to Ether.

Let's look at how you can increase and decrease your prana according to each element, according to the senses and your action:

**Earth:** Living in nature recharges you naturally. Live in a house on the ground or connected to the earth and build the house from natural materials such as wood, mud or other natural products to benefit from the prana of earth. When you enter such a house, you feel very good, because you sense the earth around you. Walk barefoot among the trees or work in your garden. Enjoy essential oils that come from plants and other natural substances. The sense of smell gives you prana from the earth.

Conversely, you drain your prana from a lack of connection to the earth element. Living in a high-rise building far above the ground or in a city far from trees and nature or in a building made of artificial materials like concrete, metal, or modern plastics and glues, you will only smell artificial, unnatural smells. Living in artificial environments and smelling these synthetic scents decreases your prana. In these environments, burning high-quality natural incense and using natural essential oils can help reconnect with prana. Abstain from using chemical perfumes. Connect to the prana from earth through natural scents.

Through the action of eating, you expend or gain prana. If you overeat, or eat unhealthy food, a lot of energy will be spent to digest and eliminate that food. You can develop constipation, IBS, and other digestive disorders. It is important to have a healthy, sattvic diet taken in moderation so the waste can be eliminated easily and regularly. By eating sparingly, you will not waste prana in digestion and elimination.

**Water:** Drinking purified water, bathing in the ocean and rivers, collecting rainwater to wash yourself, living near a body of clean water, tasting food that contains water will give you prana from the element water. The sense of taste can either give you prana or reduce your prana. You can increase prana by drinking pure water or all natural juices, and from eating sattvic foods that are green and fresh or sweet foods, like milk and honey. Eating foods that are very dry, stale, preserved, or processed, will cause you to lose prana. Food needs to taste good — you need to like what you eat — but taste should not just be to excite the senses. For example, if you drink beverages that excite the senses—like alcohol, coffee and soda—then you lose prana. It takes much more prana to metabolize sugars and caffeine than other ingredients.

Water is connected to emotions and the function of reproduction. If you overuse emotional and sexual energy, you lose prana.

Try to conserve this very important energy or learn to channel it positively through the practice of brahmacharya. Control and sublimation of your sexual energy will save prana and it will be transformed into spiritual energy.

**Fire:** If you feel low in prana, seek sunshine, absorb the warmth of the sun and you will get a lot of prana. Eating green food and fruits give you the sun energy as well. If you are indoors, open a door or window to bring in natural light. Wearing bright-colored clothing and the energy it reflects gives you prana. This is color therapy. This is why Sivananda Yoga teachers wear white, yellow or orange. Spend time looking at bright-colored flowers and plants.

Light also conveys prana on a more subtle level. If a person smiles at you, you get prana. When you're looking at nature, you see its magnificence and beauty, you feel the comfort and the sense of connection to a higher power. The sun is the main source of fire or light and the energy that it brings directly or indirectly gives you prana.

Prana is depleted by artificial light found in many workplaces. Likewise, if you spend all your time looking at a computer or smart phone screen, your prana will be drained. Light, of course, also conveys the content of the movies that you're watching, which on a more subtle level can increase or decrease your prana. For example, if you are watching a violent, sexual, or negative movie, or negative news, this will give you negative energy and take prana away. The content is a factor when considering the benefit of prana received from light and the sense of sight.

The feet correspond to the fire element, whose function is locomotion from one place to another. Thus, you overuse the fire by over-exercising, over-exertion, and moving too much. This is why the Yogi, as much as possible, does not move. Sitting with crossed legs, the Yogi is stable and conserves energy. Limit your movement to conserve prana.

**Air:** The most important way to recharge prana is through the breath. It is important to spend time in clean air and, as much as possible, stay away from pollution. The air element is connected to the sense of touch and the skin. Wear natural fiber clothing, like cotton, so the skin can breathe and absorb and gain prana from contact with the air element. If you wear synthetic clothing, or your clothing is too tight, the skin cannot breathe and your prana is drained. Touch is a way to absorb prana. Positive touch increases prana on many levels. Negative touch or the absence of touch can greatly decrease prana and be very damaging. Therapeutic massage is an example of positive touch.

Touch can also have a deep impact on the lifelong prana of babies and children. Babies who grow up in an orphanage, without being touched, lack prana growing up. Children who grow up in a loving family, always being hugged by their parents and family, grow up to be very strong and emotionally-resilient.

The hands are connected to the air element. The function of the hands is to grasp or to give. Learn to limit grasping, in terms of losing prana from the action of the hands. For example, shopping takes a lot of prana by grasping objects. The Yogi lives a simple life without too many belongings and without taking too much. We can turn it around by giving to others. Increase your prana by charity and reducing attachments.

**Ether:** Ether is space and is connected to the sense of hearing. Listening to positive or calming music, positive stories, the sounds of nature, or silence will recharge your prana. Mantra repetition is most effective. A mantra such as *'Om Tryambakam'* or *'Om Namo Narayanaya'* can be played in your room at a low volume.

Pay attention to the lyrics of songs you listen to as sometimes they are very negative, sad, depressing, or very aggressive and these qualities will be absorbed by your subconscious mind and take your prana away. It is very easy to lose prana through the sense of hearing as there is so much negative noise. Gossip, negative thoughts and bad words about people drain prana. As much as possible, choose your company wisely so that you surround yourself with only positive influences.

Be aware how much attention you give to your smart phone, constantly chatting and receiving notifications. This incessant noise and distraction is often not important. In addition, if you live in a place that is always noisy due to neighbors, sirens, and other loud jarring noises, you will lose prana.

It is important to curb the loss of prana due to hearing. If you hear something negative, learn to turn it into something positive and maintain your prana.

Ether is connected to the tongue, the organ of speech. If you talk a lot, you lose

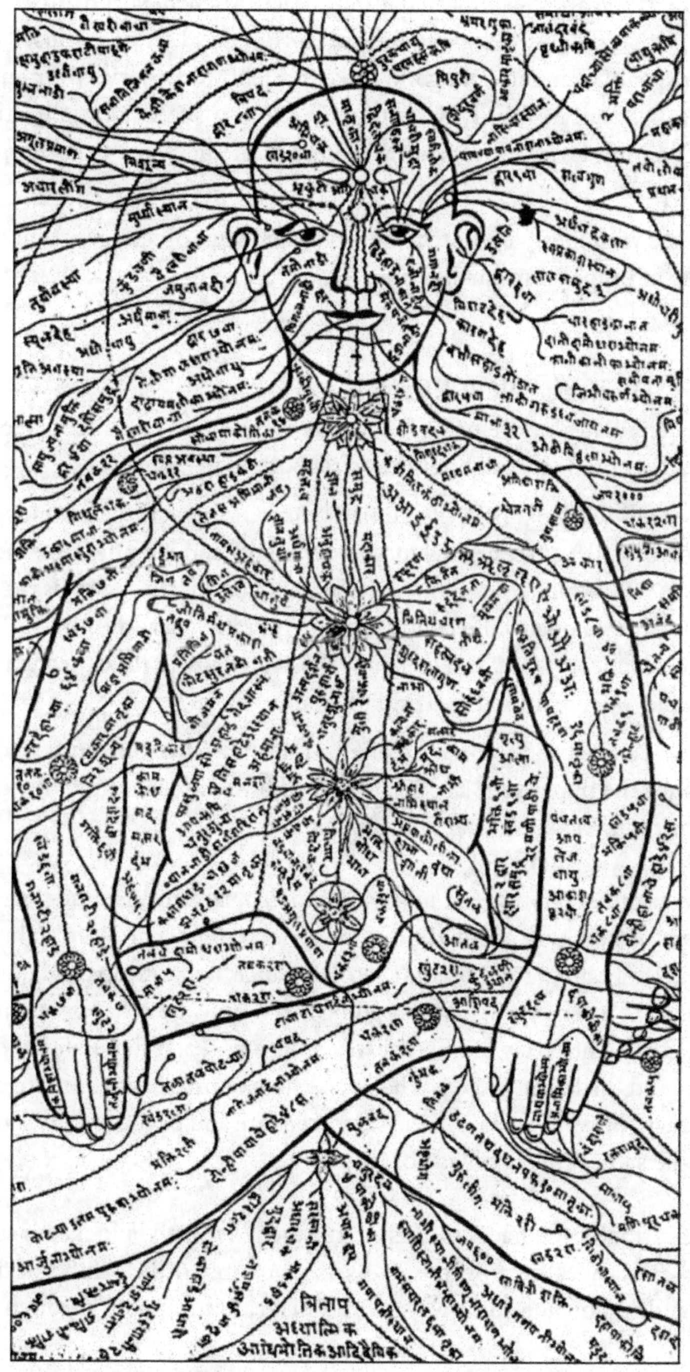
त्रिताप
अध्यात्मिक
आधिभौतिकआदिदैविक

prana, but if you control your speech, you conserve prana. The content of speech is important. If you are speaking all day long, but use beneficial, positive words to help and serve other people, you gain prana from your good service. Thus, it depends on how you speak. Generally, it's good to keep silent to conserve your energy. If you must speak, speak positively, with the intention to share and uplift, thus gaining prana. Chanting kirtan or repeating mantra is the best way to recharge using the organ of speech.

Regulate your lifestyle, control the senses and your organs of action to maximize the intake of prana from earth, water, fire, air and ether.

## 3. HOW TO BALANCE PRANA

Prana circulates in the nadis. Nadis are astral tubes or subtle energy channels that transport prana throughout the astral body.

There are 72,000 nadis in the human body. Of these, three are most important: the ida nadi which corresponds to the left nostril and channels the moon energy; the pingala nadi which corresponds to the right nostril and channels the sun energy; and the sushumna nadi, the central channel. Prana goes into the sushumna nadi when it is balanced. If we don't balance the prana, it will flow through the ida and pingala, and we remain in the world of duality.

To experience peace, contentment and healing, it is very important to purify and balance the prana so it can be channeled into the sushumna, the central nadi, where the prana or energy can flow upward.

In his commentary on *Hatha Yoga Pradipika*, Swami Vishnudevananda taught that when the nadis are purified, your thoughts no longer go from right brain to left brain, and left brain to right brain. There is balance, no more ups and downs. Usually life swings like a pendulum, one day going this way—we are happy and jumping and joyful—and the next day going that way. Like a yo-yo, it fluctuates back and forth and back and forth. But Yoga is a balanced state of mind, wherein hot and cold are the same, victory and defeat are the same, censure and praise are the same, gain and loss are the same. This is called contentment.

Purification of the nadis means to free them from any blockages so that prana can flow. Blockages form in the nadis as reactions to the taking of drugs, meat, alcohol and an unwholesome way of life. Purification happens through the practice of asanas, prana is made to flow and there is release of obstructions. Purification also happens through pranayama, controling the breath to control the prana. The most common pranayama practices are:

- **Anuloma viloma** - alternate nostril breathing [without retention for beginners and with retention following the ratio of 1:4:2 for intermediate and advanced students]. It is necessary to follow proper instructions on the technique, timing, which nostril and how many rounds to do.
- **Kapalabhati** - forceful exhalation and passive inhalation, where you recharge yourself with prana quickly, bringing about the "shining skull" state.

**Balancing Ha and Tha**

Ha is solar energy and Tha is lunar energy. When prana is balanced, the sun and moon energies are balanced and you become an integrated person. You can see the picture of Siva and Shakti as in one body.

Symbolically, Siva is male and Shakti is female. When you have balanced the sun and the moon energies, you have balanced the universal male and female energies within and you can function on a higher level. Thus, through pranayama, you can attain balance of prana, of solar and lunar energies and of the functioning of the right and left hemispheres of the brain.

Hatha Yoga is the science of balance of the two flows of energy. Prana is like electricity, but very subtle. Being mindful of the sensations from the body and mind, you can recognize which energy is operating, which energy is dominant and thus how to balance them. With this understanding, you work to balance your prana flow through correcting your living, your thinking and your actions through the practice of asanas and, more importantly, through pranayama. When you have successfully balanced your prana, you will become an integrated and a high functioning person. This will, in turn, cause your awakening to higher spiritual energy. Peace and contentment will come to you. Your happiness is no longer dependent on outside influences. It is not ego if you have self-confidence in your own Self. Confidence in the Self means that you are seeing that one Self in everything—all are one. You are truly satisfied with your life.

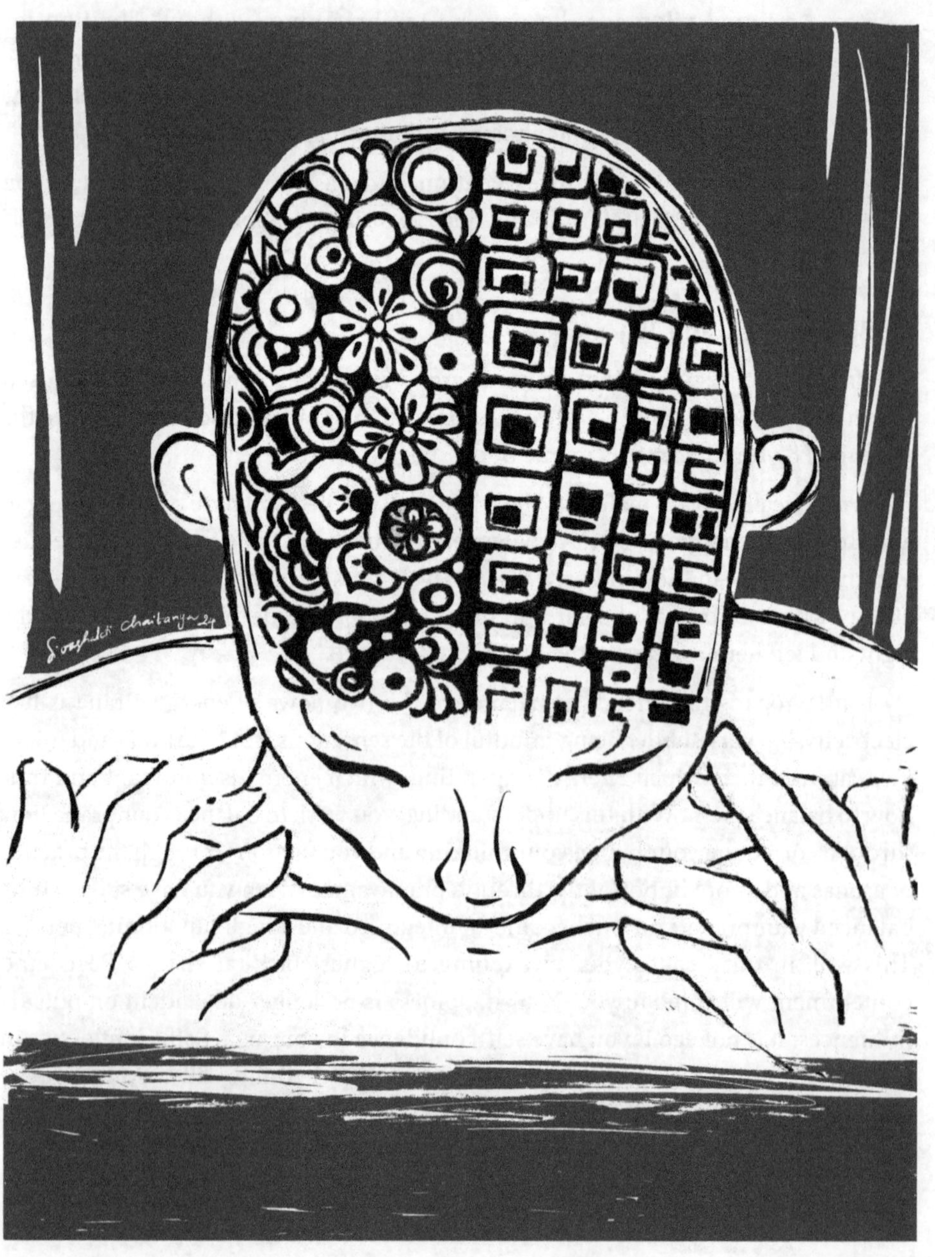

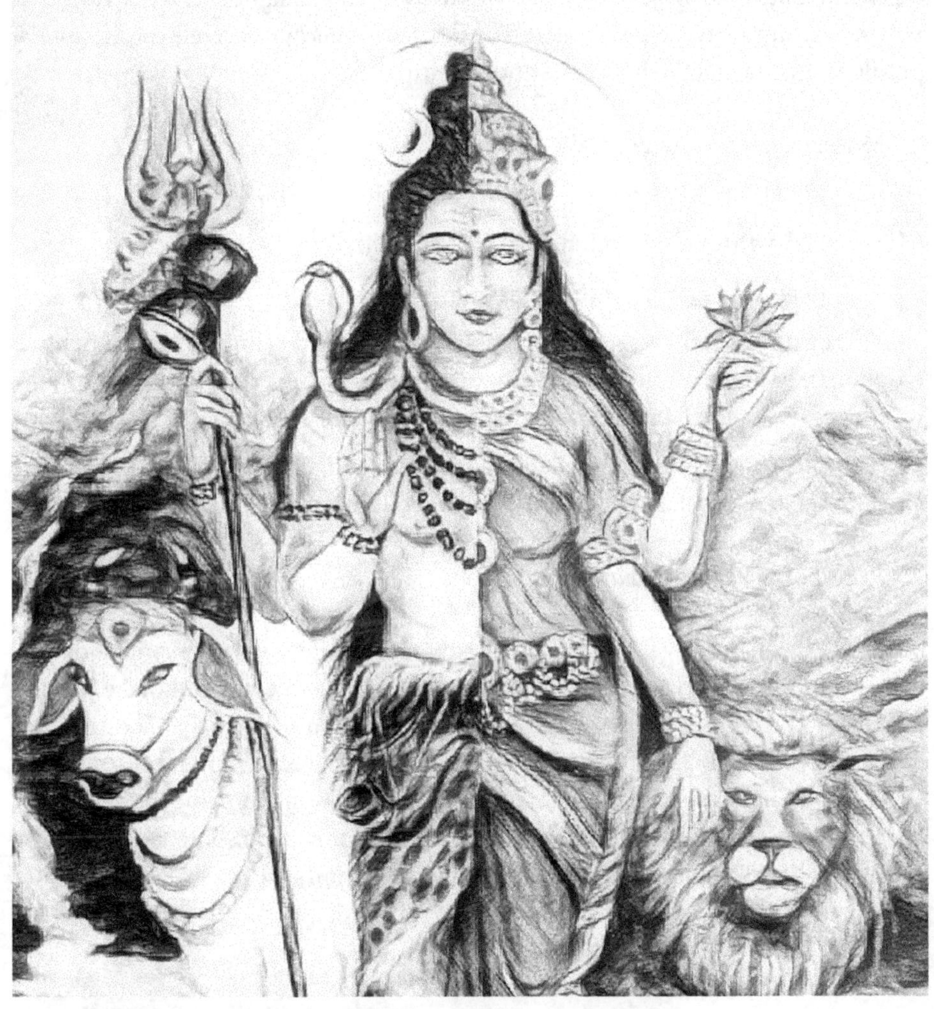

**Be aware of the two flows of energy within you**

**Sun energy = Ha energy**

- Equates to Yang energy in oriental medicine system.
- Flows through the right nostril, or pingala nadi.
- Corresponds to the left brain functioning.

This energy is hot, active, masculine, aggressive, logical, sequential, analytical, highly-intellectual, directed outwardly, rational and objective, thinking only in words, extroverted, verbose and talkative.

It stimulates the sympathetic nervous system, or the fight and flight response, making you always tense and on alert. Too much sun energy can create cardiovascular problems increasing the heart rate and elevating stress.

**Moon energy = Tha energy**

- Equates to Yin energy in oriental medicine system.
- Flows through the left nostril, or ida nadi.
- Regulates activity of the right brain.

This energy is cooling, receptive, passive, female and calming. Moon energy is emotional, indirect, intuitive, subjective, nonverbal, using visual imagery or music to express itself, quiet, introverted, creative, imaginative and artistic.

It stimulates the parasympathetic nervous system, allowing for relaxation and ease. Moon energy relaxes your system and reduces your heart rate.

*Relationships impact your balance*

If you have an active, more male or sun energy and you meet somebody that is very calm, passive, more female or having moon energy, this will make you feel balanced. Likewise, if you are passive and you meet somebody that is active, this will make you feel balanced. But if you are already active and you meet somebody that is super-active, then you become overheated and even more imbalanced. In the same manner, if you are very passive and you spend time with someone who is also passive, you will become even more imbalanced towards the passive or moon side.

*Lifestyle impacts your balance*

Similarly, your lifestyle—what you eat or drink, how you respond to the weather, what you think and your attitude about life, all of these—will be generated by either the flow of hot or cold energy and will impact your overall balance. For example, if you are already very hot, more masculine, logical and analytical and you live in hot weather, work with computers under high pressure, removed from nature and surrounded by loud noise with a very aggressive boss always pushing deadlines and high productivity, and not caring about how you feel, you can imagine you will burn so hot that you might burn out. You can balance this environment by having some nice flowers in your office, or some plants and cool natural air flow, or a picture of your family or a beautiful favorite flower or a sunset—something that makes you feel soft and relaxes you. Drink fresh whole juice and listen to calming music or soft mantra to regain balance.

Start to recognize the prana or dominant energy in yourself—and in everything you encounter in life—and how it affects you. For a Yogi on the path towards Self-healing, you must know the "pulse" of your own prana all the time and you need to know how to find balance.

## 4. CHANNELING PRANA

Prana comes with thoughts, actions and intentions. Using prana wisely, by holding pure intentions, will channel prana upwards and elevate you. You must be in charge of directing your prana consciously.

External actions by different people might be the same, but the intention behind the action will result in different types of energy. For example, the pure intention of sharing knowledge gives higher prana than the intention of displaying knowledge to impress; the pure intention of service is higher than the intention of exercising power; the intention of sincerity is higher than the motivation of pride. If the intention is pure, then the prana is converted. A sincere spiritual teacher might lose prana by using the organ of speech for hours, but as the intention is selfless service, this use of prana will make him/her gain prana instead.

A person might say, *"I don't have enough energy for my own life, so I cannot serve anybody."* This is incorrect thinking. They don't have enough energy, because the prana is stuck in thinking wrongly about who they are and what they are supposed to do in life. They worry, or think, solely about selfish activity and personal gain. Or they constantly worry that they cannot take care of their life. This kind of worry leads them to choose selfish action, leading to loss of prana. Selfless action would increase prana.

If you understand that this life and this action are not about you, and if you understand the prana you have is not *your* prana, but universal prana, then you understand how to use your prana selflessly, which will give you even more prana. You will lose some prana, because you have to work, even if selflessly, but at the same time, you exchange that lost prana with a more sublime prana, when your intention is selfless.

Prana is also the energy of consciousness. Consciously elevating your intention is important and is called channeling or using prana. Some people have a lot of prana, but are lost as to what to do with their life, how to use their prana to serve and move to a higher level. Eventually, they start to waste their prana, like a business person who makes a lot of money, but doesn't know what to do with it, and thinking only selfishly, they start to waste the money on travel here and there, or they buy a car and then a bigger car.

It is essential to understand that you need to increase and accumulate prana and use it, channel it, correctly. Your life purpose is to elevate yourself and to serve. If you don't understand this, you might use the prana you have accumulated incorrectly and waste a lot of precious time. You might lose your sense of purpose as you drain yourself of prana, become depressed and feel blocked. Rather, become a sattvic person by being selfless and channeling your prana correctly.

## 5. PURIFYING PRANA

Thoughts yield prana and prana yields thoughts of a certain vibration and wavelength. Your duty, according to Swami Vishnudevananda, is to raise your vibration by choosing the kinds of thoughts you generate and radiate around you. Every thought yields prana, but not all thoughts have the same power and value. Some thoughts are more valuable, more positive, and have more impact while other thoughts are divergent and unimportant. For example, with selfish thinking like, "I know it all, I'm the doer and without me nothing can happen," you will lose a lot of prana. In your endeavor to transform, channel and manipulate prana in daily life, learn to concentrate on the important thoughts and disregard the unimportant ones. You purify your prana when you exchange the negative thoughts for sublime, higher vibrational thoughts.

Every thought has a certain pranic or energetic content so we say every thought has a vibration. By exchanging the low vibrational thoughts for higher vibrational thoughts, you are purifying your prana.

Let's say, for example, you have one hundred one-dollar bills that have the same value as a single one-hundred dollar bill. But accumulating a stack of one-dollar bills will not give you as much money in the end as accumulating a few one-hundred dollar bills. The same is true of your thoughts. If you occupy your mind with too many unimportant, low-value thoughts — *"Should I wear this dress?", "Will it go with this belt?", "Is the color coordinating?", "Is it nice looking?"*— you are wasting your thought power. But if you think high value thoughts— *"How should I live to have less harmful ecological impact?"* and *"What kind of work should I do to become more selfless?", "What is the Self and what is not the Self?", "Whose company should I keep so I can be closer to my true Self?"* —these are very important, high-value thoughts.

Some thoughts are like gold and can change your life completely. But at other times, you can sit and think and think forever, day after day, but your life doesn't change. Your head becomes full of inconsequential thoughts, you become dizzy, stressed, and anxious, and still your life does not change. We need to constantly purify our thoughts by purifying our food, and working on improving our lifestyle so it becomes more sattvic.

Remove the tamasic thinking, activity and lifestyle, and calm the rajasic desires, impulses and actions. Nourish the sattvic activity and thoughts: repeat mantras and do more prayer; forgive other people and detach from things that we cannot control; have faith in God and know that God is taking care of things; understand everything happens for the best and the Supreme Being is omnipotent, omniscient and omnipresent, so you don't need to worry. With this understanding, you will gain a lot of prana. You will purify your prana.

- **The chakras and the journey of kundalini shakti:**

Kundalini shakti is a purified spiritual prana, lying dormant at the base of the spinal column at the muladhara chakra in the astral body. In most people, it has not been awakened. When the prana and nadis are purified, kundalini shakti is awakened, moving from chakra to chakra, each chakra representing a different level or state of consciousness. When this spiritual prana is activated or awakened *(see section on purification and balancing prana)*, we access higher levels of consciousness. The prana changes at each chakra. The lotus petals represent the amount of power and knowledge present at each level of consciousness represented by the chakra. The journey of expansion of consciousness eventually blossoms into transcendence of duality and realization of our oneness with God.

1. **Muladhara chakra,** located at the base of the spine, is visualized with four petals and is purified by meditation on the Earth Element.
2. **Swadhisthana chakra,** located at the genital area is visualized with six petals and is purified by meditation on the Water Element.
3. **Manipura chakra,** located at the navel area is visualized with ten petals and is purified by meditation on the Fire Element.
4. **Anahata chakra,** located at the heart area is visualized with twelve petals and is purified by meditation on the Air Element.
5. **Visuddha chakra,** located at the base of the throat is visualized with sixteen petals and is purified by meditation on the Ether Element.
6. **Ajna chakra,** located between the eyebrows is visualized with two petals (i.e. transcendence of duality) and is purified by meditation on the universal mind.
7. **Sahasrara chakra** is beyond the other six centers, and is located at the crown of the head. Its name indicates it has a thousand petals, representing full enlightenment, full supreme consciousness.

Once you balance your prana and bring it into the sushumna nadi, then you awaken higher consciousness. The ascent of kundalini shakti will help you to change consciousness level by level, chakra by chakra.

You can help awaken kundalini shakti and realize your highest level of consciousness by:

a. following a sattvic diet
b. exposing yourself to higher teachings, developing Satsanga
c. increasing discrimination and detachment
d. purifying body and mind through practicing asana and pranayama. The main focus is to purify the nadis. Instead of indulging rajas and tamas, you transform everything in your life to become more sattvic. When you achieve purification and balance, prana will automatically move into the sushumna nadi, or central channel, and you elevate yourself to higher levels of consciousness.

- **Awareness of subtle prana, higher state of consciousness**

To achieve Self-realization and Self-healing it is very important to feel the subtle prana. Dr. David Frawley, an extraordinary teacher of Yoga and Ayurveda, says that Yoga is an alchemical process, balancing and transforming energies of the psyche, of the mind. The subsequent teaching on subtle prana is derived from his teachings.

The subtle energies of vata, pitta and kapha are called *"prana, tejas and ojas."* Prana, *tejas* and *ojas* are subtle essence, the subtle energy of nature.

– **Prana** is a subtle energy of air, responsible for the coordination of the breath, the senses and the mind. On the inner level, it governs the unfolding and harmonization of all higher states of consciousness.

– ***Tejas*** is the subtle energy of pitta. It is an inner radiance and the subtle fire we use to digest impressions and thoughts. On the inner level, it governs the unfolding and harmonization of higher perceptual capacities.

– ***Ojas*** is the subtle energy of water. It is the basis for mental endurance. On an inner level, it is responsible for nourishing and grounding the development of higher faculties.

Prana helps you to attain the higher states of consciousness; tejas helps you to understand higher states of consciousness; *ojas* helps you to nurture and to ground these higher states, to make them more stable. All three are necessary for higher development of consciousness and they are interrelated. The most important of these subtle energies is *ojas,* as it will help you to have a strong mind, and it will increase stamina in the nervous system, which will help you to contain *tejas* and prana. Prana gives you life force and vitality, *tejas* gives you will and vigor, and *ojas* gives you endurance and stamina.

In Yoga, you want to increase all three forces—prana, *tejas* and *ojas.* You want to have high energy, you want to understand your highest state of consciousness, and you want to be strong enough to continue.

Prana will give you the enthusiasm, creativity and adaptability necessary for the spiritual path; tejas will give you the courage, the fearlessness and the insight so you can continue on your path; *ojas* will give you the peace, confidence, patience and love to maintain consistent development. Without *ojas,* we lack steadiness and calm.

Prana, *tejas*, and *ojas*, the three subtle energies, also support the immune system. *Ojas* is very important for the immune system as it affords us the potential to defend ourselves from pathogens. Tejas in the immune system will be able to burn and destroy toxins. Prana helps to activate the immune function.

Increase *ojas* through the right kind of diet, herbs, sublimation of sexual energy, control of the senses and devotion through Bhakti Yoga.

Increase *tejas* through austerity, chanting mantra, concentration and through self-inquiry or Jnana Yoga. You increase prana through pranayama, Hatha Yoga and Raja Yoga, and by combining the yoga of knowledge and yoga of devotion.

Basically, the five points and the four paths that we have discussed will help to increase prana, *tejas*, and *ojas.* The practice needs to be balanced—not too much prana and not too much *tejas.* The *ojas* needs to be supportive and contain both prana and *tejas.* If you do too much intense pranayama, for example, and too much self-inquiry and you don't have the *ojas* to sustain the practices, then you will become impatient, unhappy, discontent and cynical and it will become a problem in your spiritual path. It is important to keep these three in balance. You need to be strong to hold the prana and the *tejas.* Any time you want to do intense yoga practice, you need to ask, "Do I have enough *ojas* to sustain it?"

High vata will dry up the *ojas* like the wind will dry up water; it will weaken the digestion and deplete the prana. High pitta will burn up the *ojas*, it weakens the prana and damages the *tejas. Tejas* is courage, pitta is anger and when pitta is in excess, then the higher qualities of *tejas* cannot manifest. You might become angry, but not necessarily courageous. In general, young people have high prana and sometimes *tejas*, but they lack *ojas.*

Most meditation disorders, according to Dr. David Frawley, are caused by the imbalance of prana, *tejas* and *ojas*; the main cause is insufficient *ojas*. For example, if you do too much meditation or mantra repetition without sufficient *ojas, tejas* can burn up the nadis. Likewise, if you do excessive practice of pranayama and you don't have adequate *ojas*, you also may burn up the nadis and the prana will move in a disorderly manner.

**To summarize,** a Yogi on the path of Self-healing needs to:

- consider these five actions to manage prana: increase, conserve, balance, channel and purify.
- understand the functions of the three subtle pranas: prana, *tejas* and *ojas* and how yoga practices increase and balance them.
- understand the lifestyle conducive to having a high level of consciousness.
- understand the process of awakening kundalini shakti.

## QUESTIONS

1. *What is prana , what is the relationship between prana and thought?*
2. *What actions help you to increase prana through the five elements?*
3. *What actions cause you to decrease prana through the five elements?*
4. *Describe briefly the 5 aspects of prana management.*
5. *Describe Ha and Tha and why it is important to balance them.*
6. *How do you awaken Kundalini shakti?*

*INSPIRED STORY*

**Crippling fear of death**

*One of the Yoga Health Educators told the story of meeting a group of seniors on the beach. In the group, there was a lady about 70 years old who was a retired journalist and could barely walk. She almost drowned two days before, fainted, and was transported to hospital. After the medical exam, the doctor said that she had trouble with her parasympathetic nervous system and gave her some medicine. For two days, her condition did not improve. She was almost paralyzed, and could not grasp anything with her hand. She was stiff, weak, and cold, not able to move, not able to sleep, even though she took sleeping pills. She could not do anything by herself and had to have help 24/7 by her bed.*

*I assessed her 5 koshas, the body and mind, and deduced that she was suffering from high vata derangement, due to fear of death, panic, and high stress, when she was drowning. I advised her to eat and drink ginger to warm up and taught her a chair yoga class including self-affirmation at the end during savasana. She was able to relax and slept well without medicine.*

*The next afternoon, she was able to walk with help about 500 meters to go to lunch. Slowly she became active again to the surprise of her group of friends who were very grateful and happy. In this case, I did not think too much but there was a very quick thought appearing in my mind that all her systems and organs and her life rhythm were out of sync, her breath, her prana flow, her nervous system, her digestive system, respiratory system, her fight and flight system are all disturbed. I knew my goal was to help bring back natural harmony by coordinating movement, breathing, and relaxation the yoga way, and at the same time help her to have the feeling of peace, reducing the fear by having faith that she will be able to recover. And she did.*

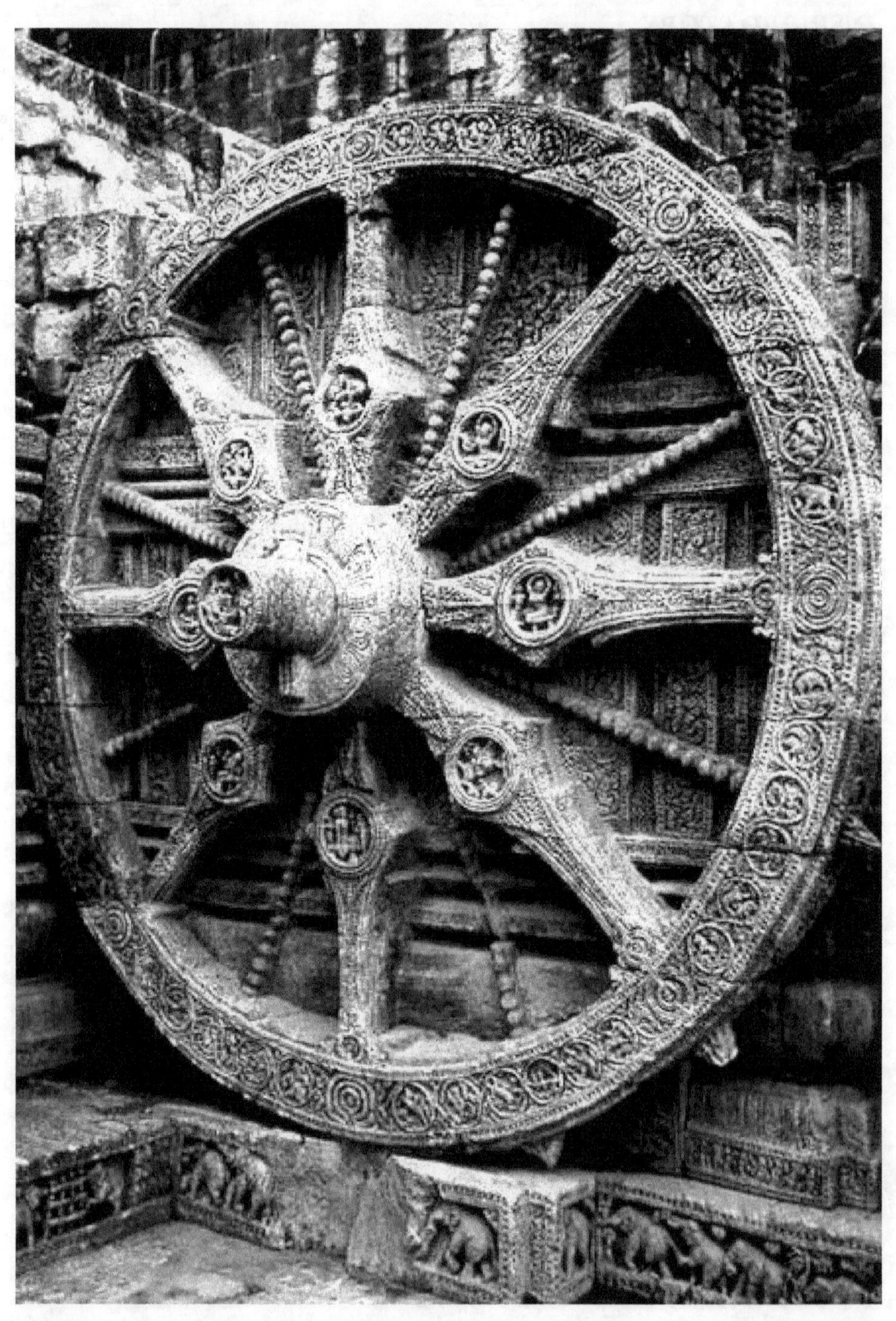

THE WHEEL OF KARMA

## CHAPTER 6

# Learning the Lessons of Karma

***"Thought is karma. Thinking is the real karma. Thought molds your character. If you allow the mind to dwell on good, elevating thoughts, you will develop a noble character , you will naturally do good and laudable actions."***

*SWAMI SIVANANDA in Bliss Divine*

The topic of karma is very important and explains many problems in life. We have talked about life and how life is a struggle. We have talked about stress and how stress is constant. We have also talked about how karma creates stress and how stress is often caused by our karma. Certain areas of life in which we struggle are not easy to deal with because they are caused by karma. This makes getting to the root of a problem and resolving it all the more difficult. Karma creates stress, because it's not easy to understand.

### 1. WHAT IS KARMA?

Swami Sivananda taught that karma is not only action, but also the result of action. The consequence of an action is part of the action itself. Action here includes physical action, mental action and emotional action.

The Law of Karma means the law of causation, or the law of cause and effect. Swami Sivananda said, *"Wherever there is a cause, then an effect must be produced, like a seed is the cause of a tree, which is the effect. The tree produces seeds and becomes the cause of the seeds. The cause is found in the effect, and the effect is found in the cause. The effect is similar to the cause which is the universal chain of cause and effect that has no end."*

Further, he said, "*No event occurs without having a positive definite goal at the back of it. The breaking of a war, the occurrence of an earthquake, the breaking of an epidemic, the disease of the body, fortune, or misfortune all have definite causes behind them.*"

Within the law of cause and effect—the law of causation—there are three laws: the law of action and reaction, the law of compensation and the law of retribution. The three laws come together in what is called the Doctrine of Karma.

- **The law of action and reaction:** Everything that happens will have a reaction of the same nature and the same force. Let's say you broke someone's leg in a past life. Then in this life, you're out walking, and suddenly a branch falls from a tree—and breaks *your* leg. The reaction is of the same nature and the same force. You break a leg, your leg gets broken. You did not have to amputate your leg, but you incurred the degree and type of injury from the prior broken leg. Nobody broke your leg, it happened by the natural falling of a tree branch. So, the set-up of the event is different, but the consequence is the same. Because you broke somebody's leg in a past life, you would have to experience the pain of a broken leg. The law of action and reaction teaches us relentlessly that for every action in the universe there is an equal and opposite reaction. Swami Sivananda said the law operates everywhere with "unceasing precision" and "scientific accuracy." It operates on the physical plane and also on the mental plane. If you create suffering for somebody, you will have to bear the same kind of suffering at another time.
- **The law of compensation:** The spiritual law of compensation is a universal principle that governs the relationship between effort and reward. It states that everything we do creates an outcome equal to the effort we put in. It suggests that what we give, we receive in equal measure. By focusing on providing value and contributing positively to the world, we can attract abundance and prosperity in our lives. Everything is balanced in nature. If there is extreme cold somewhere, there will be extreme heat somewhere else. If there are ten negative people in a place, there will be two sattvic souls to bring balance. The law of compensation keeps the balance and establishes harmony in nature. It operates everywhere in the phenomena of nature beautifully. Basically, you will not be able to understand your karma if you don't understand the bigger picture of your life. You will have to take into account the widest angle of view of the life of the soul.
- **The law of retribution:** Every wrong action will have its own punishment. Nothing happens by accident in this world. There is a direct connection

between what is being done now by you and what will happen in the future. If you always sow seeds which will bring pleasant fruits, then you receive pleasant fruits and it will make you happy. But, if you sow wrong actions, then you will receive some negative consequences.

We have to learn our karmic life lessons in the middle of conflicts. The famous discourse between Arjuna and Krishna in the Bhagavad Gita is being taught in the middle of the battlefield. This symbolizes that the lessons of life, the lessons of karma, are being learned right in the middle of living. It is exactly in living this life that we learn the lessons we are meant to learn. We must understand the workings of our psyche and the inner conflicts we carry. Though the psyche is often quite deep, if you gain understanding, then it's easier for you to face the issue.

Karma is often understood wrongly. We think that karma relates only to bad things happening. This is incorrect. Karma is everything about your life; you are born out of karma. The present life and all its aspects are the accumulated results of past karma.

## 2. THREE KINDS OF KARMA

Even though only the present exists, understanding of three kinds of karma—past, present and future —sheds some light on our current state of affairs. We inherit circumstances from the past karma, and have the choice of paying off karmic debts or reproducing the karma in the future.

***The three kinds of karma are:***

1. **Sanchita karma** is all of the accumulation of all of the actions that you have done through all past lifetimes. These karmic impressions carry forward into each new incarnation.
2. **Prarabdha karma** is that portion of the sanchita karma coming to fruition in this present life. It takes many lives to pay up all the karmic debts from the past, so we have to be reborn and live through many lifetimes to exhaust the sanchita karma. The prarabdha karma is inexorable; it is impossible to stop, avoid, or prevent. What we are experiencing now is a consequence of our past actions and we cannot really escape it. We can, however, learn to understand it and how to deal with it. There are many causes hidden in the past which explain what happens in this life. There are conflicts whose roots are very deep in the past.

3. **Agami karma** is the karma we create from our actions in this present life. If you are wise, as you deal with the prarabdha karma in this life, you will avoid creating new karma for the future.

## 3. WHERE DOES KARMA COME FROM?

Karma comes from *avidya* or spiritual ignorance, not knowing the truth of who you are, projecting different ideas about yourself, and believing these false ideas of yourself. The root cause of karma, the main cause of karma, is desire. Because you don't know your true Self and have incorrect understanding of who you are, desire arises and compels you to seek happiness in external things.

Due to karma, you are born in this body with this mind; you project different desires, then run after them to realize the Truth and exhaust the karma. The journey is endless. Desire is insatiable. Satisfaction of one desire will inevitably bring about new or more intense desires. The fact is, you are looking for peace and happiness in the wrong place.

## 4. TWELVE AREAS OF KARMA AND HOW TO HEAL THROUGH AWARENESS AND REMEDIAL MEASURES

Karma governs every aspect of our life. In the science of Vedic astrology (Jyotish), the science of karma, different karmas are grouped in twelve areas covering all aspects of our lives. The position and disposition of the planets in these areas indicate the specific karmic lessons. Being aware of them helps us to cultivate detachment. These areas of karma come from the framework of Vedic astrology. Of course, this is only a guideline, considering the multitude of ways and scenarios karma can play out. The remedials are suggestions.

1. **The body, yourself**

    The body is like a battlefield on which the karma is playing. You're born as a male or as a female, tall or short, black or white, beautiful or handicapped, with a lot of prana or innately weak—whatever it is, it's part of the setup of the karma. The body is limited and can't do all that you want. It goes through the process of growth and of aging. The body is an instrument and it serves the purpose of your birth.

    **Remedial:** Accept the body and cherish it as your precious vehicle to fulfill your purpose, your dharma. Honor the body and do not mutilate it. You are not the body, but you need to take care of it. Endeavor to increase prana in the body and conserve prana for a long meaningful life. Try not to over-care for the body, not over-identifying with it, not using it for wrong purposes. With the body, you have the organs of action whose function are elimination, reproduction, moving, grasping, speaking. Use the organs of action and organs of perception, the senses, correctly. Do not over-use them.

2. **The family of origin, your relatives, your financial resources, your mouth, your speech**

Your family of origin can be supportive or you can be deprived of family support. The way you eat can be supportive to your life or it can be problematic. Your speech can be supportive to you or not. You can be deprived of financial resources to sustain your life or you can be wasting your money.

**Remedials:** Nurture healing voice (connect your voice and your soul and express it, like when chanting kirtan), healing speech (you heal yourself and others through speech, not aggravating relationships), healing food (honoring the body, not harming it), use financial resources for healing purposes. Be grateful for support received. Give support to others, even when you have not received support. Remedy the karma of not having money by donating money. Then money karma can no longer be a criteria to make you suffer—by your feeling either greedy, needy or feeling lack. Be free of the idea that money is the purpose of your life. Do not waste money in search of sensual pleasures. Learn to think about money correctly to work out your karma.

3. **Communication skills, your own self-will, the way you express yourself, your relationships with your siblings**

Some people have problems in communication and expression, some have extraordinary skill of communication, enjoy themselves and give joy to others through their communication.

**Remedial:** Practice compassionate communication skill. Learn to honestly express your needs and listen to others. Surrender to God's will and see the big picture about your life and the life of others to remedy blockages in communication. Help to connect or network people for a higher purpose, seeing the sacred and the divine all around.

4. **Your core heart and your peace of mind, your happiness, what makes you happy, your relationship with your mother, your home, your house or property**

   Your heart and peace of mind can be disturbed. You can be sad, depressed, angry, restless, needy, emotional, isolated and have emotional difficulty and a bad relationship with your mother.

   **Remedial:** Practice openness of heart, learn to love, practice contentment, open your heart and have a loving disposition. Resolve your difficult relationship with your mother, and thus with your own emotions, by devoting yourself to the Divine Mother. Heal all your heart wounds, forgive, forget and keep loving and being at peace with yourself and with all. This is the key to liberation from karma. Avoid being fearful, victimized, defensive or manipulative of emotions.

5. **The way you use your intelligence to follow dharma, your creativity, your education, your children**

   Use your intelligence to understand how the universe works in order to follow your dharma. You might have the karma of good education, good intellect and have power of discernment and discrimination coming from past merits. You might inherit blockages in your secular and spiritual study, coming from past demerits (wrong thoughts from before that block your knowledge now).

   **Remedial:** Care to follow guidance, ethics and dharmic behavior, spiritual education, and study of scriptures. Purify your intellect by chanting mantras. Take care of your children as instruments of God's creativity and not as your possessions.

6. **Your obstacles and overcoming obstacles in terms of your own weaknesses, creating debts, enemies or diseases**

   Because you have weaknesses, you create obstacles for yourself. These obstacles can create debts, enemies or diseases to yourself. Everyone has weaknesses, more or less pronounced.

   **Remedial:** Face and strengthen your weak area to overcome obstacles, proactively practicing the guidance of Yoga Life (understanding the law of nature) and the four paths of Yoga to self-develop, self-discipline, and achieve self-purification thus diminishing the impact of weaknesses.

   See obstacles, conflicts and diseases as an opportunity to review your lifestyle and negative thinking. Learn the principles of health and live according to the law of nature, which is the divine law. Learn to work selflessly (doing Karma Yoga), to give instead of to consume, to be disciplined instead of being indulgent. Learn to see your own *atman* in others. Stop fault finding. Learn to forgive and have the vision of unity. Turn your weakness into strength.

7. **Your enjoyment coming from good or problematic association with partner in business or in life**

You might have a good marriage, a good lasting association with a partner or a problematic one. You might have the karma of rejection, a story of abandonment, a story of disloyalty, unfaithfulness, betrayal, treachery, infidelity, or untrustworthiness. You might be abusive or a victim of abuse in relationships. All these are manifestations of the karma of your relationship with the partner or with the other.

**Remedial:** We are One, so try to see unity and solve the problem of attraction, rejection and split in partnership. Learn to see the Self in others, treat others as you would treat yourself. Learn detachment instead of passion. Learn to honor commitment and responsibilities and control your lustful tendencies.

8. **Karma with the hidden forces in the psyche and the astral world**

The karma here will manifest not in your life, but in your mind. The working of your psyche can bring spiritual insight, intuition, and enlightenment, revealing the way to liberation, leading to freedom from suffering. Or you can fall victim to dark forces in your mind that bring miseries to you and others.

**Remedial**: Learn to uplift yourself through the power of Satsanga and association with wisdom, wise people or good people, so you can get out of your psyche. Purify. Become aware of the mind and the subconscious. Renounce siddhis, occult practices, dark associations, hidden secrets and exploration of astral realms.

9. **Your good fortune and luck or lack of blessings and luck coming from your good or bad association with spiritual or religious teachers, karma regarding your religion and your faith**

You might receive good dharmic guidance or bad guidance. You might have a good relationship with your father or father figure. You might have a good mentor or Guru. Or you might have difficulty in finding spiritual guidance. You might be a good teacher yourself, with elevated and expanded consciousness that you inherited from a good, blessed and lucky life.

**Remedial:** Cultivation of respect for teachers and spiritual traditions, practice of humility in the pursuit of Self-realization. Discrimination in the choice of teachers or guides, avoiding tamasic and rajasic teachers and methods. Abstain from guiding people, not having purified yourself first. Become a sattvic teacher and a sattvic student. Replace a negative relationship with your birth father with a positive relationship with the Divine Father. Cultivate trust, faith and security of being protected, remove doubts and anxiety. Remove fanaticism in the matter of religion. Remember that, *"Paths are many but Truth is One. Names and forms are many, but God is One."*

10. **Karma about work and career, about acquisition of name and fame or lack of recognition, about positive or negative contribution to the welfare of society**

    You can derive either satisfaction or unhappiness from your work, have a sense of purpose and mission or lack a sense of your place in life. You may lack fulfillment and recognition, not knowing what your ideal career is.

    **Remedial:** Develop a sense of selflessness through the practice of selfless service (Karma Yoga) as a remedial to purposelessness. Patanjali said that non-acquisitiveness, absence of greed or realizing that material possessions are not the end and goal of life will help you discover the purpose of this birth. Name and fame are illusory, so renunciation of ego and name and fame will help you to counteract that karma. Become the instrument to Higher Will instead.

11. **Karma with your community, society, environment, your friends and your gains and success in life**

    Your environment and community can either be conducive to your growth, success and fulfillment or it can be detrimental to your growth and success in life. It might be that you will meet with unfavorable environments and society, or the opposite, you will be favored by the circumstances and connections.

    **Remedial:** Be an honorable contributing member of the community, care for the environment (nature, people, animals), care for friends and connections. Respect the web of life. Avoid taking advantage of the society or environment, people and friends. Avoid unethical behavior to gain financial success at the expense of others.

12. **Karma with losses and unfortunate events**

This is a story of suffering coming from material losses or separation from loved ones, a story of losing yourself to addictions, pleasures and expenditures. It includes lack or loss of self-confidence, lack or loss of success and fulfilment. These losses might lead you to hospitals, jails, ashrams, or make you go into exile or foreign countries.

**Remedial:** Instead of losing yourself in a negative manner (addiction, indulgence, expenditures), lose yourself in a positive manner (through charity and selflessness). Counteract the losses, through the active practice of humility and charitable actions. Volunteer losing the ego through selflessness and charity, volunteering in hospitals, jails, ashrams, or service to the forlorn, the downtrodden and the homeless.

There are many combinations of karmic situations possible. Different areas of karma are connected to each other.

## 5. KARMA LEADS TO DHARMA

Vedic teaching says that the way to be free from karma and suffering is through the observance of dharma. Dharma is right conduct, right understanding and comes from karma, wrong conduct, wrong understanding. Remember, karma comes from desires. Through elevation of consciousness, we are freed from making the same mistakes and being reincarnated again to face the karmic results.

Let's say you have a certain desire; you want to have a child. Then you have a child, but you find you don't want to have a child anymore. The desire is gone, but you still have a child to take care of. You have to carry on with the result of your desire and do your duty towards the child. This duty is called dharma. Dharma is a duty that you need to fulfill. Everyone has a duty towards their father and mother. If you are a father or mother, you have a duty towards your child. This is dharma.

Everyone has their personal dharma (swadharma). The basic dharma is towards your body. When you take care of your body and you are healthy, you are fulfilling the dharma with your body. Like it or not, you have this body in this life that comes from karma, but now you have the dharma to take care of it.

There are different kinds of dharma, but the dharma with your relationships is very deep and, since you are born in a certain environment, you also have the dharma with your society and your community.

### How to progress in life between karma and dharma

There are many stories of people wanting to pursue Yoga and meditation and not being able, as their karma/dharma takes up all their energy. Karma is constantly changing and bringing new challenges. Dharma keeps us very busy paying his/her karmic debts.

You want to progress in life. You want to know yourself. So, what do you need to do? Between karma and dharma you need to squeeze in the Sadhana. Sadhana is a conscious practice of daily Yogic life routines (asana, pranayama and meditation) for you to gain awareness—in the middle of the battlefield of life.

## 6. SUMMARY OF TEACHING ON KARMA

- Karma is action and the consequence of action.
- Karma comes from past wrong thoughts or emotions.
- Wrong thoughts repeat themselves. Karma repeats itself. Thoughts repeat themselves, right or wrong. The groove becomes deeper and deeper. They become karmic patterns.
- Karma is difficult to resolve, because the karmic patterns are quite deep.
- These wrong thoughts or selfish thoughts are like karmic seeds; they always create new situations.
- Specific karmic seeds produce specific trees. The seed of the banana tree creates a banana tree. Life unfolds exactly according to what we need to experience.
- There is no good karma or bad karma. Depressive thoughts come from a lack of acceptance of karma. We experience this life and wish it could be different. We hate our bodies. We hate our minds and our emotions. We wish life were different, but it cannot be different because it depends on the karmic seeds.
- There are no accidents. Everything happens for a reason, according to the law cause and effect.
- Life is a school. Feel that you are going to school and every event is a learning opportunity.
- Our actions in the present create our future. All we need to do is take care of the present.

*A beautiful young lady was my student in Yoga and meditation. She was excellent in asanas, and she performed all advanced postures beautifully. Also she had lots of devotion to Lord Krishna.*

*One day she discovered she had a brain tumor. She couldn't do asanas anymore. She had to switch to other kinds of practices, chanting kirtan, painting sacred art.... The nice thing about her was throughout these many years of struggling with her disease she was always very positive. She never complained or blamed. She did what she could and she was always smiling.*

*One day she left the body.*

*I believe that she had paid her karmic debts nicely. When she had the disease, she did a lot of introspection and a lot of dreams came to her. She told the story that she remembered her past life. She was a slave. In America there were slaves not long ago. She was a slave and she was being mistreated or beaten because she did not work enough. She then committed suicide. She told the story of many lifetimes of suicide.*

*These are attempts to not accept the karma and escape. In this life what happened? She had a very good family condition, a perfect beautiful body, perfect mind, and then she got brain cancer. In past lifetimes, she committed suicide because she did not accept her condition. Now in this life, all the conditions were perfect but she was going to die of disease. In this life, she learned to surrender and lived her life bravely and positively to the very end.*

Swami Sita

- Control your emotions and reactions. Our common mental pattern is to like something and dislike something else. Whatever you like, whatever you dislike, is all karma. There is no good karma, nor bad karma. There is no good life, nor bad life. There is no lucky, nor unlucky, life. There is only karma and freedom from karma. Being a prince or princess in a royal family is not necessarily lucky; often kings, queens, princes and princesses are actually miserable.
- Do not desire the karma of someone else and mind your own business. You are better off with your own karma than someone else's. The answer is within. You do not really know what is inside other people's minds and karma, and no one can really know yours. Practice gratitude and peace every day, because we are growing in greater awareness through the challenges and the lessons we're learning.
- Life, your life, is an opportunity for growth. You dissolve your karma by right thinking and right action. Acceptance of our life circumstances, and having positive thinking and positive actions, will free us from karma. We are not victims of our life condition. When we feel we are victims, we blame other people. At that time, we are not understanding our karma. We are not understanding that karma itself created something that we did not understand about ourselves. We do not understand our weaknesses. Then we blame other people. Unfavorable conditions are stepping stones to great growth. Weakness attracts negative conditions to think about and make you grow stronger in the future.
- We can change our destiny by self-effort. Amidst favorable or unfavorable conditions, we can learn to be responsible for our minds and actions and emotions as well. Human life is the result of mixed karma, good and bad. Do not expect heaven, but learn to bear difficulties and detach.
- We cannot escape our karma. Some people want to. They cannot accept the challenges, difficulties and conflicts with themselves or other people. They don't want to live their lives. They don't want to fight the battle and they run away. Escaping takes place in the form of depression, addictions, unceasing traveling, constant busyness, irresponsibility and the like.

## 7. KARMIC INNER CONFLICTS

Inner conflicts are deep and difficult to resolve, coming from the long-term pattern of past lives.

We often identify with these mental impressions, which makes it more difficult to detach from them. You will have difficulty changing, because you think you are the mind and the mental impressions. The first step in paying karmic debts is to step back from your mental patterns, recognize your mental patterns, recognize your weaknesses and try to train yourself into new habits of thinking and new behaviors. Study of Vedic astrology *(Jyotish)* as a science of karma helps bring awareness of these patterns. Yoga is the remedial measure par excellence. Self-healing means that you need to train yourself consciously into a new attitude, into new thoughts that counteract your mental tendencies.

***Six types of karmic conflicts***

1. **Conflict between self and others**

   You are a free spirit, the pure *atman*, but you go through life believing that you are this limited body and mind and you feel separation. You always see yourself as different from other people. This is the first karmic conflict. Some experience this karma between self and others very acutely as repeated relationship problems. The only possible way to be freed from that karma is to transcend the idea of yourself as your body, and the idea of other people separate from you. Only when you realize the oneness of all will you free yourself from this karma. This Karma is very difficult to reconcile. On the one hand you always think of your needs and reject others, while on the other hand, you reject yourself and always think that others are more important than you. That's why, in Vedanta, it is said that you have to learn to see other people as your own self. You have to see God in yourself and in others. You have to humble yourself, and sometimes you have to deny your own needs. You have to self-sacrifice to find the Self that is uniting all. There are many lessons here to learn from this one karmic conflict. Sometimes it takes a lifetime to understand all the dramas that happen in a family, within a couple, or between friends. Emotional conflict and people blaming each other is very common. *"You don't care about me; you only care about yourself."*

2. **Conflict between material security and seeking the truth**

   You never feel you have enough money or material support and you never feel secure materially. And you certainly don't have time for Yoga and meditation and seeking the truth about yourself. You say, *"Later, when I'm more secure financially, then I will meditate."* But this is a karmic conflict, an illusion. You can never feel secure materially, because security comes only from inner knowledge of your eternal Self. Security cannot come from transient material objects. If you have material things, like houses and cars, the tendency is to want to have more houses, better houses, better cars, and a better job, so you can pay for a better car and better house. The more you think of material growth, the more spiritual growth is tempting. You feel some kind of nagging feeling inside that you are missing something, you are needing something. You go to study Yoga and take a course on meditation. But then you say, *"I have no time to meditate, because of my job, so maybe later."*

The opposite also can be true. Somebody will go into spiritual life, but neglect the material. This also does not work. It creates a lot of conflict. Then your father, mother, and family say, *"Stop meditation. Stop the Yoga life. You better go find a job."* So you go find a job, but it doesn't feel meaningful. You go back and forth between material- and truth-seeking. It is very difficult to resolve this karmic conflict. You have to accept these conflicts and do your sadhana, no matter what the physical conditions are. Recognize this kind of karmic conflict, do sadhana and eventually dissolve the karmic conflict.

3. **Karmic conflict between self-will and God's will**

You always want to follow your own will, but it never really works out. You realize you need to think of something bigger than yourself to be really successful. If you think only of "my idea," "my will," "my preferences," then you cannot be truly successful. You forget God's will—something bigger than "my eyes" can see. You will inevitably encounter obstacles. Something will not work out. You can take all kinds of initiative. You can work very hard to be successful, but it will not work out. Eventually you will have to understand there's something else called God's will. If you don't fit in that picture, it will never work out. You have to slow down. You have to be humble. You have to become more tuned in to listening to God's will. You understand eventually, that it is a waste of time to put so much energy into something that will not work out. You learn to put the energy into listening to God's will. This is termed sadhana. Make the effort, but at the same time, relax and surrender. Yoga promotes both effort and relaxation. We have this conflict, because we have an ego that wants us to do only what it wants. We do not want to listen and surrender. Learn to surrender and to accept, to conform to a larger picture. Be ready to receive guidance. If you are very attached to your "I-ness" and "my-ness," you will reject any guidance you receive. Learn to consult with others; this is not easy. When you think you know, you never consult others. You think you're independent. You don't have to report to anybody.

The other scenario can also be true. In this case, someone is constantly looking for a perfect teacher and changes teachers all the time, finds fault with a teacher or has multiple teachers. They reject their own will and constantly wait for guidance from the teacher.

To resolve that karmic conflict, you need to study spiritual books and teachings to grow in maturity and be able to match your self-will and God's will. At that time, you can slow down, accept, surrender, and listen to your own inner guidance.

4. **Conflict between your private and public recognition**

This is the conflict between the private feelings of your heart, your soul, and external recognition. Some people work to get recognition and neglect the soul's voice in the heart, but you cannot try to make other people happy and not make your own heart happy. Some people just follow their heart and cannot hold a job or they compromise at work. You have to reconcile your heart and your work for public recognition. Name, fame, position and recognition are illusions and will never be enough, so you swing between that and your inner spiritual life.

To reconcile this, you can live and work at home, dedicate your life to making someone happy, while following your own path to help and contribute to society.

5. **Conflict between your inner personal success and outer societal material success**

Spiritual success is not measured by outer gain. Spiritual evolution depends on your inner knowledge, no matter your external gains. You have already attained a certain level of spiritual evolution from your past exertion. You have inner wisdom, but the conflict comes from not knowing how to make true progress in this life. We call it inner achievement and outer achievement. This life is part of a chain of lives. Material success and spiritual success are interconnected. You might think that your material success and your past merit are completely disassociated. You can swing between rejecting the world and being driven to spiritual knowledge *or* being driven to material gains and neglecting your inner wisdom voice. Dedicating yourself to the guidance of spiritual teachers and having a steady routine of spiritual practices will help you get out of this dilemma.

6. **Conflict between your struggle to improve and the temptation to indulge your weakness**

   Weakness comes from not being able to recognize karma and not having connection with the Self ever-present within you. There is an innate desire in everyone to lose themselves. You can lose yourself in a correct way or in an incorrect way. The incorrect way would be to become a victim of your weaknesses. The correct way would be to consciously offer yourself up through spiritual practices or Karma Yoga. There is, on one hand, the difficult struggle to improve yourself and, on the other hand, the temptation to escape in tamas, addiction, sleep, disease and other indulgences. The best choice is to do selfless service (Karma Yoga). Do charity of time and money, lose your ego step by step by renunciation of the ego and in selfless action. Do meditation and self-enquiry to rectify your thinking. Follow the ethical guidelines of Yoga's Yamas and Niyamas (restraints and observances) carefully, if you have this tendency.

   Struggle to counteract your own weakness and limitations, stop blaming others for your problems, and become stronger. Focus on your own self-improvement and do not lose yourself in other people.

   An example of weakness is having a tendency toward violence or impatience. You are easily irritated, are quick to judge and condemn others. You use tough words and fight with other people. You hide from your weakness, not being sincere and truthful. Instead, you play games and manipulate. You have to recognize this as a karmic tendency. That's why Yoga teaches ahimsa, non-violence, and satya, truthfulness.

   Another example of weakness is if you are frequently proud, jealous or envious; it's part of your character. Or you often reject discipline and indulge in sensual pleasures. Or you are driven by greed and accumulation of material objects.

   To counter these weaknesses, you have to purify these tendencies by Yoga practice, practice of austerity, practice of contentment and gratitude. You have to do self-observance, self-study and study of scriptures to return to an undistorted view of yourself.

There are many facets and degrees of manifestation of these six types of inner conflicts. They can manifest in "karmic relationships" or in terms of "karmic diseases," where your system breaks down. You have to stop and ask yourself big questions to correct the course of your actions. In the Self-healing journey, develop a positive attitude toward disease. Wake up and recover yourself from karma.

## 8. THE WHEEL OF BIRTH AND DEATH AND HOW TO BREAK THROUGH IT

How do we break free from the chains of karma? The wheel of birth and death is depicted as a circle, where we go around and around, a cycle. In one life, you learn from your karma, but as you are learning, you are also creating new karma—so you will be born again. You will be reborn to learn from that new karma. It is like you keep repeating classes in school and don't get to graduate. The idea is you have to graduate at some point, which means you have to free yourself from the cycle of births and deaths through ceasing to identify with your body and mind. Once you realize your true identity, you can live out the karma in this lifetime without creating the karma of rebirth. This is a simple explanation of how we can increase karma or decrease karma using the example of a bank account with debits and credits.

In one column, your karmic debts are registered. In the other column, your karmic credits are registered. When you know that you are constantly adding to your karmic debits, you become mindful to check your actions and thoughts in order to rectify your course of thinking. Using the metaphor of a bank account, you are constantly aware of whether your debts are being paid off as you are eager to come to a zero bank balance when you no longer have debts, i.e. the state of liberation.

## KARMIC BANK BALANCE

| Karmic debts<br>Debit (-) | Karmic credits<br>Credit (+) |
|---|---|
| - - - - - - - -<br>- - - - - - - - | + + + + + + + +<br>+ + + + + + + +<br>+ + + + + + + |

**Karmic Debts:**

- Impressions from past lives at birth. If you act unconsciously, according to those impressions, you are in a tamasic state of mind.
- Experiences from childhood and youth without self-awareness. You follow the desires and act in a rajasic manner. You seek name, fame, success and pleasures and you do not care to improve yourself spiritually.
- Negativities, impulses, selfish desires, tamasic and rajasic thoughts
- Actions harmful to yourself and others
- Unconscious actions in thought, word and deed, reinforcing your negative mental patterns

**Karmic Credits:**

- Becoming conscious of your own karmic tendencies and starting to change and become a more sattvic human being
- When you become positive in karmic situations, in karmic diseases, in karmic relationships and in karmic conflicts
- Selfless actions and detached conscious actions and feelings (Karma Yoga)
- Doing sadhana, turning inwards and calming the mind through meditation, yoga asanas, pranayama, japa, Bhakti Yoga, Jnana Yoga
- When you no longer blame others or circumstances and you take responsibility for your life and for your mistakes
- When you become forgiving
- Surrendering to the karma, and gratefully accepting your life and understanding that it is all good

- Remembering the *atman* through self-study, scriptural study or Satsang which reminds you of the true picture of yourself
- When you renounce temptations and control the mind
- When you become contented
- Seeing unity in diversity

**Bank balance:** If you spend your life increasing karmic credit, you will become wiser, more peaceful. You are actively paying your debts. When you no longer add to the debt column and only add to the credit column, you will be free of debts. Your accumulated credit can be so much that you are able to pay the debts altogether at the end of life. In this case, it is said that you are free or have attained *moksha*.

### *First example of karma: Karma of love and relationship*

Relationships and marriage karma are opportunities to learn about love—true selfless love which includes all.

A woman married early, romantically, and encountered violence in her marital relationship. Finally, she divorced, but her karma of relationships was not finished. She did not want to marry again, but a second marriage came to her, unsought, due to karma. This time the husband was very compatible and treated her well, but then he died in an accident. The first time, she walked out of the marriage, then she had a seemingly perfect marriage and the husband died. Is the karma finished? No. Why? Because the true lesson of karma is you have to find the one Self, one Love that transcends the split of Self and others. If she still thinks happiness comes from external sources, the karma is not finished. She still thinks it's the husband who gives her happiness. Having had both experiences—a violent husband and a sweet husband—she still did not realize the True Self through the relationship, therefore the karma is not over. The karma will dissolve only when she realizes that love and happiness come from the *atman*, from the Self. Then, whether she marries or not won't matter.

But, when the karma is still there, either she runs away from the husband or the husband runs away from her or toward her. All these karmic situations will only help you refine your understanding about your Self and others.

***Second example: Karma with power***

As an employee, you worked hard and were abused by the boss. You quit the job and opened your own company and treated your employees well, as you treat your own self. This is karma with power. You understand that nobody is superior to another and we are one. The other person is my own Self. Then the karma is over.

***Third example: Karma with family***

Karma with family is more difficult to recognize, because you are born into it and identify yourself with it. It is said that the soul chooses the birth family and the circumstances of life before reincarnating. To change the karma, it takes detachment from the family of origin and the adoption of a conscious family.

***Fourth example: The story of Swami Sivananda***

Swami Sivananda was considered to be a saint. He was already exceptional when he was born, and was considered very generous and loving. He was a medical doctor. He did many good things for other people, and then became a monk. People came to him to learn Yoga and Vedanta. He accepted people into the ashram and didn't ask for anything in return.

And yet one day, a man, a resident of the ashram, wanted to kill him. Because of what karma in the past we don't know, this man came with an axe and tried to hit him over the head. But Swami Sivananda did not have the karma to die at that time. He remained calm and responded to violence with detachment, forgiveness, love and understanding.

These are just some examples. Karmic situations can happen unexpectedly. You don't know what you have done in the past, but you can recognize the karma in the present and you can consciously avoid creating new karma for the future. According to the scriptures of Yoga, the best way to avoid creating new karma is to do everything as Karma Yoga; do the actions which fulfill your dharma and renounce the results of your actions. Accept whatever happens in life and do the best you can. Do your duty, but let go of the results of your actions. This means that you don't have expectations of results attached to the actions. Your ego doesn't expect it. You can go through your whole life offering everything in your life to the Divine. Do your duty, and let go of results. This is the theory and the philosophy of Karma Yoga. Approaching life this way will free you from past karma and future karma, just by having a proper attitude in the present. Karma Yoga is not only selfless service, it is resolving all the karmic debts resulting from past thoughts, desires and actions by not continuing to desire, expect, and act out of ignorance. Karma Yoga is one path of Yoga that helps you resolve the root cause of karma in this life.

### 9. GRACE AND DESTINY

Swami Sivananda taught that you need to always make self-effort in this life. Self-effort is called Purushartha. What happens in your life, what you call your destiny, is called prarabdha karma. Prarabdha means the karma of the present life, but it is only the results of self-effort in the past. Because you did self-effort in the past, you receive destiny in the present. The self-effort of today becomes the destiny of tomorrow. Self-effort and destiny are one and the same, just as the present becomes the past and the future becomes the present. In reality there is only the present. There's only self-effort. The only thing you can do is self-effort. Whatever the circumstances, you can change your destiny through your free will to act, your self-effort. This is your new angle of vision.

Swami Sivananda says in *Bliss Divine*, *"A glorious and brilliant future is awaiting you. Let the past be buried. You can work miracles, destiny is your own creation. You have created your destiny through your own thoughts and actions, so you can undo it—by right thinking and right action. You can nullify destiny. Do not just cry, karma, karma, my karma brought me like this. Whatever, just do Purushartha, do self-effort."*

We are masters of our own destiny. Remember the law of karma. Remember, if you create suffering for somebody, you create suffering for yourself. If you create happiness for somebody, you create happiness for yourself.

## *INSPIRED STORY*

**Forgetting self for others**

*Diana is a woman around 50 years old, with a 25-year history of high blood pressure. She took medicine to regulate her blood pressure for 15 years. She has difficulty keeping her balance and is easily dizzy when she suddenly changes position or when she exerts too much. She was exhausted when she came to the ashram—her blood pressure was so high that she couldn't even stand by herself.*

*As it turns out, her family's living conditions had pushed her into high-stress mode. She had been living with her husband and his family for nearly 30 years since getting married. She felt not free, frustrated, secretive, unable to be herself, and blamed her husband. Her life was always busy and revolved around caring for others in the family. However, she felt her help was not enough and felt guilty for not being able to bring happiness to family members. On the contrary, the whole family had been depressed for a few years, and the home environment was suffocating. She always felt lonely, having no support and having to cope with everything alone. As a hobby, Diana often read scriptures and taught vegetarian cooking.*

*After three days of studying at the ashram, her spirit and face were bright and cheerful. She loved the community of the ashram and understood that she had to take care of herself first, understand her own needs, respect and love herself properly—to know how to love others. Illness is an opportunity for spiritual growth, so it is necessary to practice mindful living, act slowly, think slowly, and feel right. We must understand that we can't be responsible for everyone's life, so serve and accept the results. Otherwise, we become susceptible to having high blood pressure.*

*The advice she received was to teach adaptative yoga for people with high blood pressure at the Yoga Center, and practice savasana for 15 minutes a day at work. Maintain the habit of cooking and sharing, remember to do it for fun, without stress, and attend Satsang at the Yoga Center once a week to reduce loneliness and have an active community. Now, she invites her friends and family to practice together and makes sure to have fun and stay positive.*

**Mind is ready to let go, but the body is not**

*A 25-year-old woman presented with panic attacks, which triggered the memory of childhood sexual abuse at age eight. Her parents had separated; she felt they didn't have time for her and was angry that they had left her with a questionable male figure. Now anxious and lonely, she held tension in her body—especially her hips—and cried often. She said, "My mind is so ready to let go, but my body is not." Our first yoga session together began with some simple arm movements coordinated with breath—an opportunity for proprioceptive sensing and free choice.*

*She was sitting on her heels. Inhale hands off the lap a few inches, exhale, palms back down. Other options were offered which included larger movements—arms out to the sides and back, or hands up overhead and back down. She could explore any of the options for as long as she liked. After what seemed like ten minutes of experimenting with only those movements, she finally placed her palms back on her thighs, paused thoughtfully, and declared, "I take up space!" (This was present moment awareness.)*

*We continued with a gentle class. She was uncomfortable with breath retention, so we did the simplest version of anuloma viloma. She practiced viparita karani and restorative fish to help release tension, then single-legged forward bend to help her feel safe to go inside. The final postures included a hip opener and a standing balance pose for focus and stability.*

*Over our remaining sessions, in addition to asana/movement practices, we discussed forgiveness and whether she felt safe to let go. (I encouraged her that it wouldn't matter what it looked like or sounded like.) Her recommended protocol included mantra practice to steady her mind and find the haven within, leading to self-reliance. That day, when she dared to "take up space," she took a step toward claiming her life back, making peace with the past, and shining light into a brilliant future.*

**Disease of stubbornness**

*I accepted this Yoga student, because someone asked me for advice. I knew she had brain tumors. When I did the health intake with her, I found her to be very stubborn. The message I wanted to convey was, "Because you are so stubborn, there is a problem with your brain." But I couldn't say it like that, I had to be very gentle with her as a friend.*

*Every day she asked to go to the ashram and refused to practice online. But at that time, the ashram was closed due to the ongoing Covid pandemic. I just advised her to "try hard; a little practice is fine." This lady was very sick, thin, and showing bones, yet she decided to fast for 14 days without going to treatment. I still worked hard to teach her a class for beginners.*

*I wanted to give up many times because of her stubbornness, but I continued to be patient. But then, after four sessions, she started to accept my Yoga instructions. After seven days, she practiced the whole series like other people. From her history, I realized the problem started in childhood. When she trusted me more, I asked her, "Do you think it's because you are so stubborn that you have a brain tumor?" She agreed, laughing. Then she started to listen to more philosophy and even to receive the spirit of selfless service and humility of Karma Yoga.*

P.

**QUESTIONS**

1. *What is karma? Where does it come from? Please explain.*
2. *What are the three kinds of karma?*
3. *Explain how one can turn karma into dharma.*
4. *Explain the wheel of birth and death (samsara) and how to break free of it.*

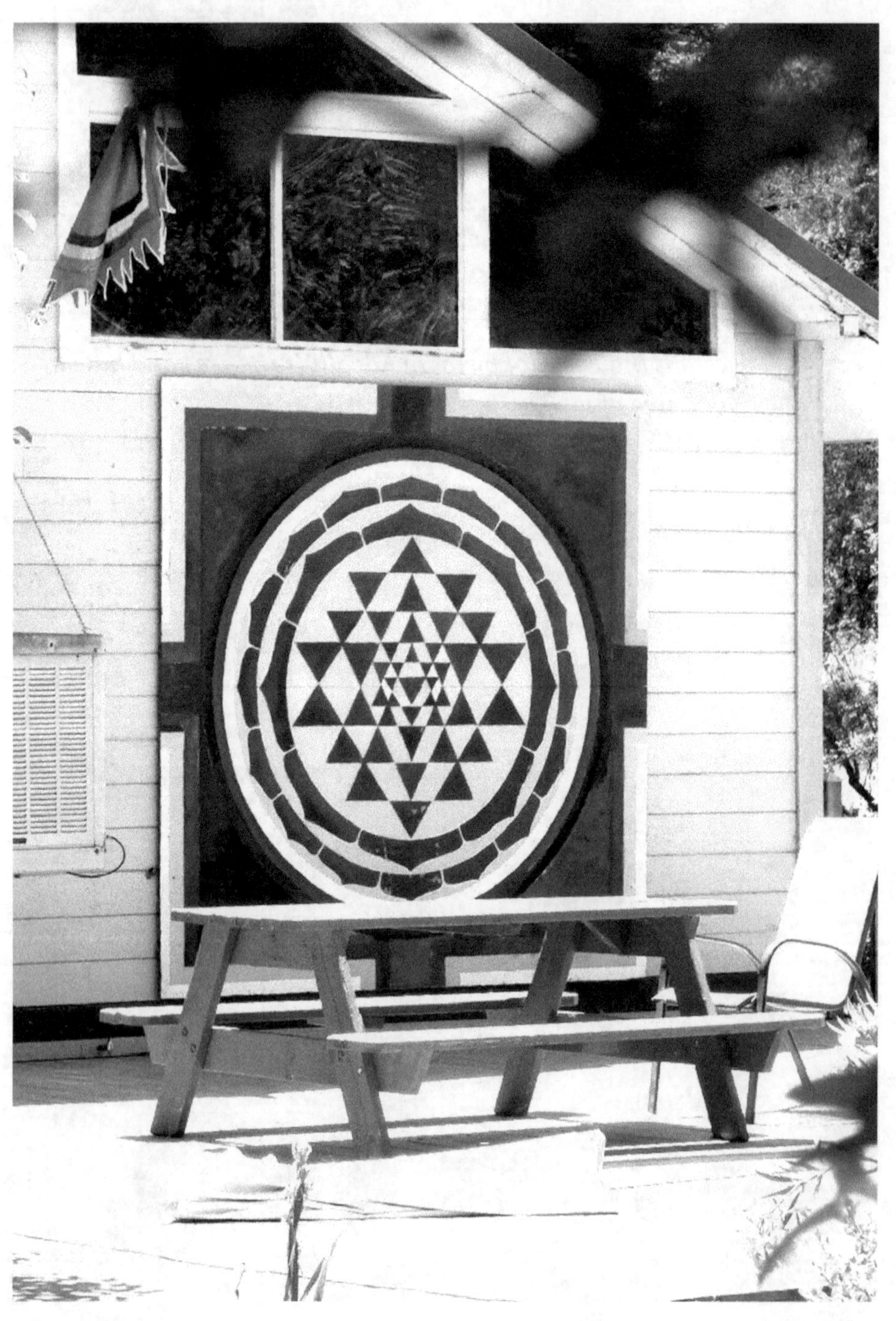

PERFECTION OF NATURE

## CHAPTER 7

# Going to the Root Causes of Suffering

***"For a man of discrimination everything gives pain. Birth is suffering. Disease is suffering. Death is suffering. Union with unpleasant objects is suffering. Separation from the beloved objects is suffering. Ungratified desires are suffering. Only he who has withdrawn himself from external objects and meditates on the Inner Self enjoys eternal Bliss."***

SWAMI SIVANANDA in *Sivananda Upanishad*

We have already talked about the idea that Self-healing, in the spiritual sense. It is a journey of returning to the Self. Self-healing and Self-realization are the same. We have also talked about holistic healing, the idea that true Self-healing encompasses the body, mind and spirit. Spiritual healing is more important, overall, when we consider our whole being and not just the physical body, which is what most people think of with respect to health. We talked about stress and its resulting strain on our minds and spirits, which can lead directly to physical ailments. And we have talked about the Yogic lifestyle and how to manage our prana. We will now examine the root causes of our suffering and clarify our approaches to alleviate suffering.

## 1. WHY DO WE NEED TO BE MORE AWARE OF THE ROOT CAUSES OF OUR SUFFERING?

**In Sanskrit, the word for suffering is *dukkha*.**

- We do not seek Self-healing unless we are suffering.
- We do not seek to change our ways if we are not suffering.

- The more we understand suffering and its cause, the more we understand the seriousness of the training, which is intended to help us escape suffering.
- Suffering can be physical, emotional, psychological or spiritual.

According to Vedantic scripture, **the first cause of disease is the disease of rebirth**. Thus. suffering includes the discomfort and pain that we experience throughout life due to birth and the resulting tribulations of living—sickness, old age and death.

**The second cause of suffering is change.** This can be an actual change in life, but in a more subtle way, it is a disconnect between the world we experience and our expectations. When we cling to impermanent situations and things, expecting them to be permanent, we know intuitively that we will be disappointed and eventually suffer as a result. Even our ideas about "who we are" are changing constantly.

**The third cause of suffering is our karma.** We exist in our specific body-mind vehicle and have to endure the fruits of our karma.

Swami Sivananda explained suffering concisely and simply when he said, *"Suffering is the gap between what you want and what you have."*

In the *Yoga Sutras,* Patanjali Maharishi, great sage and teacher of Yoga, noted that suffering begins even before this change, this disappointment of expectation. He said, *"Every action brings pain(suffering) due to the anticipation of resulting loss, new desires or conflict arising out of the interaction between the mind and the three qualities of nature, the three gunas"* [*Yoga Sutras* II:15].

As a simple example of this type of conflict, let's say a tamasic person has to live with a rajasic person. Just by the difference of their natures, there will be conflict as a result—and thus suffering.

Patanjali also said, *"The misery that has not yet manifested should be avoided"* [*Yoga Sutras* II:16].

In *Bhagavad Gita,* a scripture in Yoga, Sri Krishna said, *"Endure the pains, the pairs of opposites, from contact with the sense objects. Everything has a beginning and an end* [II:14] *...stand up and engage in the struggle with your own lower tendencies and karmic results with equanimity"* [II:38].

Also in the *Bhagavad Gita,* Krishna said, *"He who neither rejoices, nor hates, nor grieves, nor desires anything, renouncing good and evil, and who is full of devotion is dear to me"* [X:17].

## 2. THE FIVE CAUSE OF SUFFERING ACCORDING TO PATANJALI

According to Maharishi Patanjali in the *Raja Yoga Sutras*, there are five causes of suffering or *kleshas* (literally "poisons," "afflictions") [ II, 3].

The five *kleshas* are:

1. ***avidya*** - spiritual ignorance
2. ***asmita*** - egoism or I-ness, sometimes also described as *ahamkara*, the individuation or development of ego
3. ***raga*** - attachment
4. ***dvesha*** - repulsion; *raga-dvesha*, together, refer to the swinging of the mind between likes and dislikes, love and hate
5. ***abhinivesha*** - will to live or fear of death

### 1. *Avidya*

The first *klesha* is *avidya*, or spiritual ignorance. We forget our True Nature as the immortal, unchanging, pure consciousness that is the *Atman*.

Consequently, we mistake the perishable and illusory external world as being real, true and eternal (permanent). In this state of ignorance, we do not understand our True Nature as the *Atman*. We mistake our body and mind to be our True Self. We do not know the difference between that which will bring pain and that which will bring eternal bliss and immortality. This ignorance of the truth, this avidya, is said to be the root cause of all other afflictions.

If the ignorance of our True Nature is the cause of our affliction, then the cure, intuitively the opposite of ignorance, is Self-knowledge. The teaching of Vedanta is about Self-knowledge. In the context of this approach to Self- knowledge, we call it Self-healing, or Self-realization, or liberation.

What do we mean by liberation? Liberation is not like you fly up in the air, or you run away from this life and its responsibilities and go on a permanent vacation. It is liberation from our self-imposed limitations, due to our own ignorance of our True Nature. We are suffering from our negativity, from the imperfections we perceive in our own mind, activities and lives. As a result, we have lower self-confidence, lower self-esteem, we feel insecure. Why do we feel like this all the time, not knowing who we are? Vedanta says it is because we identify with the body and the mind, together known as the *upadhis* or limiting adjuncts. Our mind and our physical body are limited; they are mortal, with a beginning and an end. They are impermanent.

We have three bodies: the physical, the astral and the causal body, with five sheaths or koshas: annamaya kosha, pranamaya kosha, manomaya kosha, vijnanamaya kosha and anandamaya kosha *[see definitions in chapter 2]*. When we identify ourselves with the body and mind, we identify with our instruments, not our True Self. This false identification means we believe ourselves to be our body and our mind. Because of this, we construct our identity through our relationships with objects and others in the outside world: "I am this," "I am not that," "I have this," "I do not have that," and so on. We are the subject, but through this process, we believe ourselves to be the object. This mis-identification is the fundamental problem; forgetting our True Self is a core cause of our suffering. So correcting this misidentification with our imperfect, impermanent body and mind is the way to liberate ourselves from this suffering; it is the way to the blissfulness, the Self-healing we seek.

Once you understand that the cause of your suffering is ignorance, you need to focus a lot of energy in cultivating True Self-knowledge by practicing Self-remembrance, which is the path to *moksha* or liberation. So, if Self-knowledge is the answer, you must remember that nobody outside can help you. The teacher and the teachings can only remind you of your True Nature, they cannot liberate you. The teacher and teachings can guide Self-reflection and Self-remembrance, but you will have to do the work. You will have to recognize, through this contemplation and reflection on your True Self, that the Truth is within you, not outside.

When we are unhappy, we usually try to make a change in our lives, in the world, to make ourselves happy. We change our job, we go somewhere else, eat new kinds of food, seek new kinds of excitement. But the teachings tell us that no amount of external action like this will ever make us happy, because the fundamental mistake is the ignorance of our True Nature. Yes, we can ease our pain a little bit through sensual pleasures, entertain the intellect and satisfy our desires, but all of these are impermanent and temporary and will not last. So, we become unhappy, again.

This is why the teachings say that the only proper solution, if we truly understand the real problem, is to replace *avidya*, spiritual ignorance, with vidya, or true knowledge. There is no other solution. We must move from the darkness of ignorance into the light of Self-knowledge.

So, if we feel limited in this life or feel that this life is not what we expected it to be, we need to understand that this feeling is the result of our false beliefs, our *avidya* about our True Nature. It is only this *avidya* that creates the sense of bondage to suffering. To know our True Self, we must seek within. If we try to use our senses, we will see only our external body and the objects it can interact with. The body is not our True Self. It changes all the time and yet the Self remains the same. We cannot use the mind and intellect to know the True Self. Scientists have developed fantastic models of anatomy, physiology, psychology, but these, too, are imperfect—being only models of the impermanent and ever-changing world. They provide no knowledge about the True Self. There are no modern sciences that sincerely focus on knowing the True Self. But the Yogis and the teachings of Vedanta, existing from ancient times, offer a developed science of Self, a science to guide you to realize your True Self.

Currently, most of us do not understand our True Self, which is within. Only we can uncover it. As an analogy, when the sun is covered by clouds and the day feels dark and gray, less vibrant than usual, it is not that the sun has changed or gone anywhere. The sun is still shining brightly behind the veil of clouds. In the same manner, our True Self is always there shining within us, vibrant and full of light, purity and bliss. But our understanding is incorrect, something in our understanding is veiling our True Self so we can't see it. We merely need to remove the veil of clouded thinking that is our mistaken belief, our avidya. When we remove this veil, we will find pure consciousness, pure bliss. Consciousness is light itself; it is all-knowledge and all-pervading. That consciousness is our own Self; that consciousness is our True Self.

### 2. *Asmita*

The second *klesha*, *asmita* is a powerful cause of suffering and is born directly from the first *klesha*, *avidya*. We have forgotten the nature of our True Self. It is easy to see how ego arises. If we do not know our True Self, we will look outwardly, using our mind to position ourself relative to other things in the world. Patanjali describes the cause of asmita very simply and concisely. He says, *"Egoism is the identification of the seer with the instrument of seeing."* The ego and the intellect are only the tools which we use to know the world, but we believe their claim to be the Self.

In Vedanta, when describing the mind, egoism is referred to as *ahamkara*. *Ahamkara* is this process of identifying ourselves with the body and mind, in opposition to everything else in the world. It is essentially the development of 'I-ness,' that egoism which is connected to the intellect.

Swami Sivananda uses different words to describe the same idea. He says, *"The ego is the self-arrogating principle of the mind."* So the ego is self-asserting, self-claiming itself to be the center of the universe, insisting that it is separate and limited. It attaches to its own ideas, desires, actions, and creates pain as a result.

*Asmita* is a source of much of our suffering. It is an illusion, a mistaken identification. Due to egoism, we have anxiety, pride, selfishness, arrogance, conceit, and lust, anger, delusion, greed and jealousy. Egoism is also the root of our swinging between our likes and dislikes. The ego is attached to the idea of itself. It doesn't like criticism, but loves praise. We are a constant slave to this ego, trying to make our ego better, trying to celebrate the falsely-identified self. It thus removes our sense of peace, leaving us constantly longing for more support, more pleasure. It always compares itself with others, always wanting to be as good as, or even better than, others. This is called self-aggrandizement, the idea that I'm big, I'm important—but I need to be even bigger and more important. It is endless.

This ego, this "I", is very habitual. Sanskrit for "I" is *aham*, the root of the term *ahamkara* used above, so *aham* is very habitual. We find it impossible to get rid of. Whether it brings joy or pain, it is always there. People have a sense of love and hate for themselves constantly. Sometimes, if this hate grows too large, they cannot deal with it and become suicidal, thinking that getting rid of the body-mind is the best way to get rid of the ego, the 'I'. But according to the teachings of Vedanta, this is a mistake; the only way to get rid of the ego is to thin it out and start seeing the *Atman* as the real "I." Thinning it out means gradually removing the attachments and the identifications the ego has made, making the ego less important and thus reducing the self-arrogating habit, lessening the ego's grasp.

The Yogic way is the journey of transformation of the tamasic ego to rajasic ego, to sattvic ego.

- The tamasic ego hates itself, hates other people, and is completely in darkness. By entertaining positive thoughts of ourself and by positive thinking in general, we can thin out the tamasic ego.
- The rajasic ego is thinking that we are different and better than others; it is very proud, has a lot of vanity. It is vain about wealth, thinking I need to have lots of money and a bigger house than anyone else. It is vain about beauty and the body thinking, *"My nose is better than yours, or I'm stronger than you."* Even if you have virtues, the rajasic ego comes up with competitive thinking, for example, *"I am more generous than you are. I am a nicer, more loving person. I really am such a good person. The world should praise me, if they only saw how good I am."* This is the rajasic ego.
- The sattvic ego becomes thinner and wiser as you purify, thinking less about itself, less about attachments and vanity.

  There are Yogic methods to purify and thin out the ego, reduce the egoism and the identification with the delusions about the Self. Of course, a subtler egoism is more difficult to eradicate than the grosser ego, so the challenge will grow as we progress. For example, the grosser ego would say, *"I am my beautiful body,"* while the subtler egoism says, *"I am a good person, I am a good Karma Yogi, I am a meditator, look how hard I work to be a good Yogi."*

Bhakti Yoga thins the ego through devotion. Karma Yoga helps thin the ego through selfless service and self-denial. Our body and mind literally become a tool of service, thus removing any identification with the results of our actions, and any sense of doer-ship or separate "I". This helps to thin out the habit of self-arrogation. We can also do this through self-denial. Jnana Yoga uses contemplation and self-study, slowly removing all that is not the Self. It thins out the ego by saying, "I am not this body, I am not this mind, I am not these senses." Instead, we identify with the *Atman*, the Supreme Self, concentrating on, "I am the all-pervading Self, I am the *Atman*," and take refuge in our own True Self. These are a few examples of simple methods from the four paths of Yoga that help to thin out our ego.

Thus, *avidya* and *asmista* are the first two causes of suffering: one, not knowing who we truly are, and two, believing that we are something that we are not.

### 3. Raga / 4. Dwesha

The third and fourth *kleshas, raga and dvesha*, are taken together as a pair. "*Raga*" refers to attachments or the tendency of the mind to gravitate towards things it likes. "*Dvesha*" indicates repulsions or the mind's tendency to move away from its dislikes. We use the analogy of a pendulum in a grandfather clock to illustrate the mind's tendency to swing back and forth between likes and dislikes. When the swing becomes stronger, the pair of opposites becomes stronger. The likes and dislikes become extreme. Love will swing to hate. Sometimes we get what we want, but this attraction helps shape the repulsion, and we will meet with something that we dislike. Life is back and forth between what we like, that which excites us, and what we dislike, that which makes us unhappy. Life is a roller coaster, up and down—with a mind swinging back and forth between extremes. Therefore, Yoga encourages us to cultivate equanimity and calmness of mind.

Patanjali says about *raga*, "*Attraction is that which dwells on pleasure.*" [II, 7]. That is why you keep going there. If you eat ice cream and you like it, you want it again. This is the way your mind works. The idea of ice cream becomes a very deep groove in the mind. Having continually repeated the desire and satisfaction of the desire, we become trapped in it.

Patanjali says about *dvesha*, "*Aversion is that which attempts to avoid pain*" [Sutra II:8]. So aversion, or dislikes, includes things that cause discomfort or pain. *Dvesha* is fertile ground for development of fears. Attraction brings pain eventually—or even immediately, if you cannot have what you are attracted to—and aversion also brings pain. In the end, they are the same, both bring pain. Attraction is running towards something and aversion is running away from something. Both, what you are attracted to and what repels you come from the unique makeup of your mind. What you like and what I like and what you dislike and what I dislike are not the same. *Raga* and *dvesha* come from the intrinsic nature of the mind. They are the illusions of our own ego. Whether we get what we want or not, both will result in unhappiness. We have these illusions of the mind, we are lost in the ocean of samsara, lost in the waves of likes and dislikes. The question is, what to do?

**Five kinds of attachment**

Attraction brings about attachment. We would not be born in this life if we didn't have any attachment. We all have attachments.

- The first attachment is the attachment to our emotions, to our passions. We are afraid to let go of our emotional excitement and emotional fulfillment. We are very attached to these feelings. If it gives a sense of pleasure, we become attached to it. We need to learn to calm these emotions; reduce the excitement caused by them, reduce the sense of pleasure they bring us. This goes for both *raga* and *dvesha*. Don't allow yourself to get too attached either to your likes or your dislikes.

  When attachment grows, we spend a lot of time thinking about it, dreaming about it, talking about it, fantasizing about one day having it. We know if we fall into attachment, the mind is deluded and then we lose ourselves. All of us, at some time, do the wrong thing and suffer out of attachment, because we think that if we satisfy the desire, if we get what we want, it will bring happiness, it will last forever. But it's never like that. This idea is an illusion which ultimately leads to unhappiness.

- The second kind of attachment is attachment to action, attachment to work, attachment to what we do, as it flatters the ego. We are very attached to the things that we do and we like to be perfect. We think, *"If I am perfect in this, then I am a better me."* From this attachment to what we do, to who we think we are, to our ego, we also have a sense of accomplishment and praise. Action and accomplishment give us some sense of satisfaction, but this will not last long. When people come and change or destroy our work or criticize us for the way we did it, or say it could be better, we become unhappy. Our ego is insulted. This is why the teachings of Yoga say to be detached from our actions. We have a certain skill, a certain temperament and certain desire to do things in this world. However, offer the result of your actions. Try not to be attached. Otherwise, you will be disappointed. Detachment towards our actions and the result of actions is called Karma

Yoga. If we can feel that we are not the doer, and if we can manage that the action is not a reflection of our ego, then we can move toward detachment. Best is to forget the ego entirely and think, "I am only the instrument." But if we cannot let go of our identification as the doer, then at least detach from the result in order to avoid suffering.

- The third kind of attachment is attachment to things and situations, thinking they will last forever.

  For example, we have a house, or a car, or a relationship, or any object, and we think it will last. But we know that nothing is permanent. When things change, we are unhappy. Nothing ever stays the same—house, car, body, friendship, career—everything will change in time. Buddhist teachings talk about the truth of impermanence, contemplating on how everything changes. If we attach ourselves to anything, we know, in time, we will suffer. We may even suffer immediately if we recognize that thought. We might get attached to something that we love right now. However, it is going to change. It is impermanent. This is the partial meaning of the saying that you need to live in the present and not get attached to memories of the past or to projections of the future. Live in the present and be free from this cause of suffering.

- The fourth kind of attachment is attachment to the objects of our senses.

Here is a story to illustrate this attachment that comes from the senses.

> *There was a woman who was mending clothing with a needle and thread in her house. At some point, she dropped her needle. Her house had no electricity. She went outside and began to look for her needle desperately. Eventually, her neighbor asked, "Can we help you?" She replied, "I lost my needle so I am looking for it." The neighbor asked, "Where did you drop your needle?" She replied that she lost it inside the house while she was sewing. Confused, the neighbor asked, "Why are you looking for the needle outside, if you lost it in the house?" She replied, "It is too dark inside, outside there is light!"*

This is a metaphor for our life. We lose our True Self inside, we lose our happiness, but then we turn outward in the world of the senses to search for it. It is all an illusion.

The practices of Yoga are designed to help us turn away from the external sensual world and turn inward, the place where we will find lasting peace and joy. The pranayama practice, for example, will help to purify the nadis. Nadis are the astral nerves that affect the mind. The practice helps us calm the mind and the emotions and turn inward. The answers lie within. When we become anxious, for example, we need to sit down and turn inward. If we can truly turn inward, turn off the world, turn off the senses, turn off the source of anxiety, then we will feel fine. We will see that all is okay, it was the pull outward that caused us to become unsettled. We need to look for peace within. The five points of Yoga are there to help us to do this. They help us detach from the external world and from the senses and to feel that we are completely fulfilled from within. Eventually we might come to feel that we do not need anything. The idea that seeking outwardly can help is an illusion, a mirage of the mind, concocted from the fleeting glimpses of pleasure found while looking outward.

Here's another story to illustrate this point:

> *A man was walking in the desert, thirsty and hot and finally found some shade, a location of respite and peace. As he stood under the tree and looked out into the desert, he saw that maybe 15 minutes away it appeared there was some water. He was very thirsty, because he had walked so far in the hot sun to find this shade, this oasis of peace. He valued the shade, but the temptation to find water only 15 minutes away made him leave the shade. However, 15 minutes later, the water still appeared 15 minutes away and the shade now was 15 minutes back. He decided to go 15 minutes further and the shade became 30 minutes back. Thus the illusion and the mirage continues: 15 minutes to find water and now 45 minutes to return to shade. He ran towards the water and lost his shade, exhausted himself and collapsed. The water is still just 15 minutes away. If he had stayed in the shade and dug under the tree, he would have found water.*

This story illustrates the pattern of our mind continuously pursuing the external happiness, continuously convincing ourselves and making efforts in the wrong direction. We have difficulty detaching and renouncing the sensual allurements and the promises of our mind. We have difficulty staying still, looking within and finding that peace and happiness that is only found within.

- The fifth kind of attachment is attachment in relationships. This is a very big, very deep and subtle topic, because throughout life, we are in all types of relationships. We become very attached to our relationships: to our parents, and then our family, and friends and even more deeply to someone we love, our partner, our children. So the teachings of Yoga and Vedanta say, "There is no other." What does this mean? It means that everyone is, in reality, your own Self. There is no other, so find your Self.Do not expect to find true happiness in the company of others. When you have relationships, often there can be a problem of attachment and repulsion. You "fall in love" and you "fall out of love." You are too attached, or there is uneven attachment from the partner, etc., thus you are met with disappointment and resentment. Best is to see your own True Self in others and stop trying to find your own ego-self in others. Stop trying to complete your egoistic self through relationships. Instead, see the underlying consciousness of your own Self present in others. That's what the saying, "There is no other" means. In fact, there is only your own Self appearing in front of you. So focus on seeing your own True Self and turn inward.

Realize that attractions and aversions (*raga/dvesha*) come from spiritual ignorance. For Self-healing, we must confront that root cause.

Our attachments, our likes and dislikes, what our mind thinks will make us feel fulfilled, are constantly changing form. We attach, then we detach and attach to something else, and so the pattern continues. But what is driving these attachments and detachments is the changing ideas that the ego and mind present to you. It is an illusion of our mind and it is born of ignorance or incorrect understanding. We are attached to ice cream, but one day we don't like it as much, so we detach and then attach to milk tea or something else. The ice cream is still the same and the milk tea is still the same. The only thing that has changed is the mind. Our mind projects different ideas, therefore the objects are impermanent, unreal, temporary illusions of the mind. Our mind is constantly seeking happiness and peace, but it is running after its own delusions; it is looking in the wrong direction.

We might grow detached from this husband, but then get attached to a new husband and so on, based on the new sense of our ego-self. When discrimination is lacking, the delusion will continue, and we fall again in the trap of likes and dislikes, of happiness and unhappiness in relationships. When the discriminative intelligence awakens and we develop the intuitive capacity to know the difference between the Self and the non-self, the real and the unreal, we will free ourselves from suffering, as we gain more and more control over our own mind and see through the patterns and repeated illusions it has created.

A story of being lost in attachments:

> *A tiger was walking in the forest and came to a place where some leaves had just fallen. They still had sap on them, so they stuck to the tiger's feet. When he realized the leaves were stuck to his feet, he sat down to remove them. But then the leaves stuck to his butt. So he laid down on his back to remove the leaves from his butt, but then the leaves were stuck all over his back. When he rolled to his side to remove the leaves from his back, he realized that the leaves were stuck all over his body.*

This story shows that our lives are full of attachments, wherever we turn. We cannot free ourselves from attachment by attaching to something else. We must use our discrimination to see the root cause, which is forgetfulness of our True Self. Only when we remember our True Self, will we find true happiness, which is not from any attachment in this world. It is very difficult to detach and see our True Nature as *Satchidananda* (existence, knowledge and bliss absolute) and develop contentment in this life.

**Four ways and methods of detachment**

Detachment is the way to be free from *raga/dvesha*, the swinging pendulum of the mind. It is the way to find peace of mind. There are different approaches to detachment, depending on the Yoga path you practice.

- **Detachment in Karma Yoga:** Do selfless service, offering your efforts and the results of your efforts unconditionally. Detach from doership.
- **Detachment in Bhakti Yoga:** Convert emotions to devotion and attach them to the Divine, to the Truth within. Practice humility, and surrender to a higher power. Devote yourself completely to it. In this way, you detach yourself from your emotional identification.
- **Detachment in meditation (Raja Yoga):** In meditation, we detach from our thoughts, sensual impressions, and distractions. As thoughts and distractions arise, we continue to concentrate on a higher ideal. We concentrate on our mantra, detaching from everything else. When we detach from the thoughts in meditation, there will be an uninterrupted flow of pure consciousness. When we are completely detached from the thoughts, then we experience the bliss of the Self. In the beginning of the meditation practice, concentrate the mind on your breath and the universal, sacred sound OM. Continue to bring the mind back towards your chosen sacred

and uplifting object of concentration. When meditating, detach from the past and future.

- **Detachment in Jnana Yoga:** Detach from the unreal and the impermanent with Jnana Yoga. The unreal means anything that is changing. Attach to the eternal Truth and detach from the unreal phenomena. To do this, we must ponder what is impermanent and what is permanent. Ask the question, "*Who am I?*" and reject the identification with something that is not permanent. This is the practice of neti neti, "*Not this, not that.*" In this practice, we detach from the not-self. We detach from our desires, we detach from any sense of lack, or our feeling of incompleteness. We detach from memories of our past losses. We detach from the body, which we eventually will lose in death. Nothing really belongs to us, even our bodies will not last forever.

Detachment is the way out of this ocean of samsara. Samsara is the never-ending wheel of life, the wheel of birth and death. The ultimate detachment is freedom from the cycle of reincarnation and from karma.

### 5. Fear of death or abhinivesha

The fifth cause of suffering in Patanjali's list of five *kleshas* is called *abhinivesha* in Sanskrit, literally meaning 'the will to live.' It refers to our attachment to life and fear of death, they are actually one and the same. Swami Vishnudevanandaji often asked the question, "*What is the difference between today and yesterday?*" Do you have an answer to this question? Swamiji's answer for a non-yogi was that today you are one day closer to death, because the body will not last forever. But for a person who practices Yoga and Vedanta, then each day of practice brings you one day closer to the total detachment towards body and mind, one day closer to immortality.

The fear of death is present in our lives and attachment to the body causes us to suffer. It is constant, reinforced by the instinct of preservation and survival. We need to face death and understand it for what it is. Swami Sivananda said it is most important that you understand death in order to understand life, as life and death are two sides of the same coin. They are not separate experiences, they are aspects of the same experience.

Swami Vishnudevanandaji said, "*Death is, in reality, not what you imagine it to be; this is not a scary end of life, because after death, the astral body and the causal body continue to exist.*" The astral body includes the ego, the mind, the memories, everything continues to exist. It is just the physical body which returns to the five elements of nature—earth, water, fire, air and ether. Death is this decomposition of matter our physical body is an aggregate of the five physical elements. Our body is a temporary vehicle in which we learn our lessons in life. When we finish our lessons the body dies and returns to nature. If we have karma remaining and lessons to learn, the soul will be reincarnated in a different body. While living this life, it is important that we do our duty, experience the karma, and learn the karmic lessons as well as possible. When the karma is over for this life, the body will die one way or another and the soul will continue its journey.

Swamiji also said, "*The bondage of the soul is death.*" It is a different definition of death and life. If we live in the body, but we don't know ourselves, life is a misery. But if we realize our True Self which is eternal, it is conquest of death, i.e. realization of our immortality.

Another way to free ourselves from suffering is to have a bigger picture of our life. We live more than just this life; this life is one small phase. Due to the continuous chain of karma, this life is like one chapter of the book of our existence. Reincarnation gives us opportunities to purify ourselves. Therefore, do not be afraid of death—and also do not run away from life. Rather, focus on living well. Detach from the body and learn from your experience, work out the karma, and realize that you are the immortal *Atman*.

We are attached to life or we fear death—either way, we do not understand the true picture. Life is precious. Your life in this human body is the first precious gift you received. Why is it so precious to be born as a human? Because, in the human body, we are equipped with intelligence and self-awareness. We are not born as a cat, a pig, or a bird. We are born as a human, equipped with awareness and the capacity to know the Self. See that this life is a precious gift, feel blessed. Be grateful for what you have. When life feels overwhelming and depression lurks, remember that the pain you feel is a reflection from this sensitive tool we have been born into. It is an opportunity to care for your body and mind so that you can continue to use them well.

The second gift is when we have the desire to know the Truth. All sincere readers of this book are blessed with this second gift.

The third precious gift is that, having the first two, we encounter a teacher who can guide us in ways of Yoga and Vedanta, who can guide us to find the Truth within.

## 3. QUALIFICATIONS AND PREPARATIONS FOR SELF- KNOWLEDGE

The *Yoga Vasishta* describes four qualifications necessary to follow the path of Self-knowledge. Development of these qualifications prepares the aspirant to avoid the errors and distractions we face in our sadhana.

1. **Equip yourself with *viveka*,** or discrimination; we have to learn how to see and think correctly. Our intelligence is not given to make us more materially wealthy or to make us more physically beautiful. Intelligence is to be used for Self-Knowledge. Intelligence and discrimination should be applied to uncovering our misunderstandings, and to see the difference between what is true and not true; what is permanent and impermanent, what is our True Self and what is not the Self. This is what is called *viveka* or discriminative intelligence.
2. **The second qualification is called *vairagya*,** which refers to dispassion or the faculty of detachment—detachment from the unreal or from what by nature is changing and is not true. Simply, if you know something is unreal, that it is going to change, then you must detach from it, otherwise you will experience suffering. Don't identify yourself with whatever it is. All is changing—be it an object, a person, an emotion, or our own ego. Therefore, cease to believe that it will give you the permanent happiness you seek.
3. ***Satsampat*** gives six virtues of the mind to cultivate. Vedantic scriptures outline these six qualities to consciously develop to make our mind stronger and fit to realize the Truth.

    i. ***Sama*** is serenity, calmness and tranquility. It is the ability to maintain a state of equanimity. If our emotions are always up and down, happy and angry, upset, hateful, full of emotion, crying, etc., then we are not ready. A mind like this will not reveal the True Self, who you truly are. The mind is like a mirror, and all these emotions are like dust on its surface, it will never reflect the Truth. The mind needs to be clean and stable. Then, we can see the inner beauty that is the True Self. The mind is not the Self. Actively try to make the mind sattvic. Heal yourself. Cleanse the past impressions and impurities. Release expectations of the world being the way you want and getting upset and angry if it is not. A mind like this can never reveal the Truth. Instead, it will reflect a distorted vision of the Self. Keeping the mind calm will make the mind ready for liberation from suffering.

    ii. ***Dama*** is control of the senses. As part of cleansing the mind, and returning to the source of Consciousness, as part of the process of Self-healing, we need to have control over the senses, which are outgoing by nature. The senses work with the mind in tandem, they show us the changing illusory world (the *maya*). As the practitioner develops discrimination between the real and unreal, they see that the senses will only lead the mind externally to the world of names and forms, the illusory world of objects. To have control of the senses means to be successful in turning the mind inward so that the practitioner can inquire more deeply into their True Nature, instead of constantly being led astray by sensual promises of external happiness.

iii. ***Uparati*** is satiation, meaning having enough of external pleasures. On acquiring *uparati*, the mind is ready to turn inward, away from the allurements of the senses. This state of mind is closely related to the idea of controlling the senses. With *viveka* (discrimination), the practitioner sees that the Truth is not in the outside world, not in this body or this mind, so they resolutely turn inward to see the Truth. All practices of Yoga are designed to help you turn inward.

iv. ***Titiksha*** is endurance. As the practitioner turns inward, there are several more qualities to develop. The mind needs to be strong, able to endure, able to persist in long-term spiritual practice. Yogic practices and the meditative path are not easy and quick. Patience is needed. Patience is dependent on endurance, or the strength of mind, to keep the practice going. Also, endurance means to undergo the results of past karma, to accept all the contradictions in the mind—the conflicts and challenges in life—as they are part of our journey of purification.

v. ***Shraddha*** is faith. Faith is a necessary preparation for Self-knowledge. Have faith in yourself. Have faith that you are heading in the right direction. Have faith and patience to keep following the path. The practitioner needs to stay focused on the goal. It is a long journey, so many things happen in life. Keep your focus and avoid distractions, which only draw the attention outward and back to the ups and downs, the tribulations of life. Secondly, have faith in the teachings and the teacher and the Truth they are trying to convey. The faith needed is not blind faith, but is based on direct experience of the benefits of the practices added on to an inner knowledge that doesn't need to have proof. Until direct knowledge comes, we have to have faith to walk the path of the unknown.

vi. ***Samadana*** means balance with attention. This is the culmination of the previous qualities, when the mind no longer gets distracted or lost and no longer loses balance and is always focused on the goal.

4. ***Mumukshutva*** is desire for liberation. In order to realize the Truth, we need to have a desire for it. The stronger the desire to know, the sooner we will know.

*Mumukshutva* can be mild, medium or intense. Remember the past sufferings, exercise discrimination and self-inquiry. Continue to seek wisdom and knowledge that will free you from suffering. Continue to seek the Truth, even though you might feel alienated from your peers and your social environment. Continue to seek the knowledge of the scriptures. Swami Sivananda says, *"A brilliant future is awaiting you!"*

The desire for liberation (*moksha*) is unique to the individual seeker and cannot be comprehended by other people, so stay firm in your efforts in sadhana. Remember, "If you are thirsty, you need to drink for yourself, no one can drink for you." Sadhana needs to be kept up steadily with forbearance, against temptations to settle down, to be complacent and to stop the practice.

In order to find the Self, according to the teaching of Vedanta, there are three actions we need to do:

- The first is called ***sravanam,*** or hearing the teachings. It connotes listening to the teachings with the heart. We must expose ourselves to the knowledge that comes from the scriptures and the guru, as a way to remember who we are. We can actively attend Satsangs or take wisdom courses or read books and writings of the wise, and thus regularly and steadily stay exposed to knowledge. We must create many opportunities to expose ourselves to the knowledge of the teachings, so our doubts can be removed.
- The second action we need to practice is called ***mananam,*** or reflection. We need to reflect on the teachings so we can understand our current wrong ideas and replace them with correct understanding, true knowledge, and a correct understanding of who we are. For example, a seeker may have wrong ideas such as: "People don't love me, because I'm not pretty," or "People don't respect me, because I am not powerful or rich." They may visit a beauty parlor in an effort to look more attractive, or seek out a new job to gain more wealth or start pushing their will on the world to become more powerful. But in the end, the person will still feel the same.Love and respect cannot be acquired externally. In reality, the problem lies in the false internal belief, internal wrong-thinking about the Self. With true knowledge and wisdom,

we will understand that beauty is our True Nature, and that our True Self is powerful. There is nothing we can do to make people love us. Instead, we understand that love is our True Nature and we start to love our own Self. In summary, when we apply the teaching, the second step is to contemplate, so we can recognize our mistaken understanding.

- The third action, ***nididhyasana,*** is closely related to the second. It is deep meditation or long deep contemplation about the Truth and our True Nature. After reflecting on the teachings and understanding that there are wrong notions and wrong beliefs, the third step is Self-realization or experience of the Truth of our own Self. The Vedantic scriptures prescribe contemplating deeply and unceasingly on the thought, "I am Brahman, I am pure consciousness." After some time, realization will dawn. If the practitioner just sits there and says the words, the words will just be words, thought waves in the mind. The practitioner must purify themselves in order to experience it directly. Much preparation and purification are needed in order to truly and directly realize the *Satchidananda Atman* nature.

**Qualification of a spiritual aspirant**

*On my spiritual journey, I was introduced to four qualifications for the attainment of Brahman and why being devoted to the search for Truth means progressing on the right path in life. I was tackling a problem in my marriage with a lower mind driven by emotion and instincts, based on preconceived ideas about a perfect relationship. As much as I had faith in God, I did not surrender completely or turn my thinking around to understand that the cause of my problem was not in others, but in myself. When I hit rock bottom, I realized that I had been addressing the problem in the same manner over and over again.*

*Resenting the marital relationship hurt my health. I was unable to come to terms with my ignorance, until my deteriorating health led to surgery. After a moment of awakening post-surgery, I began to contemplate differently on my pain and sufferings over the last sixteen years. There must be a reason for the positive things happening in my life; I received the right help at the right time, even though the situation at home was not amicable. Through the Sivananda Yoga Teacher Training Course, my spiritual journey towards Vedanta took off. By improving my discrimination skills, I was able to identify the reality, understand that the self in me is the self in all, and cease to identify with my projected idea of a perfect relationship.*

*During situations of overwhelm or driven by desires, I learned to take a step back and evaluate whether I was doing the action with love and devotion and a sense of non-doership. I treated household chores as Karma Yoga. This resulted in my letting go of the sense of attachment to material things; I was able to make a conscious choice between the needs and wants in my life.*

*I slowly cultivated the necessary virtues cited in the scriptures (Satsampat or six virtues).*

*I kept my mind calm by doing mantra Japa meditation. I no longer scratch every itch.*

*I practice pranayama regularly and turn inwards more. Building this into a daily routine helped me immensely. I started responding to people and situations by listening and compassion, rather than reaction. Now when a disturbance occurs, I turn inward to see the message that the experience is giving me. What lesson is it teaching me? What opportunity do I have to learn and grow?*

*I learned titiksha, or endurance, and bearing people's questioning of my sadhana and my choices. I am able to resist my habits and choose detachment vs attachment. I learned to bear the differences of opinions and life goals between my partner and I. My faith increased with my daily routine, not just with asana, pranayama, and meditation, but also with such devotional activities as puja and chanting slokas/mantras in a disciplined manner with utmost devotion.*

*The practice of Hatha Yoga helped me turn inward and stay stable. I developed the acumen to zoom out of a situation and understand the perspectives while dealing with the pairs of opposites.*

*I desire earnestly to rediscover myself by dispelling my ignorance through this spiritual journey with the spiritual support system I found to reach the goal of life, which is realizing Brahman.*

---

**QUESTIONS**

1. *Name the five kleshas. Write 2-3 lines to describe each.*
2. *Name the 4 Qualifications of the spiritual aspirant.*
3. *Give one example of your practice of viveka and one example of vairagya from your life.*

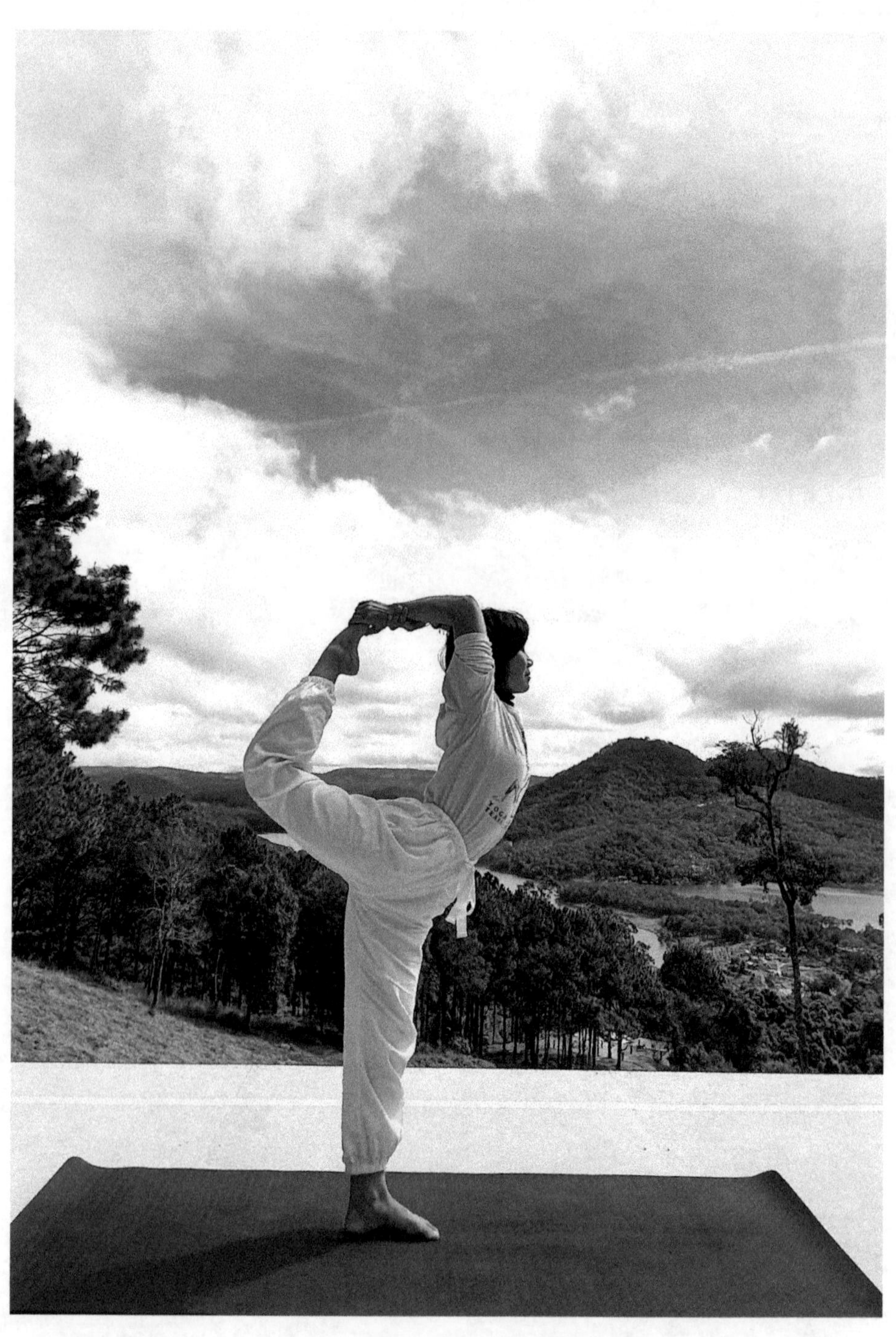

ASANA WITH THE MOUNTAIN VIEW

## CHAPTER 8

# Sadhana: Conscious Training

***"In the beginning of your Sadhana, you will encounter various difficulties. You will not be conscious of any spiritual progress, but you will be conscious of your failures in your attempts in meditation, the resistance you meet, your defects and weaknesses."***

– SWAMI SIVANANDA in *Sivananda Upanishad*

### 1. WHAT IS SADHANA?

In the last chapter, we talked about suffering and the causes of suffering according to Patanjali. Now we will talk about conscious training, or sadhana, to free ourselves from suffering and to maintain spiritual health.

Patanjali Maharishi said, *"Heyam dukham anagatam,"* the misery that has not yet manifested should be avoided [*Raja Yoga Sutras* II:16].

The tendency of the mind is to look for happiness outside. According to Yogic teaching, the world is illusory and will only bring you suffering. Not knowing who you are is a mistake in your thinking and will bring you suffering. Suffering that is yet to come is to be avoided. To do this, we consciously train ourselves in Yoga practices to change the habitual patterns of our mind and learn to make conscious choices.

The collective practices of Yoga, the spiritual practices that foster spiritual health are called sadhana. Yoga practice is not like medicine—you take it for a short time and then you are healthy. The moment you stop your Yoga practice, you will fall back into familiar illusions, wrong thinking and old habits. The practice needs to be constant, constant, constant, in order to stay healthy. This practice is called sadhana.

When you do sadhana correctly, you achieve spiritual health by getting in touch with your Self. When you are spiritually healthy, you will also have mental and physical health. The shift between positive health and ill-health, spiritually speaking, is very rapid; it can change in a moment. You are healthy because you have the right conception of yourself. But you can become sick and unhealthy in a moment, because of one wrong thought and you fall back into your old habits.

Spiritual health is attained by constant sadhana. Until you establish yourself firmly in this new way of thinking, feeling, and behaving, in this new way of seeing yourself, you will need to practice regularly and continuously.

Swami Sivananda said that sadhana is a spiritual movement, consciously systematized. Sadhana is the purpose for which we have come to the earth plane. The reason you were born into this physical body and this mind is to practice sadhana. Spiritual movement is a very slow evolution forward. In fifteen years, or maybe even one lifetime, you will learn one or two lessons and you will make a lot of mistakes and create a lot of karma—to resolve at a later time.

Sadhana is a conscious practice; you know you need to maintain your positive outlook. You know what suffering is and where it comes from; you don't have to wait for more suffering to appear to convince you. You are intelligent and you know if you continue following the old patterns, you will again find suffering. Now, you consciously choose to move forward, to practice Yoga in a systematic manner, repeating the winning formula over and over again. Yoga is a system of spiritual practices designed for you to find liberation from suffering. Concentration and commitment are needed in this journey.

### 2. THE EIGHT LIMBS OF YOGA

Patanjali's main teachings are, in a nutshell, "*Yoga chitta, vritti nirodhah,*" which translates to "*Yoga is restraining the activities of the mind*" [chap 1–2]. The eight limbs of Yoga (Ashtanga Yoga) outline the necessary steps to control the mind. When the thought waves are stilled, the perceiver rests in his own True Nature" [chap 1–3].

The eight limbs are like steps on a ladder, to climb up gradually from one to eight, one step at a time, evolving from one to the next. They also can be considered like the wings of a Chinese fan with branches touching, to be practiced together, one merging into the other.

The eight limbs are:

8. **Samadhi** - superconscious state (ref. the *Atman*, see chapter 17)

7. **Dhyana** - meditation (see chapter 16)

6. **Dharana** - concentration (see chapter 8)
5. **Pratyahara** - withdrawal of the senses (see chapter 13 )
4. **Pranayama** - control of prana (see chapter 5)
3. **Asana** - steady pose (see chapter 4)
2. **Niyamas** - observances (see chapter 8)
1. **Yamas** - restraints (see chapter 8)

## 3. THE KEYSTONE PRACTICE OF CONCENTRATION

**What is Concentration ?**

It is being able to hold one thought in the mind for a period of time. It is reducing the number of thoughts in the mind. "*More thoughts, less peace. Less thoughts, more peace,*" according to Swami Vishnudevananda.

Concentration is the mental process of gathering the thought waves and focusing the prana on something—in this case, on your spiritual practice. In other words, you let go of distractions. The mind is very active and always changing. We need to consciously and constantly make the effort to calm the mind, so we can come to a concentrated state.

**There are five states of concentration:**

1. The dull state of mind when the mind is tamasic
2. The jumpy state of mind when the mind becomes restless and unhappy
3. The gathering state of mind when the mind experiences some peace
4. The one-pointed state of mind that brings some level of happiness, being "in the zone"
5. The merging state of mind, where there is bliss

Yoga psychology says that if we can sustain that concentrated state, we will eventually attain the *ekāgratā* state, the one-pointed state of mind. Concentration is, in fact, a constant practice. You must practice repeatedly to keep building the muscles of the mind from the early stage of being dull, to being gathered, to being concentrated, to being one-pointed. You must recommit again and again to choose the practice of discovering your true Self, as opposed to the distractions and the illusions. Your mind will constantly gravitate back to the old samskaras, the habits of wrong thinking about yourself. You need to bring it back to the present again and again, until your mind is concentrated steadily in remembering the true Self. That is the *ekāgratā* state, the state of single-pointed focus on the true Self.

**Concentration practice:**

- steadies the roller coaster mind.
- calms the mind and allows it to be still, thus revealing the happiness already there. It is termed "concentration-ananda." When the mind is focused, we derive joy and contentment.
- pacifies the tendency to go to extremes, swinging between likes to dislikes. Like the pendulum of a grandfather clock, which can become still, the individual enjoys the bliss within and will not be subject any longer to the illusions of happiness from external objects.
- makes the mind stronger. (The mind is like a muscle, it can be exercised and made stronger. Like when lifting weights, it must be incremental.)
- simplifies life. You choose to say yes to some thoughts, and no to others. The thoughts that remain in the mind become very powerful, as there are less distractions. The mind can be trained to gradually become contented to function in a concentrated manner, and run in narrower and narrower circles, like a sheep enjoying eating grass in a smaller and smaller field, as the rope which ties him to a post becomes shorter and shorter.
- saves money. The mind is going inward more and more and turns away from the illusion that happiness comes from changing external objects of affection. For example, the new diamond ring of Liz, the famous actress, ceased to give her happiness after a short while, and had to be replaced with other promising objects of attention. But, in fact, her happiness depends on her own concentrated state of mind.

## 4. SPIRITUAL HEALTH AND THE YOGA OF CONSTANT PRACTICE - ABHYASA

A spiritually-healthy person is one who is steady in wisdom. We need to exercise the mind to remain established in steady wisdom. You all have wisdom, or glimpses of wisdom. It comes and goes. But even with this wisdom, the fact that you have reincarnated shows there are lessons still to be learned, past karma to work out. Looking to the world for happiness and thinking that we are this ego-self is to live in an imperfect way. Whether you are conscious of it or not, the search for the Truth is happening, and at some point, there will be awakening.

Awakening comes with a sattvic lifestyle and will lead you to health. If you persist in the sattvic way of life and balance, you will become healthy in body and mind, and, eventually, healthy in spirit. To be healthy in spirit is to have wisdom. To be healthy, you have to know how to remove the darkness and bring back the light, know how to maintain your Self-knowledge which dispels ignorance.

The Yoga tradition has many methods of practice, very well thought out and systematized, to achieve and maintain health. It takes time to apply the teachings. You apply the practices and teachings again and again, so that in time you will see your mistakes and make adjustments to your practice.

You may become bored with the practice and feel you cannot do it anymore. You have the temptation to be distracted. This is not a flaw of the practice, but rather, this is the heart of the practice. This is your opportunity to recommit yourself to practice more and to deepen your understanding of the practice. This is called *abhyasa* Yoga. *Abhyasa* literally means "constant practice."

**How to Practice**

You need the right mindset to practice *abhyasa*. Let go of expectations. *Abhyasa* changes your consciousness, but not according to any external goal. You are turning inward, seeking the beauty of your true Self. Practice with faith, but without expectations. You are, after all, seeking for something you knew, but have forgotten.

Sadhana, consciously training our minds, our body, our heart and our spirit, is a lifelong process. Every day, every hour, every minute is an opportunity to advance towards your true Self. Swami Sivananda said, "*The obstacles are innumerable on this great journey.*" Mere curiosity will not help you to attain spiritual progress. You need to have real spiritual hunger; good intentions will not do. Strong self-discipline is absolutely essential.

This does not mean suppressing, but taming, the lower nature within. Swami Sivananda captured this beautifully when he said, "*The journey is the humanization of the animal nature, and spiritualization of the human mind.*"

All of us have a lower animal nature, as well as a higher human nature. We must elevate the animal nature to become human, and we must elevate the human nature to become divine. That is our journey of Self-healing. The spiritual path is thorny and precipitous, high and steep. The causes of suffering must be weeded out with patience and perseverance. On this journey, some of the thorns are internal and some are external. We can become stuck or fall off the precipice and return to our lower nature, as a result of internal and external obstacles. The internal obstacles include lust, greed, anger, delusion, vanity. External obstacles can be experiences of economic collapse, financial loss, national wars and political conflicts, negative influences from friendships or family, addictions to all forms of technology and obsessions of technology and media.

## 5. YAMAS AND NIYAMAS: GUIDELINES FOR SELF-HEALING

Practice of the yamas and niyamas, the observances and restraints, guides us towards good health. A thorough understanding of what wrong thought tendencies are, as outlined by Patanjali Maharishi, is necessary to find ways to alleviate them. Basically, all wrong thought tendencies stem from desires. Desires are the root of all karma. Karma, action and the consequence of action, comes from desire. Desires stem from *avidya* or ignorance of our True Nature that is bliss and fulfillment. Desires, being illusory by nature, are insatiable. If there is no attempt to control them by right understanding, they can lead to stress, loss of prana and exhaustion. Repression of desires is also not advisable as this leads to ill health. A correct understanding of the root cause of desire and the ways we can get back to our True Nature constitutes a spiritual remedy to ill health.

Recall that the teachings of Ayurveda say there are three reasons for ill health:

1. *Avidya*, forgetting our True Nature as Spirit
2. Misuse of the senses; improper use of the intellect; wrong identification with objects
3. Time and use of the body; the body is a manifestation of the karmas ripening from the past. Karmas come from ignorance, desires and aversions. Experiencing the karmas and reacting to them accelerate wear and tear on the body and bring about the aging process.

The yamas and niyamas transform our long-term negative mental habits. Diseases arise as the result of steering away from Nature and disconnection with our pure Self.

Indulging in negative thoughts results in wrong actions and poor choices, pulling us further away from health. Some of these mental distortions and tendencies run deep and are difficult to change. A person identifies with and attaches to the tendencies as being who they are. These repeated negative tendencies block the flow of prana and then disease manifests in the physical body. The physical body is the gross counterpart to the subtle astral body (pranic or mental body). Repeating negative tendencies leaves subtle impressions in the astral and causal bodies that are carried from lifetime to lifetime.

These are the seeds of our karma which bring about unhappiness and disease. Disease is an opportunity to re-examine our thought patterns and to free ourselves from karmic tendencies. Observing the yamas and niyamas in daily life, either in the diseased person or for the prevention of disease, is the first step in the ladder of Yoga or the ladder of Self-healing.

Physical health and mental health are inter-related. Any physical action (physical karma) originates with mental action (the karma of thinking). If we want to be physically healthy, we need to cease wrong thoughts and wrong actions, which are based on our egoistic tendencies. We need to proactively observe a certain discipline to keep our mind in check. Thus, the yamas are abstentions from things that we are prone to indulge in, but which is preferable to abstain from for our own physical and mental emotional health. The niyamas are the observances, the things "to do" in daily life in order to purify and progress. Yamas and niyamas work together and reinforce each other. While watching and abstaining from the old negative habits, we also need to observe certain practices in daily life that will prevent our mind from falling back to past negative habits. These are psychological guidelines, but can also be considered as behavioral guidelines that lead us to health and healing. The yamas and niyamas need to be practiced in thought, word and deed, as they represent the different levels of transformation and purity. First, we refrain from indulging in negative physical observable action, then refrain from expressing with words (speech) about our negative actions, and then refrain from negativity altogether at the level of thought. Physical health and mental health are interrelated. We cannot expect to be physically healthy, if we are not tackling our wrong thoughts and habits as well.

We need to proactively observe a certain discipline to keep our mind in check. Thus, the yamas are abstentions, addressing habits that we are prone to indulge in, but that are detrimental to our physical, mental and emotional health. Abstention from these habits allows our healing. The niyamas are the observations, things we must do and observe in daily life in order to remain on the path.

The yamas and niyamas are guidelines consciously applied to transform our negative long-term mental habits. The primary causes of disease are the vasanas, or mental thought waves. Diseases arise as the result of steering away from Nature and disconnecting with our pure Self. Disease is an opportunity for spiritual growth; we are more inclined then to examine the predominant karmic tendencies in the mind. Even though the disease exists in the physical body, we can still slowly change our way of thinking. Yoga gives clear guidelines to alleviate our conditions and maintain our health.

**The Five Yamas**

Yamas, or restraints, are all the things that we should avoid doing. Implementing the five yamas will improve our life and help to remove the long-term obstacles we encounter in our karmic tendencies, our character defects, and negative habits. Further, they address our fundamental egoistic and desirous nature.

1. ***Ahimsa*** is the practice of non-injury or non-violence towards all living beings. It addresses the emotion of anger. Anger comes from selfish desires or expectations that are unfulfilled. Selfish desires come from our failure to recognize our true Self. Selfish desires result from attachment to the ego (false sense of self) and the mistaken thinking that this creates. Attachment arises when we invest our happiness in external objects and situations. *Ahimsa* means to restrain our desires and any resulting anger when those desires are unfulfilled.

   It's very difficult to refrain from anger. Therefore, we practice refraining from the reactive tendency that moves us to anger when desires are not met; refrain from the tendency to abuse others or enter into conflict and inflict harm merely to fulfill our own selfish desires and needs. The antidote to anger is contentment, santosha, and letting go of expectations. There are many methods to control anger stemming from the classical four paths of Yoga.

2. ***Satya*** is the virtue of truthfulness. It is very easy for people to tell lies and to modify the truth to suit their own wants. Yoga teaches us to remain in the truth, to be truthful in every way. We talk a lot about revealing our true Self; this certainly cannot be achieved if we lie.

   *Satya* is the practice of sincerity and honesty. We fear not living up to the image we want others to have of us. This feeling of attachment leads us to wanting people to have certain thoughts and opinions about us. It becomes a source of anxiety and fear, which may push us to be untruthful sometimes. But in reality, we cannot gain or lose anything—name, fame, position, love—because we are always perfect. We apply the principle of *satya* to refrain from our tendency to exaggerate, to manipulate others with lies and non-truths in order to achieve our selfish goals. It is far better that we remain sincere, honest, and straight-forward. The mind will become simple and clear and will bring us inner peace.

3. ***Asteya*** literally means "non-stealing," but the term also embodies the idea of non-covetousness—not stealing with your mind or eyes, not desiring something that is not yours. For example, let's say you see your neighbor has a nice car. Every day, you come home and see the car and think, "*I*

*wish I had that car,*" or "*I deserve that car more than he does.*" Or maybe he has a beautiful wife and you think he's not very nice, and you find yourself thinking, "*I would be a much better husband for this woman.*" Covetousness is to constantly think you should have something that is not yours. You can covet wealth, objects, people, talents, intelligence, looks—anything that belongs to somebody else. Again, the root cause is desire and manifests in jealousy and envy. Failing in asteya means you are not accepting your own karma. *Asteya* counters the incorrect idea that satisfying desires is the goal of life and Self-realization is possible through satisfying material desires.

Practice contentment and know that what is supposed to come to you, by your own karma, and merits will come naturally without your intervention.

4. ***Brahmacharya*** is sublimation of sexual desires and sensual energy. It deals primarily with the emotion of lust. To practice *brahmacharya*, we restrain the mind's tendency to seek sensual pleasure as the goal of life. *Brahmacharya* guides you away from desires and away from the tendency of seeking sensual gratification. It aims to channel sexual energy into spiritual energy and into realizing the true purpose of our life. *Brahmacharya* serves to regulate our impulses and their associated thought waves. It serves to calm the mind and turn the prana inwards and upwards. *Brahmacharya* brings awareness to our motives and reduces the drama in our interactions that arise from uncontrolled selfish passion. By the practice of *brahmacharya*, we are able to transform our emotional and desirous nature into a fulfilling relationship with the Divine, based on devotion and pure love.
5. "***Aparigraha***" literally translates to "non-grasping" and refers to the concept of non-accumulation. *Aparigraha* curbs our tendency towards greed and counters our tendency to think that the more that we possess, the safer and more secure we are. Thus, we are guided away from forfeiting our soul for material life and do not see material gain as the goal of life. *Aparigraha* helps us cultivate an attitude of detachment towards material possessions and lead a simple life free of desires; a life of santosha. Simple living allows our spirit to remain elevated, detached, and Self-reliant. We are strong and free in our dealings with others, who may manipulate, bribe or in other ways attempt to corrupt our intentions through the promise of material gain.

**The Five Niyamas**

The five niyamas are the observances of Yoga practice. Yamas, as abstentions, are things we avoid doing; niyamas, as observances, are good activities and attitudes that we can incorporate into our daily lives for healthy living.

1. ***Saucha*** is the practice of purity, both internal and external. External purity is the easier of the two. For example, you clean your house, you wash your clothing, you bathe, you keep your environment clean. These are easy to understand and easy to practice. Internal purity is more difficult, because you have to purify the very emotions and thoughts that act like veils over your eyes. If you feel hatred toward someone, it's as if you have a stain on the lenses of your glasses, which prevents you from seeing clearly. It can be any negative emotion. You clean your glasses, or overcome the veils, by purification of your thoughts and emotions. There are many Yoga techniques and Yoga methods to help you purify.

   The practice of pranayama purifies the prana. Prana itself gives rise to thoughts and emotions. Pranayama helps to increase and balance the prana and make the mind one-pointed, serene, cheerful, strong, harmonious, loving and generous.

   According to Raja Yoga, as summarized by Swami Vishnudevananda, purification comes by the daily practice of the Five Points of Yoga—asana, pranayama, savasana, vegetarian diet, positive thinking and meditation. These lifestyle practices purify the energy in your body and mind, helping to remove blockages. Bhakti Yoga is the method to purify your heart, mind and thoughts through the development of humility and pure love. Karma Yoga purifies the ego, removes *raga-dvesha* that generates the swings between likes and dislikes and, thereby, removes attachments. Jñāna Yoga purifies the intellect through self-inquiry, guiding you to remember the pure, limitless *Atman* that is your true Self, that remains untouched by the events and impurity of the world.

2. ***Santosha*** means "contentment." Every day upon waking, we can practice being grateful for what we have, instead of being desirous for the things we do not have. First thing in the morning, bring to mind five things that you are grateful for. This will help set the tone of contentment for the day. It doesn't need to be complicated. It can be as simple as, *"I'm grateful to have this blanket and this bed so I can rest comfortably and warmly."* Reconnect with all that you have, before the mind falls back to thoughts of all that you lack. The goal is not to desire anything, to be content. You will realize peace and tranquility and will find it easier to practice one-pointed focus on your true goal.

3. ***Tapas*** means "austerity or self-discipline." This is not about torturing yourself or seeing how much pain you can endure. It is about realizing how little you actually need. *Tapas* is about being simple. *Tapas* is the practice of reducing desires and comforts that your body and mind clamor for. We are conditioned to think that the more comfortable we are, the more successful we are in realizing the goal of life. But, this again, is wrong thinking. As we have said many times, the real goal of life is to know the Self. *Tapas* helps us to avoid the entrapments of the mind and senses. *Tapas* increases discrimination, our ability to recognize what we do and don't need, asserting our supremacy over the mind and emotions. Thus, we are free to focus our prana on the practice of Self-realization.

4. ***Swadhyaya*** is Self-study and refers to the practice of introspection based on study of Vedantic scriptures. Study directly from the guru elucidates the True Nature of the Self for the practitioner to contemplate. We constantly forget the nature of the Self. In the outside world of news, advertisements and entertainment, the whole society reinforces the avoidance of telling us the truth about ourselves. Instead, we study scripture and listen to the guru to counter all the wrong ideas of ourselves that we have learned and internalized from the outside world. Scriptures tell us about a reality beyond our normal perceptions and glorify the true Self. They inspire us in our search for Truth.

A side story:

> *Sometimes I travel by airplane and I see these thick, full-color magazines in the seat back pocket in front of me. When I flip through them, I am shocked that this represents the level of our general consciousness. "These magazines are full of lipsticks, watches, jewelry, clothing, perfumes, and other objects for us to possess in order to make ourselves 'better' and 'more attractive.' Pure materialism and superficiality are displayed in these magazines by companies who spend excesses of money selling objects and ideas which are unnecessary and do not make people truly happy or healthy. A lot of money is spent on lipstick in the name of external beauty, while lies and untruths reside in that mouth. It would be better to avoid the lipstick and, instead, tell the truth and become a truly beautiful person.*

*It would be better to advertise classes on positive thinking and meditation and to support groups and organizations who care for the true welfare and advancement of mankind.*

This story illustrates the necessity for studying scripture, of true Self study. Study the writings of sages, Yogis and masters, only of those who speak the Truth.

5. ***Ishwara-pranidhana*** is Self-surrender. It refers to surrender to Ishwara, God, or the higher power or submitting yourself to the divine intelligence and wisdom. If you don't like the term "God" or "higher power," you can say the "Supreme Being." The point is to know there is a power greater than you. Ishwara-pranidhana is tuning our actions to something higher than ourselves, thus freeing ourselves from the bonds of karma. It is important to remember that this higher power exists, even though sometimes we might feel let down by it or sometimes ask, 'Why me?' Everything has a reason, but we have to look fearlessly at our own behavior and karma. The problem lies in our selfishness, our tendency to think solely with the ego and prioritize what matters to us the most. We have a tendency to think that we are the best, we have power and control over our own lives, our own destiny, and nothing should go contrary to our will. The teachings say it is better to surrender to the supreme intelligence. It is better that we accept—to know that we do not know—and it is fine to not know it all. It is not that we become weaker, we become wiser. We begin to see the complexity of everything that is happening and we see that we are not the center of the universe.

Let me share a humorous story to illustrate this incorrect focus on the ego-imbalanced self.

*A man is riding on a train with his suitcase. For some reason, the train slows down and eventually comes to a stop. The man thinks, "Maybe my suitcase is too heavy, that's why the train has stopped." So, he throws the suitcase out the window. But the train doesn't budge. Then he lifts his feet up, still trying to help the train.*

We cannot see all the factors that go into a particular situation; we always think from the perspective of the ego: me, me, me. Wrong thinking leads us to wrong decisions. It would be much better if we would calm down, be humble and be smart, and remember there is a higher power at play, something larger is taking place of which we are only one small part.

## 6. TARGETED, SPECIFIC SADHANAS

If we are able to pinpoint certain weak mental tendencies, we can address these with specific sadhanas.

1. **Sadhana to address arrogance**

   Practice humility. Swami Sivananda said, *"If you are arrogant, you will say vulgar words or think, 'Don't you know who I am? I cannot be dictated to by anybody. I have my own way and nobody can question me about anything I think or do. Why should I report to you?'"* Arrogance comes with rudeness, insolence, impertinence, being overbearing—you think your will is above everyone else and push your will onto others.

   Here is a story to illustrate this.

   > *A sadhu is sitting in the forest in meditation. He has a very disciplined practice and lots of power in his mind. One day, he decides to visit the nearby village. Just as the sadhu gets up from his seat, a bird poops on his head. He is furious at the bird and thinks, "How can you do this to me?" His eyes contain so much anger and fire (because he has been meditating for a long time) that he burns up the bird and the bird drops dead. Nobody is there in the forest to see that the sadhu killed the bird.*
   >
   > *He goes down to the village to beg for food. He stops at the house of a lady who is taking care of her handicapped husband and asks for food. She says, "Yes, but please wait. I need to take care of my husband first." The lady is taking some time and once again the sadhu becomes angry, with eyes burning. Seeing this, the lady said these words, "Please be patient. You may have killed the bird in the forest, but now be patient."*
   >
   > *Shocked, the sadhu thought, "Oh my God, how can she know I killed a bird in the forest? She must have some kind of psychic power. Who is this woman? She appears just a normal woman with a handicapped husband." The sadhu asks, "Who are you? How did you know I killed a bird in the forest? Please tell me the secret of your practice." The lady answered, "Go to the end of the village and there you will find my teacher." The sadhu walked to the end of the village searching for the teacher, but only saw a butcher shop and*

*thought, "How can a butcher be a teacher?" He went to the butcher and asked if he knew the lady. The butcher said yes. The sadhu then asked, "How do you practice in your daily life?" The butcher replied, "I do my duty. I have to take care of my old parents. This butcher shop is my family business, so that is all I do. I do my duty."*

*The sadhu immediately realized his mistake, having thought his Yoga and meditation practice in the forest was the highest way to live. In fact, under challenging circumstances, as soon as he stopped meditating, he lost patience. Yet these people who live in the world and who simply and humbly do their duty and, being challenged every day, have developed the necessary patience, perseverance and wisdom. The inner wisdom resulting from daily dedication to our duty with the spirit of self-sacrifice—without egoism or pretension—makes us achieve the highest good.*

Swami Sivananda said that, as aspirants, we need to mix with people of different mental temperaments and watch our own thoughts. When you are ill-treated, when you are disrespected or persecuted, only then will you conquer your arrogance and ego through the practice of humility, patience, kindness and love.

2. **Sadhana to address anger**

Anger comes from desire or expectations unfulfilled.

Let's say you are angry at your husband, because he did not help you bring out the garbage. How do you deal with this? As a Yogi, you know that you are practicing and working on yourself, so how do you deal with this? You have to let go of the expectation and cease complaining, "It's not fair, I do everything else already." Perhaps you bring the garbage out and realize that you are not what you do and the relationship is not about fairness, but about your own search for true love.

The goal is peace of mind and selfless love that is your own true Self. Let go of your expectations and eventually you will start to recognize that maybe the husband is doing a lot of work that you do not see. Maybe his work does not conform to your expectations, but he's doing many other things. Regardless, you are working on yourself, you are not working on him.

We can use the Four Paths of Yoga to conquer the very important and dangerous emotion of anger.

In Karma Yoga, think that:

- I do my duty and let go of the results.
- I am not in a position to judge. How can I be certain I am seeing the bigger picture?
- I offer my success or failure, and I do my duty, it is not about me.

In Bhakti Yoga, accept that:

- It's not my will, but Thy will.
- I surrender to a higher power.
- Whether my desire or expectation is fulfilled or not, I surrender to what is and remain open and flexible.
- I'm ready to adapt to all situations.
- Everything happens for a reason.

In Raja Yoga, think:

- I keep my mind calm and concentrated while engaging in life, so I can reflect upon who I am.
- My mind is getting stronger and stronger with each test.
- I remain positive in all situations.

In Jñāna Yoga, contemplate:

- I am not this body. I am not this mind. I am not these emotions. I am not this intellect. I am *Satchitananda*, eternally fulfilled.
- I am not the garbage can and I don't worry about the garbage. I can bring it out.
- I keep my mind focused on my eternal nature; I am *Satchitananda*.

3. **Sadhana to address fear and anxiety**

The cause of fear and anxiety is attachment. Anxiety can consume a lot of your energy. It is a primitive emotion. Fear can paralyze, causing you to lose your mental faculties and your ability to respond. At its core, fear causes you to feel unsafe. It can be fear of insects, fear of guns, fear of people. Swami Sivananda said that 95% of all fear is imaginary. Only 5% is reasonable fear.

Remember to cultivate the courage to face your illusions. It takes courage and honesty to see who we really are. You need courage to remove wrong beliefs and false identification. Remember that the *Atman* is always shining within. It is the illusion of our mind which creates this fear. Imagination can create even bigger fears.

Practice replacing fear with faith. There are three types of faith:

- Faith in yourself. I have the capacity. I am strong.
- Faith in Nature, in a higher power, in the supreme intelligence. Everything happens for the best. I am protected and taken care of.
- Faith in the teacher, scriptures and teachings. By putting the teachings into practice; fear will disappear.

Everything that happens is a test of faith. Practices to conquer fear include:

- Improve breath, body and mind awareness. Breathing exercises help us to slow down and restore balance to the flow of prana.
- Anuloma viloma, alternate nostril breathing, is very helpful for anxiety.
- Increase *ojas* shakti through proper food, proper rest and proper devotion. When you increase *ojas*, you increase your contentment, increase your gratitude, relaxation and faith.
- Use props to help create a sense of calm and safety: For example, place a heavy pillow over your belly while breathing in savasana. Place a heavy eye pillow over your eye-lids to switch on the parasympathetic nervous system to relax your nervous system.
- Learn to detach from that which causes you attachment and fears. Learn to let go. For example, in savasana, you let go of the body and the mind and relax deeply.
- Learn to contemplate your fear. Identify all the facets of your fear.

4. **Sadhana to address depression**

Depression is a big problem in modern life. Many people will experience some degree of depression at some point in their life. Again, we refer to the Four Paths of Yoga for practices to help alleviate depression, specifically seeking to stimulate the sympathetic nervous system.

Through Hatha Yoga and Raja Yoga, you activate the prana and cause it to move, unlocking and releasing energy through asanas. Sun salutations, backward bends and loosening exercises are particularly effective in moving the prana. Awareness is increased following deep relaxation of the body and mind. Return to balance of mind with pranayama, especially anuloma viloma, or alternate nostril breathing.

Through the practices of Bhakti Yoga, open your heart and connect to the Self by connecting to people around you. Feeling connected to others and reducing feelings of isolation is very important in countering depression.

5. **Sadhana to reduce stress and become stress-resilient**

One of the main causes of stress is lack of prana. So, to reduce stress we simply focus on increasing prana. Increased flexibility, both in mind and body, is very helpful to create stress resilience. Stress can also be managed with positive thinking. Again, the practice of faith and self-study help us understand the bigger picture of our life, not getting engulfed by the world around us. We learn to accept the karma that comes to us, adapting to situations as they are, while doing our best and detaching from the result.

## 7. PROGRESS IN SADHANA

We envision progress in sadhana as a spiral. In general, know that you are progressing in your sadhana, it just might not be immediately apparent. Sadhana will help you to evolve, to learn and grow—but not in the way you think or expect. It is not a straight line. It will spiral and undulate up and down, seemingly forward and backwards. But, if you observe carefully, the low point of the second round is higher than the high point of the first round. The low points are also enabling progress, because through them you learn to consolidate your knowledge. The overall trend is upwards.

### Signs of Spiritual Progress

Failures are said to be stepping-stones to success. So, learn and practice letting go of expectations and judgments. Swami Sivananda said, "The gradual inward progress is mostly silent, unseen, like the quiet unfolding of the bud into the flower in the late hours of the night." There is no grand announcement of the flower's arrival. It opens very slowly, very calmly, but always progressing to reveal its beautiful nature. We must have faith that we are progressing, even if very slowly. Do not be dejected. Do not grow depressed thinking you are not progressing.

Swami Sivananda also said, "*The real measure of spiritual progress is the peacefulness and serenity that you manifest in the waking state. You will find you have a healthy mind and a healthy body. Your excretions will be scanty, the voice will be sweet, the face will be brilliant, the eyes lustrous, and you will be ever calm, tranquil and poised. You will be ever-cheerful, fearless and content. You will be dispassionate and discriminative and there will be no attraction for the external world. Things that used to upset you will not upset you now. You will have an unruffled mind and introversion. Things that used to give you pleasure will produce the reverse effect. You will have a one-pointed, sharp and subtle mind, and you will be longing for more meditation. The idea that all forms are forms of the Divine will grow stronger and stronger in you. You will feel the presence of God everywhere and you will experience the nearness of God. You will have a steady asana and you will develop a burning desire for selfless service."*

Swami Sivananda also cautions that if your japa, your meditation, your Vedantic inquiry actually thicken your veil, as it did the Yogi in the story above, then, in fact, your practice is increasing your egoism. This is not spiritual sadhana. It is only a kind of occult practice. You need to watch, introspect, practice self-analysis and remove this formidable egoism. Do not stop sadhana when you get a few blossoms; continue your practice until the final beatitude is reached. Do not be carried away by name and fame. Do not let failure discourage you, but go on doing your best. Do not brood over past mistakes, but likewise do not repeat them in the future.

Strengthen yourself with new vigor. Develop virtues and build your willpower. No sadhana ever goes in vain. Entertain no negative thoughts. Be regular in your sadhana and, little by little, the power will accumulate and grow within you. Let your practice be continuous, unbroken and earnest. Meditate regularly and annihilate the undercurrents of vasanas. Start now! Do not say, *"I will start spiritual sadhana when all my cares, worries and anxiety cease, when all my children are set in life and I have retired."* You must start your spiritual practice NOW, whatever your circumstances.

To conclude, here are a few reminders to keep training and living the Yogic life without getting lost.

- Swami Sivananda says, *"Do it now!"* Do not fall victim to the illusion of time. You might say "tomorrow," but tomorrow never comes. Do it now; constantly strive to live in the here and now. Do this by keeping your mind focused and steady, detached all day.
- Try at all times to live in unity. Wherever you are, try to see unity.
- Be in the world, but detached from the world.
- Let go of control; let go of the idea that you know.
- Do everything with concentration, one thought at a time.
- Bring a spark to your practice, make it interesting; make a little adjustment and a little change in routine.

- Resist the temptation to doubt yourself, even when other people doubt you or what you are doing. Remain strong in the Truth of your heart.
- Choose well what you focus on; fewer thoughts mean more peace. Dedicate everything to the Divine, to a higher power and you will achieve emotional healing through Love.

### *INSPIRED STORY*

**Devotion to Atman/Self**

*Before I worship all Gods and Goddesses*
*Now, after Vedanta, all Gods and Goddesses*
*Are the Atman Within*

---

**QUESTIONS**

1. *What is sadhana?*
2. *Name the Yamas and Niyamas. Write 2-3 lines about each.*
3. *Describe the 8 Limbs of Raja Yoga. What is the relationship between Hatha Yoga and Raja Yoga?*

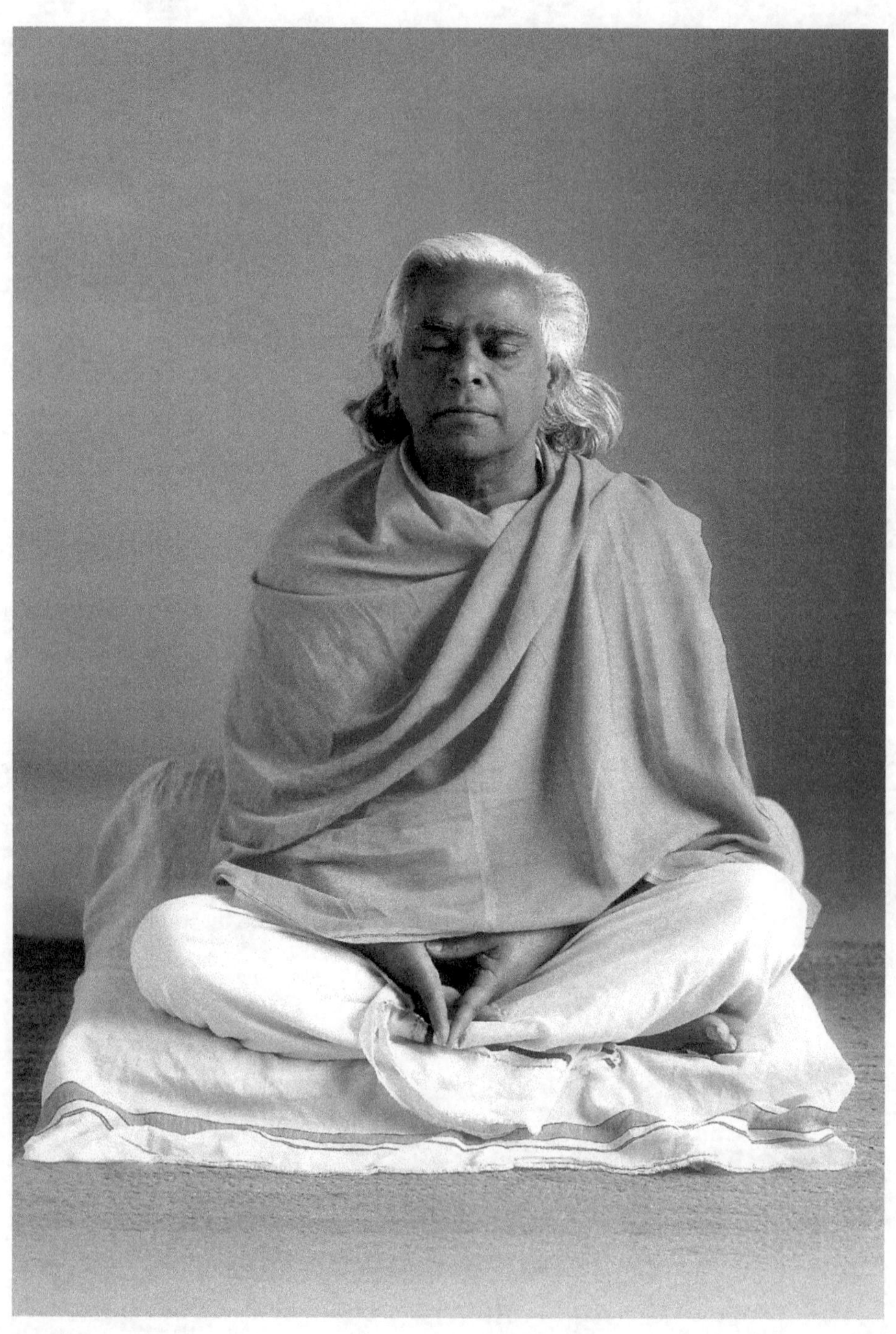

SWAMI VISHNUDEVANANDA

CHAPTER 9

# Inner and Outer Obstacles and Vedic Remedies

***"Vedic knowledge is the core knowledge of the Self and the Universe as an integrated power and presence of consciousness that is the fundamental force of creation, of prana and well-being behind the body and mind but connected to the core of our being beyond the body and the mind. It is the core knowledge that integrates and helps us understand all the levels of the universe outwardly and inwardly."***

– DAVID FRAWLEY – *Interview at the Sivananda Ashram Yoga Farm, 2014*

On the journey of Self-healing, there are numerous obstacles, both inner and outer. We can apply teachings from the Vedic sciences to help alleviate them, ease our way and live meaningfully and contribute to the welfare of others. The Vedic sciences include Yoga, Vedanta, Ayurveda, Jyotish, Vastu and the Vedic approach to the environment.

## 1. NINE OBSTACLES IN YOGA ACCORDING TO PATANJALI

Patanjali identifies nine obstacles to Yoga practice or the journey of meditation. Being aware of the obstacles and adjusting your lifestyle accordingly will help maintain enthusiasm in your sadhana and prevent discouragement and stagnation.

1. ***Vyādhi*** - illness or disease. When you are ill, your prana is lost, your motivation and discipline decline, and you lack higher goals and motivation in life. The Yogi prevents disease by living a moderate and healthy lifestyle.

2. ***Styāna*** - mental torpor, apathy, lack of motivation, disinclination. You avoid performing your duty and procrastinate. The Yogi stays alert with a balanced schedule, alternating duties with physical activities (walking, swimming, asanas), pranayama, chanting, rest, and relaxation.

3. ***Saṃśaya*** - self-doubt, lack of self-worth, low self-esteem. It can also manifest as loss of faith in your teacher or the teachings. It is a defeatist attitude. The best antidote is satsang—be in company of enthusiastic aspirants or of inspired teachers. If teachers are absent, keep company with their inspired teachings in the form of books, audio talks, etc.

4. ***Pramādā*** - distraction, negligence, impatience, haste. Counteract this by developing concentration and focus of the mind using mantra repetition and connection to God.

5. ***Alasyā*** - burnout, laziness in body and mind. If you are burnt out, restore yourself with Ayurvedic modalities, such as *abhyanga* (warm oil massage) or *Panchakarma* (detoxification process).

   Laziness comes from lack of: prana, motivation, self-will, self-encouragement and enthusiasm, due to forgetfulness of your ultimate goal. Increase *ojas* shakti by adjusting your lifestyle and diet.

6. ***Avirati*** - desires, cravings, self-indulgence, non-dispassion; lack of detachment, not being able to turn the attention inward. The mind has ups and downs. Calm the senses through sense therapy, pujas and devotion. Increase the practice of self-inquiry to increase the fire of discrimination in the mind.

7. ***Bhrāntidarśanā*** - false perceptions, delusion, misunderstanding. Satsanga, a balanced Yoga life, immersion in nature, or retreat in an ashram among other aspirants, will help bring back groundedness, balance your outlook and remove darkness and delusion.

8. ***Alabdhabhūmikatvā*** - doubting progress, lacking optimism, doubting potential for further progress. Doubts may arise after initial enthusiasm, wrong expectations and the resulting loss of prana. Renew courage and faith in the teacher, the teachings and in yourself. Have confidence in yourself and in your capacity to find the Truth.

9. ***Anavasthitatvā*** - inability to maintain stability, inability to maintain progress or gains and the tendency to slide backwards. This arises when we lack a schedule in daily life, lack self-discipline, lack steadiness in sadhana or lack control of the senses. Remember your aspirations and rededicate yourself to the sadhana.

Swami Vishnudevananda, in his book *Meditation and Mantras*, encourages you to follow a daily practice of asana and pranayama to help prevent disease and foster mental alertness. He says that doubt can be dispelled through meditation. When you feel you are not progressing, plod on; it is very important to stick to your daily routine. Remember, in the last chapter, we talked about the journey that looks like a spiral, swirling up and down in the overall trajectory of progress. The best practice for maintaining this routine is to live in a community of like-minded people and keep company with teachers or have satsanga.

## 2. HOW AYURVEDA HELPS SUPPORT YOUR JOURNEY AND OVERCOMING OBSTACLES

Here are a few important practices in Ayurveda to help keep your balance and strength.

1. **Manage your doshas through an Ayurvedic lifestyle.** Ayurveda will help you tune to nature. It will teach you to constantly manage your doshas—vata, pitta, kapha and their subtle energies, prana, *tejas*, *ojas*—and it will guide you to keep them in balance. Learn the Ayurvedic techniques to balance yourself.

   The doshas change as your activities and environment change. Yoga teaches you the virtue of balance. Vata is the energy of action and movement and the corresponding elements are ether and air. Prana, the subtle counterpart of Vata, gives you enthusiasm.

   Pitta is the energy of transformation, conversion and metabolism and its corresponding elements are fire and water. *Tejas*, its subtle counterpart, gives you strong will and the fire of comprehension and insight.

   Kapha is the energy of construction, lubrication and nourishment and its corresponding elements are water and earth. *Ojas*, its counterpart, will bring you contentment and endurance.

   Balance requires reducing excess doshas, which lead to disease, both physical and mental. Avoid too much movement, too much work and too much sleep to control vata, pitta, kapha, respectively. In order to maintain balance and manage your doshas, understand your strengths and weaknesses; understand your mind-body constitution or type. Understand the subtle energies behind everything; understand the relationship between proper nutrition, waste elimination, sleep, rest, detoxification and so on. As we saw with the Covid-19 virus, if we do not maintain balance, we will find ourselves ill and be forced to slow down and rest.

2. **Follow the natural rhythm of day and time**

One aspect of living according to your mind-body type, according to doshas, is timing actions and behaviors with the natural energy rhythms of the hours of the day. Align your daily routines with your doshas. The day is broken into segments aligning with the energies of the doshas:

- 6am–10am – kapha time
- 10am–2pm – pitta time
- 2pm–6pm – vata time
- 6pm–10pm – kapha time
- 10pm–2am – pitta time
- 2am–6am – vata time

In the ashram, we eat at 10am, because before that time, the fire of digestion is less active. We get up before 6am and meditate. By 10pm, we know we should be asleep, so the liver can detoxify.

3. **Prepare for good sleep:**

People of Vata constitution tend to need the most sleep—eight or more hours. People with Pitta-dominant traits need seven to eight hours of sleep. Kaphas need about seven hours or less—and should get up during vata time to get the most out of the day. Preparation for sleep is important. Take a hot bath and go to bed during kapha time. Turn off your cell phone and computer at least one hour before your sleep time. Practicing pranayama, meditation, and japa can help to calm the mind in preparation for sleep.

4. **Nourish yourself with a good diet adjusted to the seasons**

One factor in maintaining balanced doshas is living in harmony with the seasons and having a seasonal routine. This should be studied in more detail, but here are a few examples to briefly illustrate the point:

Spring is kapha season. The effects of this cool and moist season can be balanced by taking warm drinks and foods that are warm and dry —like legumes and vegetables. Use warming spices, as well as pungent, bitter, and astringent seasonings, like ginger and clove. Avoid sweet, salty, and sour foods, as well as dairy, and heavy, oily foods, which tend to increase kapha.

Summer is pitta season. Adjust foods to be more cooling. Eat more fruit and raw vegetables. Have light cool drinks like coconut water and lime juice. Avoid hot drinks and hot or spicy foods.

Fall and winter are vata seasons. Eat warm, moist, heavy foods, hot soups and kitchari to counteract the influence of vata. Avoid salads, raw vegetables, bitter or astringent foods and cold drinks.

5. **Managing the doshas through the six tastes**

- The sweet taste calms pitta and vata, but increases kapha qualities. The sweet taste promotes growth, strengthens all body tissue and contributes to healthy skin and hair. In the mind, sweet taste promotes compassion and love, but, in excess, creates attachment and heaviness. Examples include: grains, root vegetables, natural sugars, honey, maple syrup, milk, dates, and complex carbohydrates.
- The sour taste will calm vata and increase pitta and kapha. The sour taste energizes the body and increases the appetite. In the mind, the sour taste helps with perception and attention, as well as stimulating and energizing the mind. In excess, it will create discontentment, jealousy, anger, and overly-critical thought patterns. Examples include: sour cream, yogurt, cheese, fermented foods.
- The salty taste calms vata and increases pitta and kapha. Salty foods strengthen your *agni* (digestive fire), maintain your water electrolyte balance and help eliminate waste. For the mind, the salty taste promotes enthusiasm and passion for life. In excess, it can create greed and make us overly ambitious. Examples include: rocksalt, seaweed.
- The pungent taste reduces kapha and increases pitta and vata. The pungent taste improves digestion and absorption, reduces congestion, and improves blood circulation. In the mind, the pungent taste helps you to focus, be sharp and attentive. In excess, it can create hostility and cruelty. Examples include: black pepper, cayenne pepper, chili pepper, ginger, radish.
- The bitter taste calms pitta and reduces kapha, but can aggravate vata. Bitter taste helps to eliminate toxins, is anti-inflammatory, has laxative effects, supports the liver and acts as a digestive tonic. In the mind, the bitter taste promotes satisfaction, contentment and self-awareness. In excess, it can lead to grief and depletion. Examples include: leafy vegetables, aloe vera, fennel, green and black tea, bitter melon, sandalwood, coffee, turmeric.

- The astringent taste calms kapha and pitta, but can aggravate vata. It improves absorption, constricts the blood vessels, stops bleeding, promotes healing, and it is anti-diabetic and anti-bacterial. For the mind, the astringent taste is quieting, but too much can lead to anxiety and fear. Examples include: chickpeas, green beans, unripe bananas, turmeric, goldenseal, beans.

As an example, if you have high blood pressure, you should avoid salty foods, which increase the pitta, and take more astringent tastes, that are cool by nature; it will increase the vata and decrease the pitta and kapha.

The main objective is to see that you have to adjust your lifestyle, as well as your diet, to complement the season in order to maintain balance. Balance is the key takeaway! Know your type of mind and understand the effect of the different tastes on the mind and the body. In general, eat a sattvic, vegetarian diet, avoiding tamasic and rajasic foods.

6. **Dietetic guidelines**

For the maintenance of balance, it is also very important to know how to eat properly. Here are some guidelines:

- Say grace or a prayer before each meal. This brings mindfulness to eating food in a proper frame of mind.
- Choose foods that look and taste good; you should enjoy your food. Do not indulge, but enjoy.
- Be thankful, show gratitude for your food, and be certain that it is prepared with love. This is why it is better to eat at home with family or community rather than in restaurants.
- Always take a short repose after eating. This should not interrupt the day, just a brief rest before continuing with your duties.
- Maintain a proper state of mind and being; do not eat when you are experiencing stress or anxiety.
- Avoid distractions like television, computer, reading, intense conversations or business, etc. while eating.
- Avoid ice cold drinks with food. It will dampen your *agni*.
- Allow time to chew the food well, at least thirty times, before swallowing.
- Spices and herbs can also be used to help you balance the doshas with food. It is important to tune to the power of plants. For

example: cumin seeds provide a bitter taste, tumeric is pungent and astringent, mustard seeds are pungent, coriander or cilantro is bitter and pungent, fenugreek is bitter and astringent, asafoetida is pungent and helps the nerves, ginger is pungent and sweet. So you see, the right spices can also be incorporated into meals to help maintain internal balance and balance with the seasons.

From the perspective of the gunas, sattvic spices include cardamom, saffron, and cinnamon; rajasic spices include black pepper, cumin and asafoetida; tamasic spices include red pepper, mustard and garlic.

7. **Care of yourself through Ayurvedic treatments for the body**

Rooted in traditional Ayurvedic medicine, abhyanga body treatments help manage the health of your body. Abhyanga is a classical warm oil massage given by a trained therapist or as a self-massage. Abhyanga can be full-body or can focus on a body part—head, face, hands or feet, or wherever a person is afflicted or as prescribed by their Ayurvedic practitioner, according to their particular constitution and the season. This type of massage should be avoided when there is fever or when there are excessive toxins in the body.

Other kinds of Ayurvedic body treatments include:

- pouring oil on the forehead (*shirodhara*)
- steam bath (*swedana*)
- local oil treatment (*kati basti*)
- dry powder massage (*udwarthanam*)
- detoxification (*Panchakarma*)

Detoxification cleanses the body from the inside out, and includes rest and restoration of energy. The classic approach for detoxification in Ayurveda is *Panchakarma*. As *pancha* in the name indicates, there are five cleansing actions included in the process that aim to remove high or imbalanced doshas. There is a preparation phase prior to *Panchakarma*; the treatment itself can be seven days to three weeks. *Panchakarma* is a strong detoxification program and is usually done under the guidance of an Ayurvedic practitioner or *vaidya*. The five kinds of action included are:

– **Vamanam** (therapeutic emesis) - induced vomiting helps clear the upper digestive tract to the duodenum (end of stomach)

- **Virechanam** (purgation) - induced purgation clears the intestines, evacuating the bowels and eliminates high pitta
- **Anuvasana** (enema using medicated oil) - oil enema helps lubricate the system and remove all the lipid soluble waste to eliminate vata and also reduce pitta and kapha
- **Nasyam** (oiling of the nostrils) - nasal instillation of medicated substances helps clear the respiratory tract and sinuses. This eliminates high kapha.
- **Raktamokshana** (blood-letting) - not commonly used in modern times

Look out for ailments or signs of imbalance:

One last thing to consider is the ailments, or the signs of imbalance, so you can determine which adjustments and treatments to use to restore balance and health.

- Vata ailments include: joint problems, diseases of the colon, head colds, urinary and genital tract infections, trauma.
- Pitta ailments include: diseases of the skin, blood, eyes, liver, stomach, small intestine and any condition of increased acidity.
- Kapha ailments include: diseases of the respiratory tract or stomach, head cold, diabetes, slow metabolism, any condition of increased mucus, blockages, swelling and excess tissue.

With specific ailments, it's recommended that you consult a trained practitioner, but there are home remedies that you can research on your own. [Ref. book *Practical Ayurveda* from Sivananda Yoga Vedanta Center Penguin Random House, 2018].

## 3. HOW VEDIC ASTROLOGY (SCIENCE OF JYOTISH) SUPPORTS YOUR SADHANA

i. **Jyotish** is the Vedic astrological science of karma. Learn to navigate and work through the obstacles that come from your karma using the guidance of Jyotish. Jyotish, meaning science of light, is also referred to as Vedic Astrology, as it is based on the same Vedic principles as Yoga and Vedanta. A consultation with a professional Jyotishi, who is sattvic, can help you understand your strengths and weaknesses, your karmic path, and periods of life. A Jyotishi, or a spiritual teacher using Jyotish, will be able to recommend remedial practices based on the path of Yoga most favorable to help with your karma. Beginners should note that Jyotish is an intricate science requiring time to learn. Be patient and allow time to mature; avoid jumping to conclusions too quickly about anything. You only have a partial picture of your karma, so carry on focusing on your Yoga practice, which is the remedial measure par excellence to any karma.

ii. **Understand your sign.** Please note that Vedic astrology is calculated and interpreted differently than Western tropical astrology, as it is based on the same Vedic body of knowledge of the Self, karma and reincarnation.

First of all, look at the quality of the ascendant sign in your birth chart (your lagna = yourself, your body, your overall life, represented by the sign and the degree of the sign, that is rising at the moment of birth), the placement (the position in the chart) of the planet that rules your ascendant sign, the moon and the sun.

In general, the placement of your ascendant (lagna, 1st house) determines if you are:

- an emotional person (water signs): Cancer, Scorpio, Pisces;
- an action person (fire signs): Aries, Leo, Sagittarius;
- a practical person (earth signs): Taurus, Virgo, Capricorn;
- a thinking person (air signs): Gemini, Libra, Aquarius.

iii. **Discover your main karma**. Look at the placement of your "planet ruler", the ruling planet of the first house, which represents you. Your motivation, your main subject of concern, is represented by the location of the planet ruler in the houses.

iv. **Understanding your life motivation** through the planets' motiation. There are twelve areas of karma (twelve houses), each of which can help us to understand our motivations and our karmas. Planets situated in the houses carry the motivation of that house.

Where is your ruling planet placed? What is its motivation? Which motivations do the other planets have? Look at the placement of your planets in the houses and figure out your overall sense of purpose.

- **Dharma** motivation is to live a good, dutiful and meaningful life contributing to others, manifested through the 1st house (body, the overall personality), the 5th house (education, creativity and intelligence) and the 9th house (higher mind, spirituality and faith).

- **Artha** motivation is to accumulate wealth and financial resources, manifested through the 2nd house (support system, money), the 6th house (service, health, conflicts, weaknesses) and the 10th house (career, achievements, contribution, name and fame).
- **Kama** motivation is to enjoy life, manifested through planets in the 3rd house (communication and will), the 7th house (partnership—marital, romantic or business) and the 11th house (income, gains, community).
- **Moksha** motivation is to go beyond this life to seek liberation. This motivation is manifested through planets in the 4th house (heart, home, mother, emotions), the 8th house (transformation, deep psyche, kundalini) and the 12th house (losses or charity, indulgences or renunciation, foreign countries).

v. **What is your moon's disposition?** What is the quality of your mind and heart? By observing the nature of your moon in your chart, which represents your mind, Jyotish teaches us that we are not our mind and we cannot expect other people to be like us. There are unique combinations of planets influencing any given individual. It teaches tolerance and flexibility when trying to understand your own mindset and the distinctive mindset of other people. Being a Vedic science, Jyotish recognizes that we experience what the mind projects. For that reason, it is important to understand the quality of your moon-mind-emotions. The location and quality of the moon in your birth chart indicates the qualities of your mind. The possible dispositions include a dark moon; a debilitated and attached moon; a bright, exalted moon; a full moon; a sweet moon; an angry moon; a moon alone; a depressed moon; an oppressed moon; an impulsive moon; a fiery mind; a restless mind; an organized mind; a persevering and stable mind; a mind that gives up easily; a moon governed by favorable influences or conflictual influences; the quality of being open-minded or narrow-minded; an introspective mind; a hopeful mind with strong faith; doubtful mind; an edgy mind, losing balance easily; a delusional mind; and an ungrounded mind.

vi. **What is your sun's disposition?** The sun can represent the ego-self or the *Atman*. In Jyotish, the location of the sun in your chart helps you understand what you will identify with, as it is the disposition of yourself, your soul, and your ego. The sun is like the king, giving you self-confidence, health and vitality, as well as executive and administrative capacities. A weak sun, on the other hand, gives you lack of self-confidence, dependency, ignorance of the Self, lack of self-care and self-love, and a need for support. If the sun is very strong, your disposition may tip towards being egoistic, which can make you overly strong and abusive towards others. The house the sun is in indicates the area of life you identify with.

vii. **Understand the atmakaraka (purpose/mission in life of the soul) and the planet significators (karakas).** The planets are viewed as embodiments of cosmic energy, not just large objects in the sky. This cosmic energy influences your life. It is said that Lord Vishnu gave the planets the job of distributing the karmas, and this is the role they play in your chart. The planets each represent different energies and influence different aspects of your constitution. *Karakas* are the "significators" that determine which person or thing a planet influences. *Atmakaraka* is the indicator of the soul, the planet with the highest degree in a birth chart. What is the disposition of your *karakas* (significators) in general?

- Sun represents the Self for a spiritual person or the ego, or false self, for a non-aware person. In terms of relationship, it is your father.
- Moon represents the mind, emotions, and mental health. The position of the moon indicates what you like and are attracted to, as well as your social life and ability to connect with others. In terms of relationships, it represents your mother.
- Mars represents your energy, your actions, courage, initiative and ability to make changes in your life. In terms of relationships, it represents your siblings.
- Mercury represents your communication, intelligence, learning, analytical ability, and affinity for writing and business.
- Jupiter represents wisdom, knowledge, prosperity and your likelihood of being spiritual or your connection to the Divine. In terms of relationships, it is your guru or teacher.
- Venus represents love, beauty, relationships, harmony, social life, comforts and marriage. It can also mean devotion. It is the partner or wife, in terms of relationships.
- Saturn represents responsibilities, seriousness, hard work, discipline and detachment. It represents your obstacles, your life lessons.

- Rahu represents worldly desires, materialism, ambitions, obsessions, illusions and greed. It represents your area of being driven and is hard to control.
- Ketu represents otherworldly desire and spirituality, detachment, introspection, insight, fantasy and liberation. It represents your area of past life knowledge and mystical knowledge.

**Note:** Rahu and Ketu are not really planets, they are shadow planets, but are considered as planets for their effect. They represent the intersection point of the paths of the sun and moon. Rahu is the northern intersection point; Ketu is the southern intersection point. Rahu and Ketu are considered opposites of each other, but are always understood together. They represent difficult areas of inner conflict.

viii. **Areas of growth are represented by benefic Jupiter—and your blessings.** The location of Jupiter, in Jyotish, will help identify areas of potential growth. Jupiter is your best planet and it shows where you expand, where you grow spiritually. For example, somebody can grow from education. So the more they study, the more they grow. Some people may grow from the development of the heart by doing service for others, meditation or living in a community. The placement of Jupiter can help you understand this aspect of your blessed life.

ix. **Jyotish shows your weaknesses and areas for improvement** through the location of debilitated planets in your chart—planets in the 6th, 8th and 12th houses. Just as we have strengths, we have weaknesses. Become balanced; become stronger in your weakness and relax your effort in the area of strength. Balance the two flows of energy—sun and moon, ha and tha.

x. **Compare your innate strengths and weaknesses from past lives to the current one.** Karma is dynamic and complex. It is interesting to know your tendencies of the past and how they compare with those of your current life. Weakness in the present might be strengths of the past and vice versa, mitigating the result of the karma.

Jyotish shows that the state of your life, in any given moment, is just a small part of the continuum that is your karma across many lives. Your life is very long—with many events, much movement, and much learning.

xi. **There are "periods of your life" (dashas) unfolding one after the other representing periods of your karma unfolding.** Jyotish teaches you forbearance and hope, revealing that this cycle of karma, even though it might be difficult, is not permanent. Things will constantly change. Never despair, your life always changes for the best.

xii. **Early motivation is set at birth.** Your life unfolds as it should, from period to period as the karma unfolds. However, the distribution of planets at the beginning of life (the birth chart) will influence the overall life. It represents the karma remaining from the past and what you now focus on in the present.

xiii. **There are five qualities of light, or energy, at the moment of birth, the *panchanga*.** The essence of the *panchanga* is how the sun and moon relate to each other on a daily basis and, in particular, on your day of birth. Depending on which solar day you were born—Monday, Tuesday, Wednesday, Thursday, Friday, Saturday, Sunday—the corresponding quality and energy of the planets give added information about who we are and how we feel.

xiv. **Use practices from the four paths of Yoga to work with your strengths and weaknesses.**

- An active person can practice Karma Yoga.
- A devotional person can practice Bhakti Yoga.
- A mystical person can practice meditation and Raja Yoga.
- A physically-active person can practice Hatha Yoga.
- An intellectual and high-minded person can practice self-inquiry and Jnana Yoga.
- The synthesis of Yoga, the practice of all paths, will gradually make a person stronger in all aspects.

xv. **Choose a muhurta for auspicious timing of events.** It is beneficial to know the favorable time to start an event, get initiation, or take an internal vow. The intention at that moment will determine the outcome of the event.

Thus ends the overview of some ways Jyotish can help you understand your nature and the nature of your karma. Learn to navigate your life, alleviate your obstacles and maximize the auspiciousness of your enlightened choices.

## 4. HOW THE VEDIC SCIENCE OF VASTU HELPS TO ENHANCE YOUR ENERGY AND ALLEVIATE OBSTACLES FROM THE ENVIRONMENT

Some obstacles from the physical environment can hinder your sadhana practice and Self-healing. While Ayurveda addresses obstacles from your lifestyle and Jyotish addresses obstacles that come from karma, obstacles from your environment and external factors are addressed through Vastu.

### What is Vastu, the Science of Space?

The Vedic science of Vastu Shastra is the traditional Indian system of architecture. As Jyotish is the science of time, Vastu is the science of space. The aim of Vastu is harmonizing your living environment and your life here on earth with the greater cosmic energy of the universe. Vastu is an intricate science and, here, we will introduce a few simple guidelines, showing how it can help your journey of Self-healing.

Vastu embodies the idea of a higher cosmic energy that informs our planet, our lives, our homes and buildings. Vastu is the science of living according to natural law and principles of cosmic energy. It is the natural basis for architecture. If you live in spaces designed according to Vastu, you bring a higher energy to your home and work environment. The Vastu principles guide the orientation and organization of space and function; designs are in harmony with the cosmic energy, following a universal energy grid. A few guidelines:

1. The Brahmasthan is the most powerful and holy spot of any property or house. It is the space at the center of the house and it should be left empty to allow harmonizing and beneficial energy into the building. Specifically, avoid putting a toilet or garbage bin in this location as this would pollute the energy of the house.
2. The northeast corner, called the *ishanya*, is considered the most auspicious corner of a building or room. It is beneficial to install water here, so a well, water storage, or a fountain could be located there. Do not put trash cans or waste materials in this corner of the house. We need to respect the *ishanya,* as it is where God resides.
3. Each direction corresponds to an element. Vastu locates the spaces in the house according to the directions and then puts the activity that corresponds to the element in that space. In this way, architectural plans are designed in harmony with the larger cosmic space and energy. For example, as water is good for meditation, the altar is placed in the northeast corner of the meditation room. The southeast corner corresponds to the element of

fire, so this is the appropriate corner for the kitchen. The southwest corner corresponds to the element earth and is a good location for sleeping and, thus, for the master bedroom. The head of the bed should not face north. The western zone is good for the family room and gathering. The northwest corner corresponds to the element air and is good for children. The northern zone is good for reception and for the living room. In summary:

- Northeast corner (water) – meditation room or home office
- Southeast corner (fire) – kitchen
- Southern zone – dining room
- Southwest corner (earth) – master bedroom
- Western zone – family room
- Northwest corner (air) – children or elders' bedroom
- Northern zone – living room or reception room
- Eastern zone – study room and altar room

## 5. LIVING ECOLOGICALLY BY CONNECTION WITH NATURE – THE BIOPHILIA EFFECT

We humans have a deeply-ingrained love of nature, an intuitive and natural drive to seek connection with nature imprinted in our DNA. Our well-being and overall health can be improved by returning to nature.

- Be aware of the earth, the soil, the rocks and the mineral kingdom. Be aware of the land around you and the ground beneath your feet.
- Be aware of the plants, the trees, and the flowers around you; they are a primary source of prana.
- Be aware of the animal kingdom; feel a connection with animals. We share the same greater life force. Understand the intrinsic wisdom of this world and the cosmic powers that the creatures around you possess. They, too, are an important source of prana and learning.
- Be aware of the waters—oceans, lakes, rivers, streams—around you. The atmosphere, the wind, the clouds, the weather patterns and the seasons are also part of life on this planet.
- Be aware of the sky and the cosmos. And always be aware of the cosmic space that envelops this planet.

This is the foundation of learning to respect all beings; honor the diversity in human culture in art, religion and spirituality. Respect everyone and help to promote global peace and well-being for all. Embrace our spiritual and cosmic origins, and those of all beings around us, to bring peace to the planet.

## 6. CARING FOR ETHICAL GUIDELINES IS CARING FOR THE ENVIRONMENT

We cannot live independently from the environment. Therefore, we need to recognize that our Self-healing must, in part, extend to healing the whole earth. Here are a few guidelines for how we might extend our Self-healing to the larger being that is this planet.

It is fairly obvious to most people that climate change is a very real problem for all species on this planet. Increasing floods and cyclones and storms are a direct result of the temperature changes taking place. Humans are primarily responsible for these changes. Our intelligence comes with too much ego and a lack of tuning to the law of nature and respect for the environment.

Keep in mind that when you practice Yoga and heal yourself, you build the health, the energy and the principles to heal the earth as well; Self-healing and healing of the earth happen simultaneously.

As a Yoga teacher, you can help others to live a more contented life and this will help reduce the strain on the earth. People desire more money, more business, more consumption. This desire is the result of, and the seed of, even greater discomfort. Happiness is not found through increased consumption or increased power. Go in the opposite direction; help people become content by going inward and leading a simple life close to nature.

In this modern era of artificial intelligence, stay humble. Realize that—even though we can replicate, embellish and control everything through the computer, through the study of our brain and through the imitation of neural-networks—there is a level of existence beyond the reach of the senses and the mind. There is the eternal witness of all phenomena as revealed in sacred scriptures.

The yamas and niyamas, the restraints and observances of Yoga, introduced on p. 191, are to be observed personally and collectively to bring balance and enlightenment—here, applied toward the environment.

- The first yama, **ahimsa,** is non-violence and non-injury of any living being. This principle is the foundation of the vegetarian diet that Yogis follow. Our human body constitution is naturally equipped to be more vegetarian. The meat industry causes depletion of resources—water, land, energy—and it creates solid waste pollution and greenhouse emissions. Consuming meat is consuming energy secondhand; grass gets energy from the sun, the cow eats grass and you eat the cow. Vegetarianism is a more intelligent way to live and it is less harmful to the planet.

Drive and fly less. Buy local, seasonal, organic food or grow your own. Reuse, repurpose, recycle, compost. Buy in bulk. Clean the ocean, the land and the environment.

- **Satya,** the second yama, is truthfulness with yourself and others. It is genuine, straightforward, and honest living. Say what you think and do what you say. Examine daily choices honestly and correctly.
- **Asteya** is not stealing or coveting the possessions of others. Not taking what is not yours and detachment from the desire for things leads to a simpler life and contentment. Trust that God will take care of your needs.
- **Brahmacharya** is sublimation and control of our desires and passions by channeling that energy towards something higher such as living in harmony with the greater being that is this planet.
- Avoid consumption for vanity and sexual attractiveness. Channel this energy to a higher cause.
- **Aparigraha** deals with our tendency to be greedy and to seek things for ourselves wherever possible. Do not hoard. Give away things you do not need. Refrain from greed and corruption which is at the root of many environmentally-harmful activities. Only buy the food you need, that you can eat. Don't take too much or let resources and energy go to waste. Think about future generations; if you consume too much, you take from future generations. Live beneath your means, people usually live higher than they need or can afford.

Yoga life has the potential to help the world. By practicing the niyamas, we channel our higher sattvic energy and stay away from rajasic and tamasic energy.

- **Saucha** is cleanliness and purification. Clean your living and work space regularly. Do not accumulate things; declutter and regift to those who actually need them. Keep your body clean, using natural products. Avoid perfumes, artificial soaps, and too many beauty products.

Thought is a very powerful energy. When people think of negative things, or speak of negative things in a space, it shapes and influences the energy and will influence everyone who enters that space. In an effort to purify your body and mind, it is best to avoid negative locations like bars, clubs, and crowded public places. Avoid places where you might expose yourself to negative people; avoid people who gossip and tell lies. Avoid social media and news focusing on sensationalism, drama, and ego. Choose to spend more time in nature. Build good energy in your home. Create your private meditation room, keeping the space clean, purifying the energy with kirtan, arati, and mantra. When you go out or travel, practice using a protective mantra when you move around. Play the mantra *Om Tryambakam*, which is a protective mantra, in your home all the time on low volume; it helps to protect your mind.

- **Santosha** is contentment. Pay attention to the allurements of our consumer society, which always tempts you to consume the best and latest new product. Have a shopping list when you go shopping; shop for what you need and not what you desire. Be content.
- **Tapas** is austerity. Be aware of the temptation to have more comforts for the body and forget the spirit. Practice of austerity in all aspects of life—food, clothing, housing, etc.
- **Swadhyaya** is study of scriptures, which will help keep your priorities in the right direction. It reminds you that you are full and complete in your core Self; you cannot purchase anything outside to gain peace and happiness.
- **Ishvara-pranidhana** is surrender to God's will. It is most important for you to turn inwards, stay content, away from desires and acquisitions.

**Turning inward**

*For the past few years, I have enjoyed being by myself as I've found that I was getting very tired when focused externally and talking with people. It's been nice to know that going inwards is not being rude and helps you to understand the person in front of you better. I had two near death experiences, and each time it brought me closer to myself than ever before. I felt alive and peaceful when I gave up clinging to life on my terms.*

*I was feeling nice, being by myself but there was pressure from my family and friends to get married and have kids. I have tried a few times but, relationships didn't continue and I felt like a failure but there was this reframing when I said to myself: well now I have less to detach from, it might be harder if I were married and had children. The reframing is improving your faculty of discrimination, knowing that you come into this life for yourself or the journey of realization but you are not going to sacrifice your life progress for external relationships.*

*However, I have some strong attachments. My attachment to my parents is very strong. I have an attachment also to knowledge but when I leave the ashram to go home, at home in the city there is no knowledge because everything around me is like the corporate world and my work will not show me who I am.*

*I understand the concept of giving back to the community, of finding myself while giving to others. It is a devotional practice. I feel in my work when I dedicate to my students, it does that. It takes a lot to unbalance me. But when it happens, it feels very intense. But then I can bring it back relatively quickly. But still, you know, it is like walking on shaky ground. I've also been doing quite well, no matter what setbacks there have been, I have been continuing with faith.*

*I think I didn't process the fact that I experienced anger until relatively recently. I realize that I have pushed my anger down and so now it's kind of coming out uncontrollably at times. I did not know that anger comes from desire and expectations. I had a lot of expectations projected on people.*

**QUESTIONS**

1. *Describe 9 obstacles to your journey of self-healing from the perspectives of Yoga and what to do to prevent and deal with them.*
2. *Name 5 ayurvedic lifestyle guidelines that support sadhana life.*
3. *Give 5 examples how Jyotish science helps the Yoga practitioner to adjust and retarget his or her sadhana.*
4. *Give 5 vastu suggestions to enhance your energy in your house and improve your positive life.*
5. *Discuss how we can connect better with Nature and ourselves and how to live ecologically.*

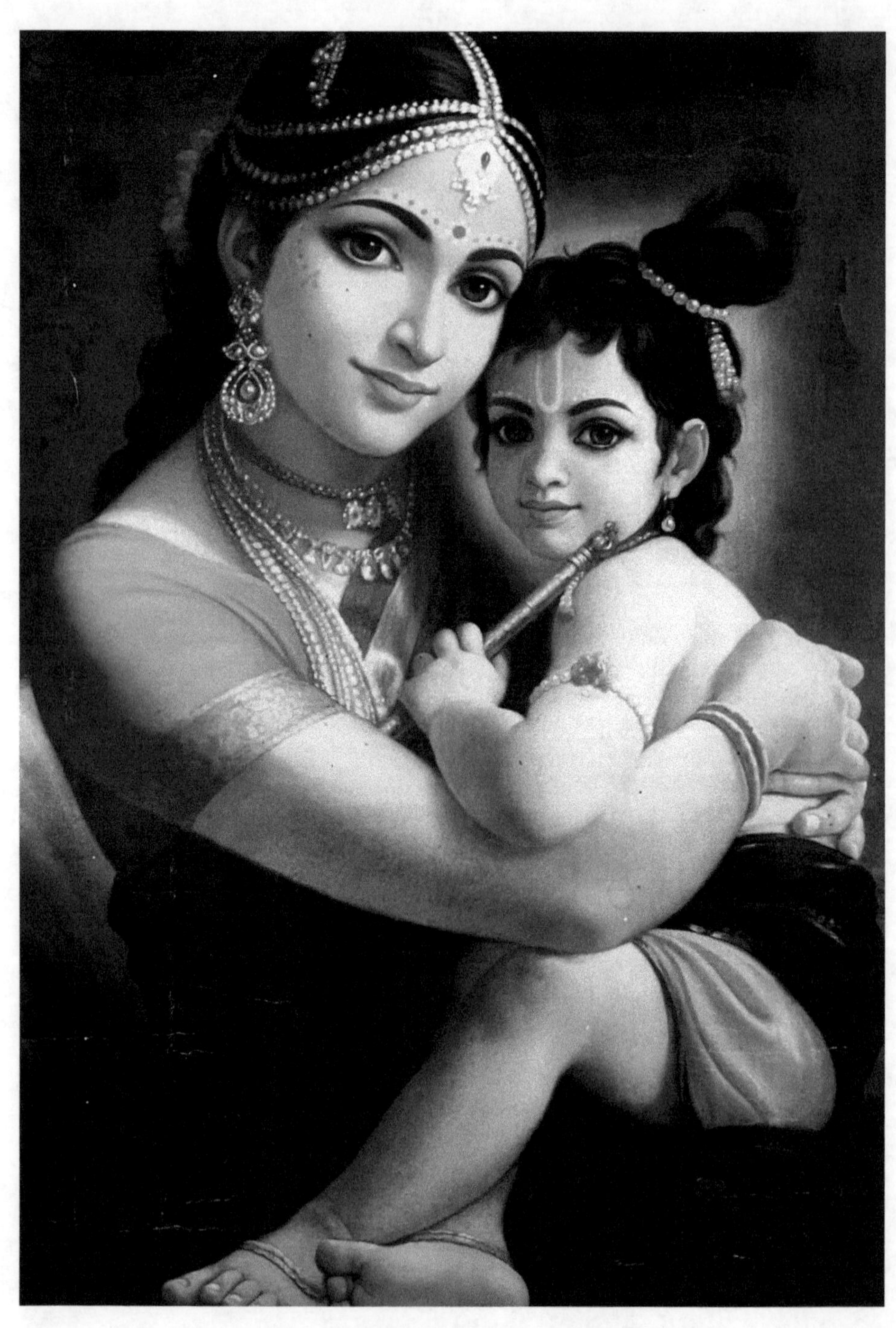

MOTHER YASHODA AND BABY KRISHNA

CHAPTER 10

# Healing Emotions and Relationships

***"The mind becomes clear through the cultivation of friendliness, kindness, contentment, and indifference towards happiness, vice and virtue ". Taming the mind requires the development of goodwill and universal love towards all. Any kind of negative feeling or identification with the dualities of good or bad destroys peace of mind."***

*– SWAMI VISHNUDEVANANDA commentary – Raja Yoga sutras chap 1-33*

Relationships can be a hindrance or a support on the path of Self-healing. Yoga of relationships is about healing emotions and enhancing relationships.

Swami Sivananda said, *"Forget, like a child, any injury done by somebody immediately. Never keep it in the heart, because it kindles hatred."*

## YOGA OF RELATIONSHIPS

We all have lessons to learn from relationships, despite their often causing heartaches and headaches. The problem is we cannot live alone; we are in a network of relationships. We are always looking for true love, which ultimately means being true to the Self. True Self-love leads to true Self-realization. In relationships, communication is often the source of defeat. Often, we fail to understand ourselves and we fail to understand "the other." This invisible wall between self and others manifests as difficulty to find ourselves. We struggle between opening ourselves up or staying in a defensive mode, repressing our feelings, and encountering internal problems. This can happen in all relationships, temporary relationships, but also fundamental relationships.

Family relationships tend to form the deepest impressions in the subconscious. We are born into them and we strongly identify with them. They can be the source of our comforts and safety or the opposite, a source of our griefs and heart knots. Intimate or romantic relationships are very demanding, requiring lots of emotional maturity. They can be either a source of suffering or a great opportunity for personal growth. This kind of relationship adds to our emotional baggage and brings back the subconscious memory of our lower instinctive and sexual nature. We yearn to resolve this deepest feeling of longing for our perfect soulmate.

In Yoga, we believe that everyone is our soulmate. Why? Because, in reality, there is only one soul. There is only one consciousness, one being, but we look for this soulmate externally. We are looking for someone who completely matches everything we seek in an ideal partner. We expect this person to make us feel complete and happy—a very heavy burden to carry. But we pay a great price for this relationship, because to get the love we seek, we have to be the same ideal for our partner.

In general, a relationship exists with each and every person we encounter: co-workers, neighbors, boss, doctor. From a Yogic perspective, we aim to see all humanity as God. We are always in relationship, giving us a chance to experience the richest kind of relationship. These connections serve as training for the ultimate relationship. Through Yoga of relationships, we understand that what happens externally in any relationship is always a reflection of what is happening internally. Relationships are one of the most important ways we learn about ourselves. The experience of separation exists for all of us; it is an existential separation. Relationships reflect our separation from ourselves, through the separation between ourselves and others. Resolving this separation is the Yoga of relationships.

**The problems we have in relationships are universal.**

- Our needs and expectations are not met, so we tend to blame, resent and be angry.
- Unhealed scars cause difficulties in communication. Communication may be insincere, even violent, or we build a wall to avoid any communication at all.
- We cannot understand the other person. We lack empathy and compassion for them, so we suffer from emotional swings between attraction and repulsion; one day we really like the person, the next day we cannot stand them. As emotional swings are happening, we experience very intense, paradoxical and conflicting feelings.

- We want to lose ourselves in love, seeking completion in our soulmate. At the same time, we want to be in control and want to have our way. As a result, we have doubts.
- We feel lonely, even though we are in relationships. We feel jealousy, envy and possessiveness. Also, we may suffer from abuse, unfaithfulness and lack of trust.

**Our goal, our ideal:**
In Yoga of relationships, we can learn how to:

- find ourselves in relationships.
- spiritualize relationships.
- transform our negative emotions into love.
- solve our problems of the split between self and others.

Swami Sivananda said, *"Life is relationships." "Life is love, God is love and God is one."* So love is our essential nature. This is what we are seeking, so we must learn how to love. We have to learn to transform our emotions into pure and selfless love.

**Vedic teaching on karmic relationships:**
All relationships are karmic relationships; they are our teachers. According to the Vedic teachings of karma and reincarnation, it is said that when we chose to be born, we chose our father and mother. Without this original relationship, we would not be here; we choose this relationship and it will have a great influence on the rest of our life.

- **Our first relationship is with our mother, our first guru.** Our mother is said to be the first God, as this relationship is so deep and impactful. A human being takes a long time to become independent; after nine months in the womb, we need to be nursed for at least two years. We cannot function at all on our own and are completely dependent on the mother or caregiver. The first suffering is the suffering of the baby. Babies try to express themselves by crying. Most of the time, the mother has difficulty understanding what her baby wants. The baby has pain, so it cries, and the mother says, *"Poor darling, you must be hungry."* She gives her baby food, which may be exactly what the baby needs to avoid. Despite the mother's care, many people, in their 30s, 40s or even 50s and older, are still suffering from the relationship with their mother. They still cry and say, *"My mother did not love me,"* or *"My mother did not love me as I expected her to love me."*

- **Our second relationship is with our father, our second guru.** Having a present father gives you some sense of stability and he becomes a source of guidance for you when you are older.
- **Our third relationship is with our teachers, our guru.** Because father and mother cannot teach their children everything, they are sent to school to learn from teachers. In ancient times, children could be sent as young as six years old to the gurukula (guru's house) to learn from the teacher.
- **Our fourth kind of relationship is with our "guest."** According to the Vedic tradition, a guest can be anybody in a relationship with the family who comes to the home. In Christianity, the word *"neighbor"* is used; *"Love thy neighbor as thyself."*

Family relationships are karmic relationships; we are learning from these relationships. We need to take responsibility for these relationships. They are no accident; they are the fruit of our own karma.

Relationships exist for us to learn our karmic lessons. We carry emotional patterns and imprints from our family and our relationships from past lives. We are born out of karma; we have certain impressions and temperaments that we bring into this life. This birth, this family and this particular situation are all there to help us resolve the emotional issues and wrong thinking about ourselves due to past karma. If we do not undo our karma through learning in this life, it will reproduce itself in the next life. The Wheel of Karma, the cycle of births and the bondage that comes from our actions during these births, is inexorable. We are born, we learn some lessons, we create new challenges, we die and then we are born again—and the cycle continues. Our karmic emotional patterns and tendencies repeat themselves and are imprinted in our subconscious. We are born to resolve them. But, because the imprints are so deep, we are not aware of them and we continue to reproduce them in this lifetime. Our new relationships end badly and we experience the same emotions again and again. For example, we may feel rejected or let down in relationships, not just once, but many times. It is a very deep wound, that is called karmic relationship.

In Yoga, we aim to stop the cycle of recurring negative emotional patterns of past relationships. This is the practice of Yoga of relationships. We have connections with others, but also a relationship with our Self, our immortal *Atman*, when we come into this life. We have certain skills, certain talents, and certain habits that we inherit from certain circumstances—a setup of the unfolding karma. We have certain character traits developed over time. When we die, our astral body and causal body will continue, along with all of our accrued karma. We take birth in another physical body and carry with us the mental impressions from the past. All the habitual patterns in our mind are carried with us into a new life.

The essence of the problem is that we did not learn to understand our true Self in the past. We mistake our character for our selves and fail to see that it is only born of past karma. We identify with the character traits and replay them in each new relationship.

When we look externally at another person, we are defining ourselves by the differences we perceive between ourselves and the other person. We see the differences and not our true Self. We see the world and we see other people through our tendencies of attraction and repulsion built over past lifetimes. This is how our perception becomes twisted.

In fact, we are searching for ourselves, but we keep projecting ourselves onto others. We see others through the filter of our mind, our preferences. We have our own mind and emotions, but we seek our complete Self in the minds and emotions of others. This is how we create suffering. We don't see ourselves, they don't see them selves, and looking at each other, we all try to see our true Self through distorted mirrors. In fact, we are trying to find ourselves by comparing ourselves with others.

We like somebody because we want to be like them, or we find something in ourselves that looks like them. Or we dislike somebody because we dislike something within ourselves that we see in them. In reality, we are seeking for our true Self. Relationships are always based on these external appearances. We are very attached to our emotions, to the swinging of the mind. These likes and dislikes will create problems sooner or later. Anything we believe ourselves to be will be challenged. But, if we are wise, we realize that it is an opportunity for growth. So, when we are challenged by someone, instead of blaming them, we should say, *"I thank you in my heart for showing me my false belief about myself."*

We have to work on our own inner self, recognizing all the deep negative impressions from the past. We need to forgive and forget. We need to let go of our attachments and replace our negative impressions with positive ones to find love for ourselves and, thus, true love for others.

So, the question is do we really love our own Self? We just described that the love of and attachment to our own character is the cause of suffering as that character keeps reproducing lifetime after lifetime. So, the question is do we really love our true Self? Or do we only love an image, a reflection of the true Self, our karmic or habitual self? When we are in a relationship with somebody, that false ego-self will be confronted. The problems in relationships come up to help us turn towards our true Self and away from this projection of ego-self. Relationship problems are painful, because we seek love, we seek to experience the sweetness of love, but when the relationship is based on the ego-self, it is founded on a false self. In order to find the remedy, we have to really understand the problem and the problem is quite deep, embedded in our karmic tendencies from past lives.

Ideally, when we encounter a problem in a relationship, we use this struggle to reinvent ourselves. We grow in a relationship by unraveling the fundamental truth about self-love. Our relationships will ideally lead us to a more honest relationship with our own true Self. We have to love our true Self. However, we need to be aware of resistance and obstacles in the journey of Self-discovery in an entangled relationship. When someone in the relationship tries to love themselves, tries to truly understand and work on themselves, the other person will think that they are losing love, that their partner is not 100% present in the relationship and they have lost something. So when a person sets out to find themselves, as they should, it becomes a problem for the relationship. A father or mother may subconsciously restrain a child from trying to find themselves, or someone will unconsciously block their partner from embarking on their inner journey.

We can continue to be that person the partner feels safe with, hoping that this relationship will solve all our problems, but we might become even more entangled. When we try to find our true Self, when we try to use the relationship for self-growth, then we start to open up and go in the direction of unity in diversity. This is what Yoga teaches. But in this process of disentanglement and finding true Love, we need to be patient, respectful and aware that our partner might feel uncomfortable or hurt facing a change in the relationship.

The truth is everyone needs to work through their relationships and create a little space for themselves. We have to spend time maintaining the relationship, because it's a karmic relationship. At the same time, we have to create the space for that relationship to open up. We need space for ourselves, space for our self-love, and we need space to build the spiritual relationship with our true Self. Tension doesn't have to become a rupture; it doesn't have to be violent. It does not need to be rejecting one thing and running towards another. It takes time and practice to act with wisdom in situations of tension and deep emotion. We have to open up by creating space. We cannot literally apply all the teachings, but it is even less wise to reject all the teachings and carry on with our old ways. We have direct experience of how our old ways have served us up to this point. To make a shift, we will need to open up, listen to the teachings, give ourselves space away from our emotions and thoughts, so we can view them objectively, with dispassion. Even if the teaching feels like abstract theory, take the time to understand it and ask how it applies to your situation. Take the space and time to step back and use the teachings as a mirror in which to examine your own emotions and actions.

The nature of attachment in love is very deep. It usually allows little or no space. So, it is critical that we create space within our relationships to breathe, reflect, and work on ourselves. If we are able to love ourselves more and our true Self becomes more real, our relationships with others will automatically improve. There will be less blame and more understanding, less judgment and more compassion. If we hate, dislike or are critical of ourselves, we will always be on guard and likely feel the same towards other people. If we're angry with ourselves, that anger will manifest with others. If we're disconnected and fearful with ourselves, we will be disconnected and fearful with others. The pattern is clear; what we struggle with internally, we will bring to our relationships and project onto others. We have to start to love our true Self. We have to work our way through the maze of our mind and emotions and sort out who we are and who we are not, explore what we believe to be true and examine whether it is true or not. Only then will we be able to see our relationships and the tensions in them with clarity.

So how does this work? If we can see ourselves clearly and honestly, and if we can uncover some ideas about ourselves that are not true and discard them, and if we can come to understand the core value of ourselves that is true, we will find that we love and accept ourselves. We will not need, and will stop waiting for, someone external to give us permission to love ourselves. We will stop waiting for someone else to validate our existence. Validation is not a bad thing, it is a mirror in which we know if our self-growth is manifested in the world. Unfortunately, we usually wait for someone external to make us love ourselves; we don't feel it is possible, unless we receive it from outside first. This is just a chain of projections that result in entanglement and misunderstanding.

Self-inquiry through Yoga and meditation helps us to recognize a higher Self, to develop our faculty of discrimination, and to detach from the false or external ideas of ourselves. The practice of Yoga and self-reflection will help us to see the world more objectively, more dispassionately, and free us to view all situations more compassionately. Self-inquiry and meditation practice help us to recognize that solutions come from within. If you have problems in a relationship, don't immediately try to "fix" the relationship. If we are too entangled, we will not see the problem clearly and we will respond with emotion and anger. If, instead, we step back and create some space to look at ourselves and solve the problem from within, then we can return to the relationship with this new clarity, with less emotion and more compassion and understanding for both sides. When we find ourselves, the tension will release nicely and automatically.

The solution to all relationship problems comes from within. Move self-love out of the shadow of your projected image of yourself, and focus on seeing and loving your true Self. To do this, you need to recognize and renounce your lower mind; bring your false ideas of self into the light so you can renounce them. When you shift your mind into a new pattern, a new gear, and you function as a different person. Self-awareness is all it takes. You don't have to force it, just practice Yoga and meditation, and this shift will occur automatically. You do not have to see who you will become, or know exactly the path that will lead you there. Just trust in the practice of Yoga, and practice conscious sadhana. Automatically, you will be free from your habitual pattern and will feel more and more confident in yourself and your capacity to be a beautiful, peaceful, loving, and happy person.

If on the other hand, we will not do this, if we just keep following our old habits and ways of thinking. We will find ourselves stuck in this expectation of something external. We will not be able to see ourselves or truly love ourselves, and the patterns and projections that got us here will only grow deeper. It is these patterns that lead people to feel unfulfilled, and with this, often come the feelings of rejection, self-rejection, existential crisis and depression.

## SELF-HEALING REMEDIES TO RELATIONSHIP PROBLEMS

There are a number of remedies to help us avoid these patterns.

1. **Try to not identify with your ego self, the lower mind**. The moment you detach from this ego self, you will quickly find the True Self. Put a brake on the ego-self. The more you don't find love, the more you replay this narrative of attraction and rejection, the more the ego-self strengthens. This is the wrong direction.

2. **Do selfless service and give yourself to others.** This will help you find yourself, because it helps you think less about the ego-self and more about others. Self-less service will help you identify less with the ego-self.

3. **Transform your emotions into pure love.** To do this, you will need to learn about your patterns of attachment and start to identify these recurring patterns in your life and relationships so you can unlearn them and focus on loving truly and purely.

4. **Identify your types of attachment**

New psychology research has identified four types of attachment. This attachment theory is a useful framework for self-reflection and developing self-awareness.

Understanding your type of attachment will help you understand yourself, your partner, and others with whom you are in relationship. For this research, babies were observed and classified by the different types of behaviors and responses they had to their mother when she was present and when she left the room.

a. **Insecure attachment**

The baby was very happy sitting on its mother's lap. But when the mother got up and left the room, the baby immediately started to cry, felt insecure, perhaps rejected. When the mother returned a few moments later, the baby began to cry even louder, not immediately calmed by her return. It was as if the baby was saying, signaling something like, "You let me down. You left me alone. Why did you do this? Don't do it again." This first type of attachment, actually the most common, is called insecure attachment. We are attached, but we know that we will be let down, that the person might leave us, so we tend to cling. These infants grow up to become insecure adults and display similar, though adult, forms of behavior. They often try to prove themselves, that they are kind and lovable, signaling, "Please don't leave me."

**Working with insecure attachments:** For the anxious-insecure type, you will need to find a stable sense of Self. Remind yourself of the inner resources that you possess and try to develop the ability to see things clearly, to ground and to self-soothe so you can govern your own emotions. The anxious-insecure person needs to have more self-acceptance. To note that self-acceptance doesn't mean that you are perfect or have no areas to improve. It is more that you can see yourself clearly, both strengths and weaknesses, and not collapse with any notion of non-acceptance or judgment.

b. **Avoidant-dismissive attachment**

These infants deliberately display that they don't need the mother who left them, albeit briefly. They, too, are hurt, but, in response, they will signal that they don't need her anyway. It is an attempt to hurt the mother in return. With this type, there is more of a shutdown mechanism. They disassociate. Everyone needs love and relationships, but the second type will not show this. The type of person who is closed off, hidden and dismissive or avoidant needs to learn to be more open and feel more comfortable and trusting in relationships. This avoidant behavior, even if it appears strong and independent, is actually founded on insecurity.

**Working with dismissive-avoidant type of attachment:** Remind yourself that we are all interdependent in nature, that it is natural and healthy to need and rely upon one another, and that it is a sign of connection and community to share resources. Be aware of the urge to leave or dismiss others, and don't take everything as a personal rejection. See strength, not in symbolic independence, but rather in shared support and compassion for one another. This involves developing a strong sense of self-awareness, allowing yourself to understand and view yourself objectively when you are uncomfortable or have the urge to leave.

c. **Insecure-avoidant attachment**

More complicated, this type is a combination of the patterns of the first two types. It is sometimes called the "disorganized personality," as it flips between the two. Sometimes insecure-avoidant people are very needy and they show strong affection in relationships. But in the next moment, they become avoidant, showing, "*I don't need you.*" It is a difficult type to be, and a difficult type to be with.

**Working with disorganized attachment:** You need help in all the areas mentioned for types one and two, as you have qualities of both at different times. The key to all of these types, but in particular this third type, is to find yourself and see yourself and the other, the partner openly, honestly, and objectively with compassion. Learn to be comfortable being uncomfortable.

d. **Secure attachment**

This type of person has emotional stability and has learned to regulate their emotions and understand that all interactions are not about them. They engage with others comfortably and, at the same time, are very secure in themselves; if the partner leaves or focuses attention elsewhere, this type will take it in stride. People who are securely attached appreciate their own self-worth and retain the ability to be themselves in their relationships. They openly seek support and comfort from their partner, and are similarly happy when their partner relies on them for emotional support.

People usually gravitate to a person with secure attachment, because they are emotionally stable. Types one, two and three need to move towards developing secure attachment. Those with secure attachment are like a beacon in the dark; a boat sees the beacon and can find its way home. The insecure person will attach to the secure person and the secure person remains the same. They guide the insecure person to feel safe in relationships.

5. **Be compassionate and patient with ourselves and others**

In the practice of Yoga of relationships, having an honest and objective perspective of yourself and your partner and creating space for yourself is critical. It is very difficult to see yourself or the relationship honestly while in the thick of the emotional entanglements that can develop. Sometimes, you have to wean yourself off of your relationships; step back and take some space so you can see things clearly. Taking space is a form of detachment. So perhaps, you start first with a Yoga class. You can leave home, take your space and do a Yoga class and your partner is okay with this. Maybe you can also take some space within the home to meditate. Create opportunities to turn inward, times when you don't talk and the partner is okay. Slowly, safely for both sides, release some of the attachment and make space so both can approach the relationship and its tensions honestly and compassionately. When you are able to approach things with compassion, it is a sign that you are not overly attached; you have the detachment to see your needs and those of your partner simultaneously. If you are loving, sincere, and respectful in all relationships, you can have meaningful relationships with everyone, and this strength will be perceived and appreciated. You will become more and more yourself in this cultivation of non-egoistic self-love and thus spend less mental energy worrying about yourself or your needs and, instead, have the energy to love and care for others.

**Summary of the remedies in relationships:**

- Cease to identify with the ego-self and the lower mind.
- Practice selfless service; give of yourself to others.
- Learn to transform your emotions and patterns of attachment into pure love for all.

- Become a spiritual seeker. Embark on the journey of self-inquiry, always reflecting on the question, *"Who am I?"* This requires constant self-observation and reflection. It is the path of Jnana Yoga, and is also fostered through self-surrender and the path of Bhakti Yoga.

6. **Nine practices of Yoga of Relationships according to Bhakti Yoga**

The Yoga of Relationships applies the nine practices of classical Bhakti Yoga to develop devotion and pure love in our ideal relationships. The meaning of "ideal relationship" can be interpreted in two ways.

First, it can be unconditional love for our *Ishta-devatā*, our personal ideal, or personification, of the Divine. This can be the Divine Mother, a divine teacher, or any of the deities like Krishna or Shiva, Durga, etc. This type of close affinity with the Divine constitutes the practice of Bhakti Yoga and is said to be the "fast lane" to Self-realization.

Secondly, "ideal relationship" can apply to the practice of divine love towards humanity, extending our attachment, our love, to humanity as a whole. This, too, is a version of recognizing a higher power and devoting ourselves to it. In this instance, humanity is our *Ishta-devatā*.

Classical texts lay out the nine modes or practices of Bhakti. Their purpose is to solve the problem of existential separation that we all experience in this life—separation from God, from others and from the world at large. The practices are about overcoming this separation, learning to become happy and peaceful and whole in all relationships. The nine practices are listed here, from the easiest to most difficult:

i. Listen to inspiring divine stories. Or, applied to humanity, listen to others and to yourself without judgment.

ii. Sing God's glories. Applied towards humanity, it means appreciating yourself and others. See the good in them and praise them. Normally, our minds are busy finding fault with people. Now we need to be busy finding good qualities in others.

iii. Remember the Lord's name in prayers. Or, applied to humanity, remember and see the Divine in others, in all your relationships.

iv. Serve with humility. Practice selfless service towards the Divine or towards humanity with humility.

v. Give to the Self and others. Give, give, give—every day!

vi. Offer prostrations. Honor the divinity and all that it is. Or, if applied to humanity, give respect, bow to humanity and the Divine within.

vii. Cultivate the feeling of self-sacrifice to God and remove the ego in all you do.

viii. Cultivate the feeling of friendship with God or with humanity. Be friendly, sincere and truthful with everyone.

ix. Complete Self-surrender is the most difficult step. It means accepting all things that happen with equanimity and calmness, overcoming your own expectations and judgments.

7. **Practice of forgiveness**

In Yoga of relationships, the practice of forgiveness is essential. Forgiveness is something everyone needs to practice.

Forgive all together and for all time, never returning to resentment. Here is a list of nine steps to forgiveness (according to Dr. Fred Luskin. Ref *Forgive for Good).*

i. Know, or be aware of, exactly how you feel about what happened. Do not repress any of the emotion or feeling, just acknowledge and understand.

ii. Commit to yourself that you will do what you have to do to feel better. Forgiveness is for you, not anyone else.

iii. Understand that forgiveness does not mean reconciliation with the person who hurt you or condoning the action that caused the hurt. What you are looking for is peace.

iv. Change your perspective on what is happening. Recognize the primary distress is coming from hurt feelings. It is not coming from the action, but, rather, from your response to it.

v. Apply simple stress management techniques. when you feel upset, to soothe your body's fight or flight response.

vi. Let go of expectations.

vii. Channel your energy towards meeting your inner goal, not waiting for others to change their actions towards you. What did you experience from the interaction? Exercise agency to realize it yourself, not through another.

viii. Remember that a life well-lived is the best revenge. Live it. Don't give another the control of your mind and emotions.

ix. Rewrite your inner grievance narrative to focus on your choice to forgive.

8. **How trauma affects relationships**

The last factor to consider is the effect of trauma on relationships. Most people have experienced some form of trauma in their lives. Basically, trauma is an emotional response to an extremely negative event, such as a natural disaster, war, violence, or the loss of a loved one. The person experiences that their life is in danger and they feel a sense of helplessness. This triggers the body's inner alarm system—fight, flight or freeze. The inner scarring from the experience interferes with the person's ability to live life "normally." Random things can bring the experience back in full force, or perhaps the person is perpetually living in a heightened state of fear that cannot be turned off, impacting many aspects of their life. Trauma and its repercussions can resurface for weeks, months or years after the actual event, often in seemingly unrelated circumstances.

The experience of trauma manifests in the body in many ways. A person suffering from trauma appears to be shaken, disoriented, often unable to respond or have a conversation; they appear withdrawn. They may have feelings of helplessness or anxiety. They may have nightmares and flashbacks. The person often feels very fatigued, weary of everything; this is a sign of reduced or blocked prana. They may have a rapid heart rate, panic attacks, feelings of emptiness or emotional numbness. They sometimes resort to substance abuse, or self-medication, to numb the pain. If pushed to the extreme, they may resort to suicide as the only way out of the pain and suffering. They may experience dissociation, or the sense of being separated from the body. All of these responses to trauma and the prolonged state of stress the body undergoes can lead to a number of physical ailments, such as heart disease, auto-immune disorders, or mental health problems. Trauma can cause systemic symptoms that appear unrelated to the original trauma. It is the trauma which must be addressed to truly reverse the problem and return the sufferer to a sense of peace and well-being.

Yoga can help to regulate the nervous system and return the whole person—body, mind, and spirit—back to health. We would have to manage all these symptoms and return ourselves to some level of control. Always keep the core trauma in mind, as it is the catalyst, the source, which must be addressed. Some techniques to help with coping are:

i. Develop a sense of self-connection and safety (through Yoga practices).

ii. Nurture understanding of the situation.

iii. Learn to respond, but not react.

iv. See the situation as an opportunity to learn.

Endeavor to understand the situation and, through understanding, slowly regain control of yourself. The first step is compassion, understanding and connection, so you can feel that you are not alone in this anymore. Develop an understanding of the ways trauma can surface in your life and—especially as we are talking about relationships—how past trauma can cause all sorts of tensions and reactions in the relationship. Recognize them as misplaced responses to past trauma, completely unconnected to the relationship or the present circumstances. This points to the strong need of developing the skills of deep self-awareness and understanding.

Trauma always creates deep wounds, touching us at very deep levels, so it is important to understand that any necessary change will take a long time. Do not expect that you can just switch your view quickly. You will not succeed and will only be disappointed, so set expectations that are honest and fair. Set expectations with the humility to know that you might not know how deep the wound is. The practice of self-affirmation and remembrance of our True Self that is untouched, unhurt, that is the perfect *Atman* is of great importance to work out this karma.

## *INSPIRED STORY*

### Healing Gut Pain

*A 50-year-old "Helicopter Mom," wanting to be everything to everyone, presented with debilitating gut pain. She had been to see several doctors, with no conclusive diagnosis and was resorting to hours of searching on the internet.*

*Only self-imposed periods of fasting gave her any dependable relief. Determined to be active and not miss any fun family activities (like zip-lining and indoor skydiving!), she would push through any pain she was experiencing. Sometimes she felt better afterward, and sometimes the pain returned with a vengeance. Our sessions together included breath awareness and regulation techniques and a slow asana sequence with lots of relaxation. They also included a fair amount of talking.*

*Over the weeks, she revealed her codependent relationship with both of her children and her parents—and her over-consumption of pre-packaged diet meals. She was not able to do the five-minute breath check-ins five times a day that she was assigned. She didn't have privacy, she was too busy, someone or another needed her... and then there was the three-hour daily escape on Facebook. Although she was evolving in some areas of her life, the habit of giving 200% to others at the detriment of herself was entrenched. No thought of self-care. She was conflicted over her responsibility to her grown children. She heroically wanted to save her parents from the effects of aging.*

*Over time, she realized she needed to speak up, set some boundaries, and value what was best for her. She became more detached, worrying less, leaving her children to solve their problems—and no longer experienced gut pain. Yes, she ceased to experience gut pain!*

**QUESTIONS**

1. *Yoga of relationships states that we try to see our own Self through the distorted mirror of other people. Comment on this according to your experience.*
2. *Describe 4 types of attachment.*
3. *What are the 9 Modes of Bhakti Yoga? How can they be applied in your network of relationships?*

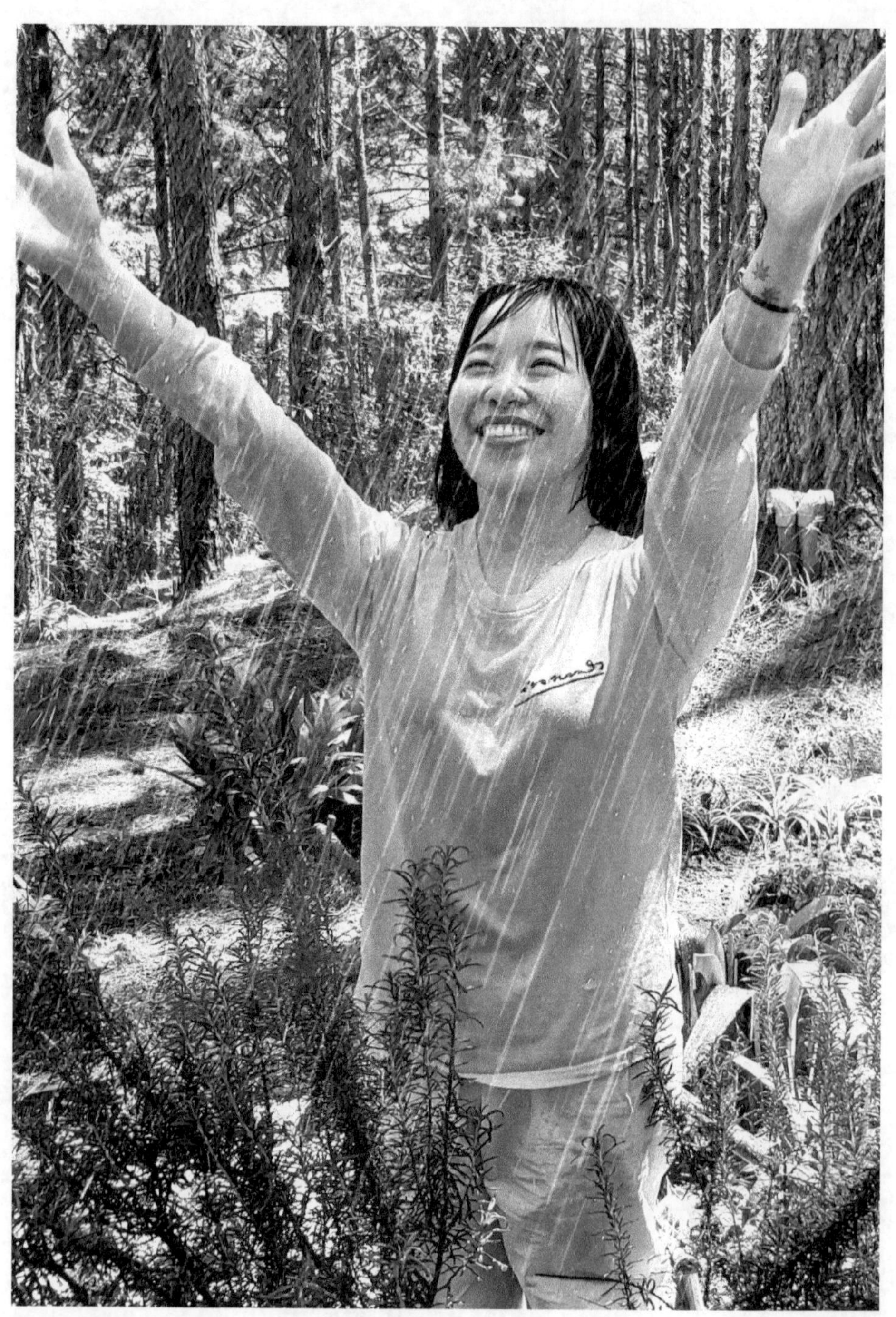

RAIN BATHING

# CHAPTER 11

# Cultivating Selfless Love

***"Love is the law of life. To love is to fulfill the Law. To live is to love. To love is to Live. You love that you may learn to live in the Eternal."***

– SWAMI SIVANANDA in Bliss Divine

This chapter continues the topic of Yoga of relationships. Cultivating selfless love means opening your true heart and learning how to love. Here, we go more in-depth on how to open our hearts and how to expand our relationships.

The first step in the development of love and the opening of your heart is to understand what is the true nature of love. Love is oneness, love is union, love is Yoga. When you practice Bhakti Yoga, you are already starting to practice selfless love.

The journey to selfless love is the journey from the subconscious mind to the conscious mind, and then to the superconscious mind.

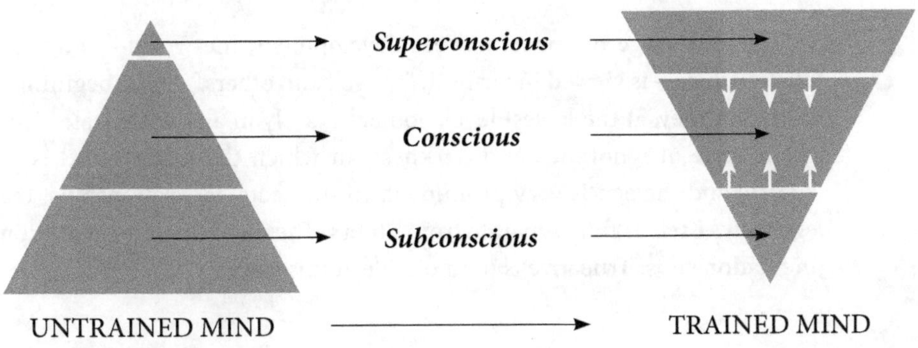

The journey to selfless love can be visualized as two pyramids, representing the development of consciousness, one pointed up and one pointed down. The first pyramid represents our state of cousciousness when untrained, when the subconscious accounts for 90–95% of the activity. The subconscious which is below our level of awareness, includes our lower emotions, our habits, our memories, and our past, as well as our animal instincts or the lower aspects of our nature. Through practice, we reduce the control of our subconscious mind and use our conscious (intellectual) mind more and, eventually, we reach our superconsciousness, or intuition, at the top.

Using the conscious mind means being more aware and using our intellect more, by reducing the influence of the lower urges and emotional responses. Before we develop our consciousness, our relationships might be based on the subconscious, i.e. based on our instincts and emotions, our likes and dislikes. A conscious relationship is one where you become aware of what you and the other have in common and you actively work on the relationship.

At the superconscious level, your mind becomes pure, with no ego, is intuitive and requires less thinking. As the conscious mind and the superconscious mind grow and develop, the subconscious will become less dominant and will no longer work contrary to the true, pure Self. At that time, you will function less from your instincts, emotions, and past habits. This evolution of the mind is the journey towards higher consciousness.

**The process of transcendence**

To understand how this idea applies to relationships, we need to look at the process of transcendence, which is the process of expansion beyond the limits of the ego or self-consciousness. The transcendent reality is the reality beyond the mind, accessible in deep meditation.

It is useful to see the evolution of the ego-self in relationship with others at each level of consciousness development.

1. **In the first stage** of consciousness development, the world—and thus relationships—is viewed in terms of "the self and others." At the beginning of the journey, at the lowest level, you are mainly in a tamasic state. This is the state of ignorance and darkness, in which the lower mind is in control and the ego is very prominent. In this state, in relationships, the ego views itself as fully separate from others. There is complete separation in relationships. True love is not possible at this stage.

**Stage 4: Oneness**
(PURE SATTWA)

**Stage 3: Together but separated**
(SATTWA)

**Stage 2: Ego exchange and bargain but the individuals are separated**
(RAJAS)

**Stage 1: Complete separation**
(TAMAS)

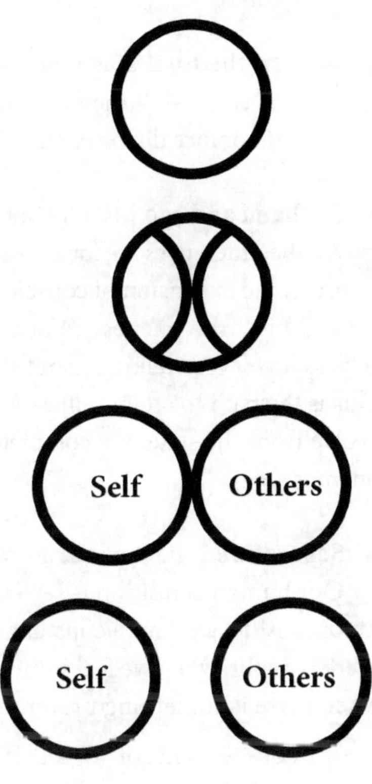


2. **In the next stage,** you enter into a more rajasic state of mind. The ego-self or "I" and the "other" connect. It is the start of relating to the other, but it is a relationship built entirely on exchange. I give you this and you give me that; we share only transactionally. I give you this much attention and love and you give me the same amount of attention and love in return. In this stage, the "I" and the "other" come closer and see each other, but are still not truly connected.
3. **In the next stage,** as you evolve, the mind becomes more sattvic. The sattvic mind is a state of more purity, harmony, unity, knowledge, and wisdom. In this stage, we can speak of "we," as the "I" and the "other" have begun to merge. We act together, we are together, we think of each other, we exist together. But, the union is not complete. There is still some separation, some independence, ego assertion and cultural differences, etc., but we think in terms of sharing and of being one collective. In this sattvic state, we are more respectful and considerate; our capacity of love is expanded. We understand the bigger picture, that we share the same humanity. We are under the wing of the Divine and are aware that there is only one world, one existence, one truth, one love. But some differences still remain between you and me.

4. **In the final stage,** or what we might call pure sattva—which is not easy to attain—all the differences dissolve. The ego dissolves; the darkness and ignorance dissolve. There is Oneness in consciousness and there is pure love.

**Sadhana and ego dissolution**

All the differences are forged by ignorance and will dissolve through our sadhana. Through the expansion of consciousness and increased purity, the ego dissolves and we will find true oneness. When we talk about opening the heart and cultivating selfless love, we're talking about this particular goal, this journey of consciousness. This is the path to attain selfless love. It is a long process and requires great effort to evolve from the state of a completely separate ego to the state of complete love and oneness.

**Separation is part of our human condition**

Our human condition is separation; we suffer from this separation and long for union. Inside, we have a constant desire for union and love. We always suffer when there is a split, when we feel some notion of duality, some notion of incompleteness, when there is something preventing us from feeling the oneness of all things.

The conscious life of Yoga, Self-healing and the realizing of our True Self help us heal this split between the self and others, between ourselves and everything that we consider to be outside of ourselves. Swami Sivananda said, *"Destroy all barriers that separate men from men. Recognize the immortal essence within all creatures. Protect animals. Let all lives be sacred."* Swami Vishnudevananda dedicated his life for world peace and unity, flying his plane over areas of active combat and offering flowers. He said, *"Cross borders with love and flowers and not with bombs."*

## FOUR TRUTHS ABOUT LOVE

1. **Love is oneness, unity, Yoga.** The simple truth is, we all want to love. Love is unity, not this vague idea of romantic love.
2. **Selfless love has to be learned.** Few understand that we need to learn how to love. The fact is, as our sense of ourselves evolves, our love evolves. It is our spiritual journey. Learning to open our hearts is a journey—moving from the lower, subconscious mind to the conscious and then to the superconscious, intuition and union with all. In the words of Swami Sivananda, *"It is a journey from diversity to unity."* Where we now see diversity in each other, we come to see unity. It is a journey from fear and hatred to conscious cosmic love. There is still much hatred and many wars

in this world. We must learn to see the other, not as separate but, as part of the collective whole, as are we. We must move from thinking in terms of the ego, in terms of "my" relationship problems, towards a consciousness of all and a love of humanity. In the previous chapter, we said one remedy for your personal relationship problems is to expand the network of relationships, learning to love other people. This does not mean expanding our group only slightly, but rather it means learning to hold compassion for all. Compassion is a term very common in Buddhist teachings, while in Yoga, we say selfless love, pure love.

In chapter 12 of the *Bhagavad Gita*, speaking on the Yoga of devotion it says, *"He who hates no creature, who is friendly and compassionate to all, who is free from attachment and egoism, is balanced in pleasure and pain and is forgiving* [XII:13], *who is ever content, steady in meditation, who possesses a firm conviction, is self-controlled, with the mind and the intellect dedicated to Me, he, My devotee, is dear to Me*" [XII:14].

Swami Sivananda advised being compassionate towards the people who seem to be lower than you, friendly towards the people who are equal to you, and respectful to people who are superior or more knowledgeable than you. We often do the opposite; we despise people that seem to be inferior, because we feel ourselves as superior and we disrespect people who we think are superior, because we are competing with them.

3. **Love is not desire.** Love is love for love's sake. Desire is an expression of ego, love is an expression of selflessness. Love of the body, of the external that you see in a person, is not love, it is passion. The love of God, the love of divinity as seen in people is called prema. It is divine or unconditional love; it is devotional love; it is pure love.

Why do we want to love so much? Sure, happiness comes from love. True happiness is not just emotional, or satisfaction of desire, it is the fulfillment of our soul's longing to be united, to be whole. True happiness is the loss of separation from others and the experience of unity with the Divine.

Krishna refers to the devotees in the *Bhagavad Gita* as "*those who fix their mind on me*" [XII:2]. This indicates that to love means to be concentrated, steady, faithful, and in continuous devotion to the Divine; this is prema. Krishna said these devotees are the best Yogis. Devotion is dedicating yourself fully with single-pointedness of mind and of heart to the highest goal. If we don't cultivate this steady, faithful, and selfless love, our minds and hearts are never steady; we love this person one day, and that person another day. We are constantly changing—and we are constantly suffering. This is the big drama of life. When there is a lack of faithfulness, there is continuous drama. We need to love the Divine that we see in other people in a continuous and stable manner.

The idea of faith is inherent here. We cultivate faith, as opposed to having doubt, which is inevitable in our journey climbing upward. We don't always have certainty, but if we are wise, we turn within and feel the truth of what we are seeking. We feel intuitively the wholeness, the completeness, the oneness in divine pure love. Because we lack that intuitive experience, we need to rely on faith in moments of doubt to give us the strength to continue our journey. Faith comes from the intuitive knowledge that the truth is there for us, that true happiness coming from pure love is attainable and we should not doubt or be depressed.

When Krishna speaks of "*those who worship me*" [XII:3], he means "those who have a feeling of love and respect for the Divine." This is the divinity we aim to see in all—our husband, wife, father or mother. But if you worship, renouncing all actions, i.e. you do everything in the spirit of Karma Yoga, without ego and with devotion, meditating on the Divine with single-minded Yoga, the Divine will become your savior.

The Divine and *prema* will lift you out of this ocean of samsara, out of the cycle of birth and death, of suffering and drowning. The Divine will elevate you, if you have love and respect for the divine in all human beings—your divine teacher, your divine husband, a divine person who is challenging you in this life. See the Divine constantly in all. See the Divine amidst the constant change. This is a very difficult thing to do. Nevertheless, it is a very worthwhile goal, given what it brings.

Sri Krishna also says, "*If you are unable to fix the mind on me, on the Divine, then by the Yoga of constant practice, do thou reach me*" [XII:9]. If you cannot see the Divine constantly in all, amidst the constant change, then you must constantly and continuously practice to do so. It is difficult, but you must constantly practice moving away from the subconscious mind that keeps you separate from others and pulls your love and devotion down to lower levels. Constantly work to lift your mind to conscious love and, eventually, to the superconscious, intuitive type of selfless love. And if you are not able to practice Yoga, not yet able to meditate and focus your energy within, then practice Karma Yoga. Learn to elevate the mind through selfless action and by renouncing the results of your actions.

Krishna also said you need to restrain the senses. If you want to attain a higher level of love, you have to constantly pull your mind inward and control the senses which lead you back to lower levels of attachment. You cannot just live an external life, constantly projecting outwardly. Attainment of pure love is not possible if you continue to see names and forms in this external world, and continue to look outward. You have to be steadfast in your journey and pull your mind inward, restraining the senses and keeping the mind even. Maintain calm when you meet something that you like or something that you dislike; always keep your mind calm and intent on the welfare of all beings. In this way, you can come closer to that state of union with the Divine, a state of true Yoga.

*"A Yogi's mind must always remain balanced in pleasure and pain, free from attachment and egoism"* [*Bhagavad Gita*, XII:13]. The teaching here is to keep yourself, at all times, detached, centered within, without egoism, and seeking true love. Do not look externally and do not be swayed by the external world. Stay balanced and calm in your encounters with pleasure and pain in the external world, i.e. detach from whatever comes your way. Don't run from pain, don't run to pleasure. Always be forgiving, always understanding that humans make mistakes.

Krishna proclaims, *"He by whom the world is not agitated, and who cannot be agitated by the world...is dear to Me"* [XII:15]. This person lives in such a way that they do not create disturbances or turbulence in this world. At the same time, this person is not disturbed by whatever happens in the world, be it drama, catastrophe, people being dishonest or cheating, etc. Their mind is not disturbed, but remains calm and clear, because they stay stable in that steadfast love of the Divine within.

*"They are detached, pure, efficient, impartial, never anxious, selfless in all their undertakings; they are my devotees, very dear to me"* [XII:16]. When you are so close to the Divine, you are willing to renounce new things that might make you happy, because you believe that God is doing everything, there is nothing you need to do.

*"He who neither rejoices, nor hates, nor grieves, nor desires, renouncing good and evil and who is full of devotion is dear to Me* [XII:17].

*"He who is the same to friend or foe, and also in honor or dishonor, who is the same in cold and heat, and in pleasure and pain, who is free from attachment"* [XII:18].

*"He to whom censure and praise are equal, who is silent, content with anything, homeless, with a steady mind and full of devotion, such a one is dear to Me"* [XII:19].

(Homeless here does not mean that you are unhoused, but rather that you're not attached to a particular location or to the particular people you live with.)

4. **Love is not attachment.** The fourth truth about selfless love, that we need to contemplate continuously, is that love is not attachment. True love is detachment. Emotional detachment does not mean rejection, it means learning to see the True Self that is Love Absolute and Bliss Absolute and feeling fulfilled in this realization. Detachment doesn't mean that you don't have feelings, it just means that you dedicate yourself to the love of the Divine in all and you don't desire anything else from the outside physical or emotional world.

   *"Peace immediately follows renunciation"* [XII:12]. This is a very important promise. We are born with the habit of attachment—attach, detach, attach, detach. Our life is not peaceful if we are not attached to something. We will lose it, cry a little bit, and then get attached to something else, and the cycle continues. The mind is addicted to attachment, but remember, *"Peace immediately follows renunciation."* If we renounce, if we truly learn to let go, then we have peace.

### Swami Sivananda's six practices to cultivate devotion

There are methods to help us cultivate Bhakti or devotion. Sivananda gave a list of six things that we can do:

1. The most helpful is the service of a Bhakta, a true devotee. When we don't have devotion, we don't see the Divine anywhere, so the top remedy is to do selfless service. Be in the company of Bhaktas—sadguru, sannyasis, saints, holy persons—and serve them. Devotion is contagious. We get some feeling of devotion when we do service of a true Bhakta, because they are always immersed in divine love.
2. Repeat a mantra or God's name; it is active remembering.
3. Practice within Satsanga or spiritual company. High-minded people will help keep your mind high and develop devotion.
4. Chant kirtan.
5. Study spiritual books to purify your mind.

6. Go on pilgrimage. Instead of traveling just to see new landscapes and tourist sights, go to places where there are sages, saints, and temples of historical praise; this will help kindle your devotion.

**Classical Bhakti Yoga's nine ways of devotion**

Nine modes are prescribed by classical Bhakti Yoga to develop devotion towards our chosen symbol of God or Ishta-devatā. Here are the nine ways to worship a chosen deity:

1. *Shravana* - listening to stories of the Divine
2. *Kirtana* - singing God's glory
3. *Smarana* - remembrance of his name and presence in prayers
4. *Pada-sevana* - service with humility, or literally "service at the feet of the lord"
5. *Archana* - worship, such as puja
6. *Vandana* - devotional gesture of prostration before a deity, guru, or a holy person
7. *Dasya* - cultivate feelings of being servant of God
8. *Sakhya* - cultivate feelings of friendship with God
9. *Atma-nivedanam* - complete self-surrender

**Bhakti Yoga applied to humanity**

If your chosen deity is humanity itself, you also need to learn to apply these nine modes of devotion.

1. Learn to listen to other people without judgment.
2. Praise other people. Look for their positive qualities.
3. Hold people you love in your heart. Be grateful for all people in your life.
4. Cultivate sacredness in relationships and serve other people.
5. Worship. Offer your time and present gifts to other people.
6. Offer prostration, give respect to other people.
7. Develop the attitude of self-sacrifice.
8. Learn to open your heart equally to all without ulterior motives.
9. Learn to accept all things happening to you or done by others with equanimity.

**Seven practices to open the heart**

(Ref. *Learning Selfless Love*, Swami Sitaramananda)

1. **Assert being love.** We always refer to being loved or loving another, but this first practice is to say, "I am love." Instead of asserting ourselves, "I am strong, I am intelligent, I am rich, I am pretty," we practice saying, *"I am love."* Close your eyes and feel the inner voice. To do that, those who are in emotional need must withdraw the emotions, feel beyond the emotional need. Assert, *"I am love."*

   For those who are more intellectual, the practice is to relax and learn to trust. Allow the soft feeling to emerge towards other people. Be aware that the intellect will block this feeling.

2. **Reduce the extremes of the emotional roller coaster.** Recognize the extremes within and find a balance between not too much hatred, not too much love, not too much passion. Free yourself from the opposites and don't allow yourself to go to these extremes. The *Bhagavad Gita* talks about the practice of equanimity. Maybe it is difficult to be equanimous, but at least we need to manage the extremes. Whether we are with friend or foe, remain the same.

3. **Seek peace of mind, as it leads to happiness.** Most of the time, we are desperately looking for happiness; we resort to our old ways and habits of finding it. But if we know happiness is temporary, we will not seek it again. Our old habits do not work to bring us true happiness. They bring a moment of respite and set us up for the next disappointment. Therefore, cease to look for happiness. Look for peace of mind. When we find peace, a gentle happiness stirs naturally. Aim to find peace, not happiness, and the happiness will happen automatically.

4. **Open the heart through forgiveness, compassion, gratitude, tolerance and a non-judgmental attitude.** Exchange judgment for tolerance. The moment you find yourself starting to judge somebody, acknowledge it and switch it to tolerance. Show generosity of heart, feel compassion for the person and understand them where they are. Feel forgiveness; it untangles the knots of the heart. Be clear that forgiveness does not mean you accept the wrongful act. Rather, you detach and see the act and the person objectively, with compassion and understanding. You forgive and continue to live your life.

   A simple practice that has been a help to many is the practice of gratitude. Every morning, make a list of five things that you are grateful for. This will help you to keep your heart open. With an open heart, you start your day in positive spirits and in a harmonious relationship with others. Notice when you get tired and the heart begins to close again. Keep opening it. Be vigilant and recognize any tendency to react when you are in unfamiliar situations or whenever defensiveness and fear are triggered. These come from the memories of the past, so be aware to not fall back to old patterns of defensiveness, fear, and hurt that stir in the subconscious mind. Approach everything consciously.

5. **Healing the emotions in order to attain pure love.** The emotions come from the subconscious mind, below the level of consciousness. We don't even always know they are there. Learn to be aware of them and heal them—fear of death, fear of being alone, fear of loss, fear of public criticism, anxiety, hatred, anger, greed, desire, lust, envy, and so on. Instead of feeling you lack something, or longing for something, feel whole and complete as who you truly are.

6. **Cultivate faith.** First, establish the spiritual ideal of love and then practice the spiritual relationship. Love your chosen ideal from within and experience the awakening of the spiritual heart, called *hridaya* in Sanskrit. *Hri* means "to give," *da* means "to take," and *ya* means "balance." Therefore, *hridaya* is "that which gives and takes in perfect balance." Dr. David Frawley says, "The soul dwells in the heart of all creatures and is the source of real feeling and knowing." This is not the physical heart, but the core of our being, which we experience in the region of the heart in the physical body. It is the magnetic force of the soul, working through our heart, which can hold us at a level where no external disturbances can reach. This is the cave of the heart; it is difficult to reach the cave.

7. **Self-love; love of the *Atman*.** Contemplate the *Atman* within. Self-love does not come naturally. Self-love and love of God are the same. Scriptures talk about the *Atman*, the True Self, which is different from the ego. Take time to hear and study scriptures, and contemplate on the True Self. Think of the supreme *Atman*—that has no separation, no name, no form, no duality—that is the Indweller.

The first step is Bhakti Yoga or love of God. The end step is love of the True Self. We practice Bhakti Yoga first to learn humility and non-egoism, then Jnana Yoga, the Yoga of Self Knowledge. Love God first, then love the *Atman*. Self-Love comes with self-discipline of the mind and the heart. All relationships, including the relationship with Nature, are relationships with the *Atman*, the Self. Assert *"I am Satchitananda, Existence, Knowledge, Bliss*

*Absolute. I am with you, I am you, I love you, no matter who you are. You are My Own Self."* Practice Vedantic or Jnana Yoga meditation, refuting the five coverings or koshas.

**Practice of puja ceremonial worship**

Puja is a ceremony through which you can express divine love by offering externally to your *Ishta-devatā* (chosen Ideal). A puja can be very elaborate (sixteen steps, taking from 1–2 hours) or simple (ten steps, taking 15–20 minutes). Optionally, the entire puja can be done mentally, as it is about your devotion and not about the external rituals. Here are ten simplified steps of a puja:

1. *Meditating* on the deity that is being invoked
2. *Aavaahana* – Inviting the deity onto the altar
3. *Asana* – Giving the deity a seat
4. *Abhishekam*– Bathing the deity with water
5. *Vasthra* – Dressing the deity in clean clothes
6. *Gandha* – Spreading fresh sandalwood paste on the deity
7. *Pushpa* – Offering fresh flowers while chanting the deity's names
8. *Dhoopa* – Offering incense at the altar
9. *Arati* - Waving a lamp to illuminate the freshly-decorated deity
10. *Naivedyam* – Offering the deity some food

The act of going through the steps of a puja purifies your heart. The invocation can be done mentally, calling in any form of the Divine.

Worship of the Divine Mother is an easy approach to the Divine. In this life, it is difficult to see God as consciousness, but it is easier to see the Divine Mother, or Shakti. We can relate to the Para Shakti as the power of the Divine, the force that creates all. There are three forms of the Divine Mother—Maha Saraswati, Maha Lakshmi and Maha Kali or Durga or Maheshwari. The Divine Mother can represent the power of knowledge, the power of prosperity, divine will, divine power—ultimately, the power that holds everything together.

**Kirtan, an effective way to uplift your mind**

Another of the nine modes of Bhakti is kirtana. We can do kirtan alone or in satsang with many people. We can do akhanda kirtan, which is continuous kirtan. Kirtan practice should not be a mere show. Kirtan is the prescribed method of devotion in this Kali Yuga (iron or dark age). Kirtan is the easiest and surest method of devotion in Bhakti Yoga.

With Bhakti Yoga, we cultivate our faith. We understand that everything is a test of faith. This is not a blind faith, or religious faith, but is spiritual knowledge, spiritual understanding. We need to contemplate to develop faith. Faith is *shraddha* in Sanskrit. Bhakti and Jnana, devotion and knowledge, eventually meet each other. Faith manifests as aspiration. A sadhaka, or spiritual seeker and aspirant, yearns to have the divine experience and always contemplates on how to attain the object of pure love.

Keep practicing that yearning, that longing and eventually you will realize self-surrender and grace. Self-surrender is the highest level in Bhakti Yoga; it is the surrendering of the separate self to God and the experience of grace. The challenge is that the ego resists the idea of surrender, but purification of ego is needed for the attainment self-surrender. There is no loss in self-surrender; we receive the whole wealth of the Lord and will be free from all desires and cravings. Swami Sivananda said, *"The Lord loves you even when you turn away from him. How much more shall he love you if you turn to him sincerely with faith and devotion? Very great is His love, greater than the highest mountains. Very deep is his affection, deeper than the fathomless depth of the ocean."*

## QUESTIONS

1. *Explain the sentence: The journey to selfless love is the journey from the subconscious to the conscious to the superconscious mind.*
2. *Describe the stages towards oneness or transcendence of the ego.*
3. *Give some practices of opening of the heart and explain why we need to heal our emotions in order to attain Pure Love.*
4. *Describe 9 modes of Bhakti Yoga as applied towards humanity.*
5. *Why does service of Bhaktas help the development of devotion?*

## *INSPIRED STORY*

**Selfless Love**

*This lady over 60 years old had a malignant soft tissue sarcoma and had her leg amputated. Her disease metastasized to the lungs and also she had lung cancer.*

*In the past, she worked in the army, so she was very active. Now she feels very hopeless. She no longer believed she could do anything. She came to Yoga to have me teach her how to breathe because this practice could improve the health of her lungs. When I started teaching her, she refused to learn, she resisted with anger. In the class, after 15 minutes, she cried: "I'm tired. Break!", even though the full class was free. At first, I thought "I teach without any money, why do I have to suffer like this". But then I saw her suffering and decided to write a diary about her.*

*Day 1, aggressive temperament, resistance, only 15 minutes of exercise. Day 2, did more exercises on the eyes and neck. Day 3, start a full workout: eyes, neck, shoulders, and even leg lifts. On day 4 was able to put her feet on the wall. After the 4th day, she started to laugh and practice. And slowly I taught the full sequence of 12 poses of Sivananda Yoga, adjusting to her health condition. After 14 days, she told herself that now she feels more in love with life. And she thanked me very much.*

*After the course with her, she became interested in practicing and wanted to practice yoga every day. In her case, I was not able to sit and counsel her until the 10th day. It was then that I discovered that she had been depressed for 20 years. Many mental issues have led to cancer. Through this case, I feel that yoga is a great tool. After the students feel well, they can begin to absorb the philosophy, become ready to listen, and ready to self-transform. The important thing I have learned as a yoga teacher is to be patient and compassionate. In such difficult times, the spirit of karma yoga has helped me a lot. I encountered many other similar cases and began to have more faith and confidence as a yoga health educator.*

**Remember the tiny flame in the heart**

*Mumukshutva, the burning desire for liberation, the desire to go beyond limitation, is it the same as my goal in life, which was to be one with God?*

*If not, how do I reconcile my desire to be one with God with an emotion-burning desire for liberation? Are they the same thing? I believe that my desire to be one with God stems from that fullness of heart that I felt when I was chanting Bhajans when I was chanting the Stotrams, and when I was chanting the scriptures.*

*At those times, I felt the fullness and the love for God and I am fixed on that. Intellectually I know that the desire for liberation is the yearning that I've experienced as a bhakta (a devotee) because I have that experience of that tiny flame in the cave of my heart, I have the experience of that tiny flame which is sometimes bigger, sometimes tinier. Even when I have that tiny flame, I know that there is something beyond the names and forms, that is bliss, absolute bliss, I know that, so I keep going. Maybe the flame is not burning brightly, sometimes burning small, but it keeps me going.*

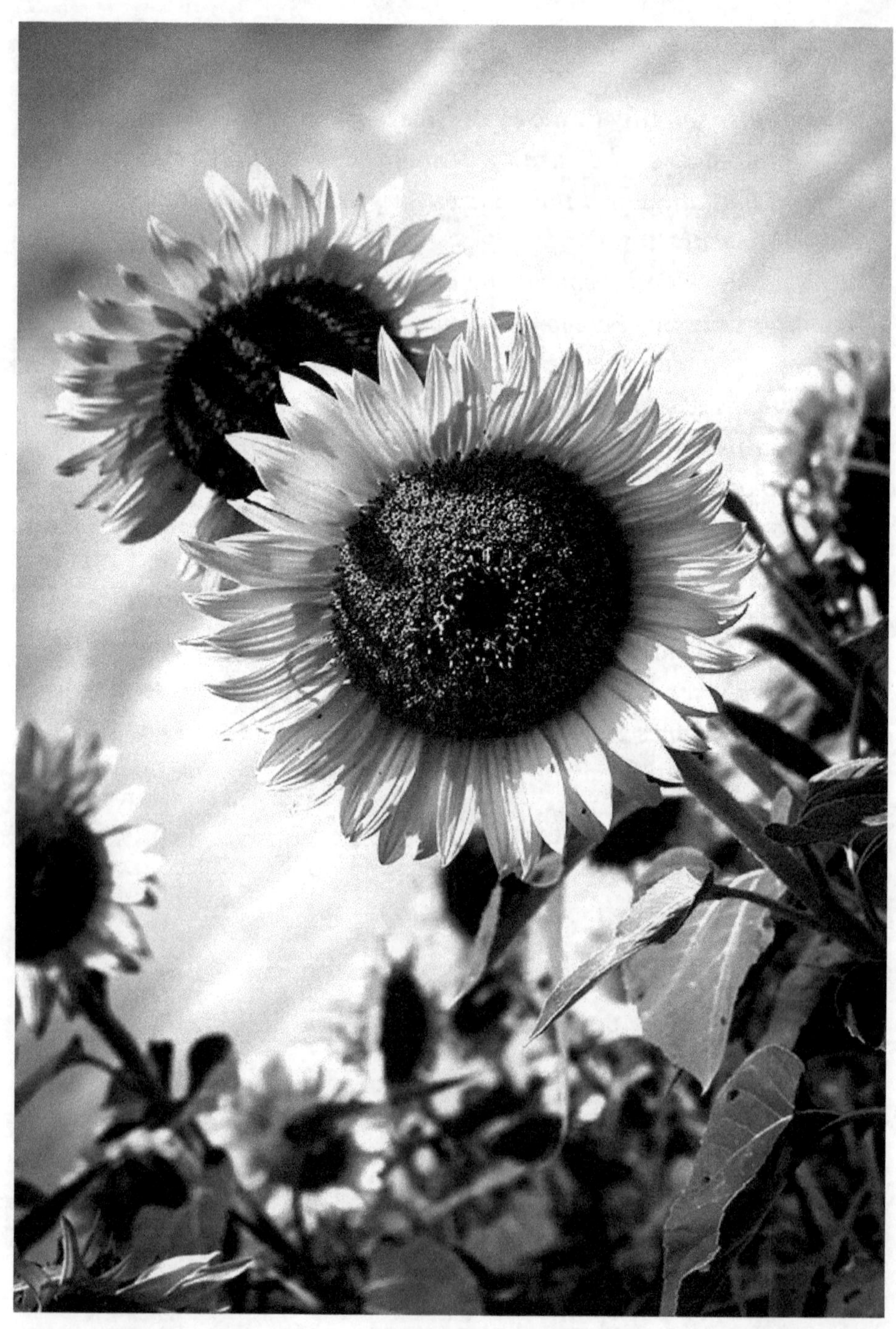

SUNFLOWERS

CHAPTER 12

# Finding Your Purpose

***"The first step in the spiritual path is the selfless service to humanity"***

*–SWAMI SIVANANDA in Sivananda Upanishad*

As in our relationships, we associate happiness and unhappiness with our work. Our career is an important part of our karma and contains lessons for Self-healing. Through our work, we seek fulfillment and realization of our potential. It is through our work, that we can fulfill our karmic debts by performing our duty. Often, however, we are motivated by the pursuit of wealth and enjoyment, instead of the desire to fulfill our duty and search for true liberation. We mistake external freedom for the internal release from karma and ignorance, which alone brings the true, highest, freedom. Ultimately, we realize that no action can fulfill us. We learn to act as an instrument, offering our actions and intelligence to the Lord of all works.

## FULFILLMENT IN YOUR SWADHARMA

*Swadharma* is a Vedic concept that refers to an individual's personal and unique duties and responsibilities, according to their nature and inherent qualities. It is derived from the Sanskrit term *swa*, which means "Self," and *dharma*, which means "duty or law." According to Yoga philosophy, by fulfilling your *swadharma*, your unique path or calling in this life, you earn good karma (merit)—and attain spiritual growth, progress, and fulfillment.

## WHAT IS YOUR UNIQUE PATH?

We ask ourselves questions such as, "*What am I going to do? What's my next step? I would like to do this, but am I good at it?*" We can feel stuck on our path to realizing our dreams, unsure how to reach our potential, while still fulfilling our duties. We then feel depressed, as we lack direction and meaning in our lives. Finding your *swadharma* means finding the occupation that brings you inner peace, contentment, and a sense of purpose. In order to find it, we must recognize and embrace our unique gifts, talents, and responsibilities, through which we contribute to the world. Simultaneously, play your unique role in society and fulfill your duties in life.

These areas of life are considered when identifying your *swadharma*:

1. Predominant guna, or temperament
2. Social group or caste
3. Current stage in life
4. Inner motivation
5. Specific karma

1. **Predominant guna**

   Understand your basic temperament, which is determined by the balance of the three gunas (qualities of nature, introduced in chapter 2). Which guna is predominant? This determines the activities that most affect you and which activities, people, and environments will balance you.

   The gunas evolve from tamas to rajas to sattva. By practicing sadhana, you can actively transform the tamasic guna (inertia, darkness, and ignorance) and the rajasic guna (activity and passion) into the sattvic guna (harmony, purity, and equanimity).

   No one is completely tamasic, rajasic, or sattvic; we are each a combination of all three qualities in varying degrees. In general, the fruit of sattvic action, good action, is harmony; the fruit of rajasic action is pain; and the fruit of tamasic action is ignorance. According to Swami Sivananda, if you are established in sattva, you rise upwards. Rajasic people stay put, and tamasic people go downwards. So, when you do sadhana and cultivate sattva, your temperament and actions become harmonious and help you ascend on your path.

2. **Your social group or caste**

   In Vedic philosophy, the concept of caste is closely linked to the gunas, your innate qualities and temperament. According to this view, humans fall into four basic categories, based on their predominant gunas. These categories are also known as the *varnas*. Your *varna* at birth—including your family *varna*—along with your gunas, will, in part, determine the types of activities you are attracted to in this life.

Traditionally, there are four types of *varna*:

- ***Shudra*: *Shudra varna*** includes the service providers or the laborers. In this varna, tamasic qualities dominate. A person tends not to ask many questions about the meaning of life or how to progress in life. Their motivations are tamasic, characterized by ignorance and inaction. They typically are content to work any particular job, make money, and simply live their life.
- ***Vaishya*:** This *varna* represents the merchants, tradespeople, and business people. The qualities of rajas and tamas predominate, characterized by passion, egoism, and lethargy towards higher pursuits. These individuals are content to focus mostly on themselves and gaining wealth for themselves and their families.
- ***Kshatriya*:** This *varna* represents the warrior and ruling class. The predominant qualities are rajasic mixed with sattvic qualities. Their characteristics are passion, energy, action, and—when sattva increases—action for the good of others, such as a community leader or selfless lawmaker, who desires to protect or change society for the better.
- ***Brahmin*:** Generally, this *varna* includes the teachers, the scholars, and the priests who possess the quality of sattva and are characterized by purity, knowledge, and wisdom. Knowledgeable and pious, they do not aspire to change society, but focus their energy on understanding nature's laws and following God's will. They lead a spiritual life, trusting that the universe unfolds as it should.

It is important to note that the *varna* of an individual is inherited from the parents, but each person can evolve and actively transform the predominant guna from tamas to rajas to sattva, through sadhana or conscious training. The birth *varna* tends to influence the individual choice of occupation, social status, and relationships. In our modern world, which is more open to having an equal chance of mobility and social justice, you can qualify yourself for an occupation or social group depending on merit and personal development, rather than on your birth or conditioning.

3. **Current stage of life**

Vedic teaching outlines the different phases in a human life, according to physical age and psychological maturity. Each stage in life comes with corresponding duties and responsibilities. These stages in life are called *ashramas.*

The four *ashramas* are:

- ***Brahmacharya,*** or the student stage, is characterized by preparing for adulthood. The student is focused on education and developing self-discipline and control. This begins in childhood from about age 6 to age 20 or 25. Traditionally, parents would send their child to study under a spiritual teacher in a *gurukula*, or "Guru's house." Under guidance, they would study, not only the basic foundations of human values, but also scriptures and basic training of body, mind, and spirit with asana, pranayama, mantra, etc. During this time, the student honors their *dharma*, or duty, to the parents and the teachers; the primary objective is learning.
- ***Grihastha,*** or the householder stage, typically begins at age 25 and lasts until around age 50. During this stage, the expectation is to raise a family, fulfill societal and family responsibilities, and accumulate wealth and material possessions.
- ***Vanaprastha,*** or the forest dweller (retirement) stage, begins at age 50 and lasts until around age 75. A person retires from professional and household duties and is expected to focus on spiritual pursuits, such as meditation, study of scriptures, reflection, and preparing for the final stage of life. At this time, material accumulation is no longer the goal or a necessity.

  In a traditional spiritual society, the main goal in life is spiritual development. So, in the retirement stage, when physical and material needs are less preponderant, spiritual needs can come to the forefront. Our birthright is to fulfill the duty of finding our true Self.
- ***Sannyasa,*** or the renunciation stage, typically begins after age 75 and lasts until the end of life. At that time, their focus is to attain God-realization and *moksha*, liberation from the cycle of birth and death. There's no other goal. The sannyasin detaches from material possessions, personal attachments, and worldly achievement and focuses entirely on spiritual pursuits.

Note that these guidelines are by no means rigid. There are anomalies and exceptions to the norm. Evolution is not a straight line. Some people may skip the *grihastha* stage and take up *sannyasa*, but they also might jump back from *sannyasa* and take up the *grihastha* stage. The famous teacher, Sri Adi Shankaracharya, took up *sannyasa* at the age of 9.

In our modern society, the duty or *varna* can be confused. Some people are leaders, but function as business people, with a strong motivation for artha (material gain). Others take up the job of the *sudra* (for example, a taxi or Uber driver) to make a living, when, in fact, they are spiritually-motivated, highly-educated, and sattvic people with the nature and temperament of a Brahmin. They cannot work in society or for unethical corporations, so they prefer to get an independent job with some autonomy, such as being a taxi driver. It is also possible that someone playing the role of a priest—which is supposed to be sattvic and selfless—acts out their motivation and character as a business person. They seem like a spiritual person on the outside, yet their motivation is for wealth and their character is geared towards business.

4. **Inner motivation**

*Purushārtha* is a compound of the words *purusha* meaning "human being" and *ārtha* meaning "purpose." *Purushārtha* can be translated as the "objective of human pursuit." Arranged in order of priority from lowest to highest, according to the gunas, the four *purushārthas* are: artha (prosperity and economic values), kama (sensual pleasures, love), dharma (righteousness and morality), and moksha (liberation from the cycle of reincarnation).

Dharma indicates behaviors that are in accord with the principles of Nature to make life and the universe possible. Dharma includes duties, rights, laws, correct conduct and virtues, and the righteous way of living. For spiritual evolution and the purpose of Self-healing, dharma must be emphasized, as well as *moksha*.

Rarely do you have just one area of motivation. Most of us have some motivation in each of the four *purushārthas*. For example, some people are motivated by *kama* and *artha* in their desire for wealth. Some people want to liberate themselves, and have no motivation for *kama* or enjoyment, nor do they have the motivation of *artha* or making money. They have the motivation to do good for society or dharma and they have the motivation to liberate themselves and to find the truth, *moksha*.

To have peace of mind and contentment, following dharma is most important. We must align our activities and decisions according to our dharma, thus fulfilling our *swadharma.*

5. **Specific karma**

   Karma is the universal law of cause and effect. It is said that our present life is the result of past thoughts and the mental imprints we have brought with us to this life. This is the idea of karma, which has been introduced in previous chapters. Over our lifetime, we experience birth, growth, change, decay, and death. We speak of karma at birth as the foundation for this life, but it is important to see how you live, and your time of death, as the foundation for the next life. It is a cycle of transmigration. Death is not the end. We will be reborn.

   You are born to pay your karmic debts. You are the immortal *Atman,* but you are born with a body, a mind, and tendencies that form your character. Your life can be viewed as a series of credits and debits in your karmic bank account.

Ideally, you increase the credit and decrease the debits as much as possible; maximize the positive actions and minimize the negative.

Knowing that your life is a series of thoughts and actions aimed at alleviating karmic debts, avoid new karma that will need to be repaid in future lives. The unceasing accumulation of karmic debts propels the wheel of birth and death. In other words, as you move through life, you perform some positive actions, thereby paying some karmic debts, and, at the same time, perform some negative actions, which increase your karmic debt. As karmic debt accrues and is renewed from lifetime to lifetime, you are born again and again to learn from your past actions and thoughts—lessons that you did not learn previously—to ultimately free yourself from all karmic debt.

## LIBERATION FROM ALL KARMAS

*Moksha* is the result of paying off all karmic debts, realizing your *Satchitananda* nature, and breaking free from the cycle of birth and death—never to reincarnate again. This is the ultimate purpose of life for everyone. It happens in stages and starts with your conscious journey from karma to dharma.

| Debit (-) | Credit (+) |
|---|---|
| – thoughts and actions that strengthen your ego<br>– selfish acts and thoughts<br>– desires<br>– anger<br>– hatred<br>– any lower emotions<br>– sensory pleasures<br>– anything that shifts your focus outward to the external world<br>– actions and thoughts that increase your ignorance of who you are | – Selfless acts on behalf of others<br>– High-minded thoughts that reduce selfishness and increase forgiveness<br>– Sadhana and spiritual practices, spiritual study<br>– Reduction of ego<br>– Understanding of karmic relationships |

## FULFILLING OUR DUTY

According to Sri Krishna in the *Bhagavad Gita*, we should perform our duty with dedication and devotion, without attachment to results.

The focus should be on the action and not on the outcome. Krishna instructs us to perform our duty, even if it seems challenging or undesirable. Indeed, we should perform our duty with detachment and without being affected by emotions or external conditions. "*Thy right is to work only, but never with its fruits; let not the fruits of actions be thy motive, nor let thy attachment be to inaction*" [*Bhagavad Gita* II:47].

## THE CONSCIOUS JOURNEY FROM KARMA TO DHARMA

The reason we do not understand our dharma is that we are functioning out of karma. We are steeped in our karma, drowning in the ocean of samsara. The degree to which you can accept and recognize your karma—and at the same time detach from it—will determine the degree to which you understand your dharma.

Devotion and commitment to your duties and actions purify the mind and reduce the impact of negative karma. The journey of working out your karma is the journey of learning to be mindful of your actions and intentions. Consciously apply the principles of dharma to generate positive karma to offset the negative effects of past actions. The intention is to honor dharma, living a dharmic life, no matter what your difficulties might be. Fulfill your *swadharma*, your specific duty with all its facets, in this life. At the same time, remember your highest duty, Self-healing and Self-realization. By fulfilling your *swadharma*, and consciously converting your karma into dharma, you find your purpose in life and become content.

**The dynamic between karmic conflict and karmic release**

There are three scenarios to illustrate our karmic/dharmic dilemma:

1. Some people feel pulled by a contradicting sense of "would" and "should." They are torn between what they would like to do—that is good for themselves—and what they feel they must do, because of duty. They know what they should do to advance themselves, but cannot do it, as they have internal and external obstacles that prevent them from realizing their potential. Thus, they are frustrated, living in a constant tug-of-war, not feeling free to do what they want. And then, if they do follow what they want, any sense of satisfaction derived from it doesn't last. This applies to all endeavors, spiritual or worldly.
2. Some seem content in their vocation. By way of karma, they have found their skills and competencies and can thus express their dharma, living life fully while growing in the process. For the lucky ones, the circumstances of their life (karma) and their inner motivations align (dharma). Only when outer circumstances and inner motivation align can we truly find our purpose in life and fulfill our potential. There are cases of exceptional people who turn unfavorable circumstances into favorable ones through strength of will and hard work.
3. Some people embrace the necessary spiritual journey and practice detachment toward all that they do. They progress in life, i.e. they consciously "pay their karmic debts." Their attitude towards their work or activities is mindful, conscious, and detached. The level at which we struggle with work and activity, remaining detached from the very obstacle and struggle, is the level at which we are "paying karmic debts" or achieving release from karma. Krishna assures us in the *Bhagavad Gita* that it is not through the non-performance of action that we will find release, but by the performance of action without attachment.

The attitude of detachment includes not blaming. If the circumstances are not favorable and you're not able to realize yourself and fulfill your dharma, you may blame the circumstances. However, you cannot blame the circumstances or anyone else. It is nothing but the result of your karma, for which you are responsible—willingly or not. Work through your karma, accepting the inherited conditions of your life. At the same time, make use of your strengths, acknowledge your weaknesses, and detach from the outcome.

**Signs that you are under the grip of karma manifesting as work, career, occupation:**

Karma indicates specific circumstances that you have to experience and learn from as a result of thoughts and actions from your past. You have had countless occupations, countless skills—and countless lives identifying with your occupation and position. When you are in a karmic situation, you are in the dark, you cannot see your dharma. But you can start to recognize the karma through these symptoms:

- The struggle manifests as changing work, changing dedication, changing moods and goals, ups and downs; happy circumstances, unhappy, then happy again for a short while. Behind this picture is your desire to find your *Satchitananda Atman*, already fulfilled and non-acting. Your sense of self is tightly linked with your position in society. You try to see yourself as the world does.
- In every new job, you are trying to apply your sense of self, your accomplishments and skills, learning from the past to be happy and fulfilled. However, you accumulated skills and accomplishments, but not wisdom. You still do not know who you are; you continue to identify with what you do and not with who you truly are.
- You are unhappy with your work, no matter what it is.
- You change your work often, but do not find contentment.
- You have difficulty finding satisfaction and fulfillment in any work.
- You are confused about your sense of self.
- You do not know how to situate yourself in life.
- You struggle to find clear motivation.
- You feel envious of other people's occupations.
- You compete with your colleagues.
- You blame your boss, your company, or your co-workers for your unhappiness at work.
- You think you are not valued.

- You think that you are not good enough for your position.
- You think that if you work hard enough, you will find satisfaction.
- You are a workaholic and overly-driven.
- You have a sense of self-importance in your interactions with others.

**Signs that you are moving closer to your dharma:**

- You become more selfless in your motivation.
- You are comfortable in any work and do not identify with it.
- You do not seek name and fame.
- You do not have a sense of your self-importance being due to your work.
- You do not compare yourself with others, do not feel envy or jealousy, and focus on doing your duty well.
- Praise and censure do not affect you.
- You forbear any unpleasant work. You persevere with patience.
- You overcome sorrow from any unfulfilled expectations.
- You have a less competitive spirit in your work.
- You do not criticize people for their incompetence, nor think yourself superior.
- You see your work as service and Karma Yoga.
- You are not burdened by your work but feel joy in serving.
- You see work as worship.
- You are calm and detached whether successful or unsuccessful in any endeavor. You do not blame others.
- You listen and follow God's will, not following your own will. You seek to understand what is asked of you and endeavor to be an instrument of God's will.
- You think obstacles to your achievements are good for your ego and act as purification as you detach from results.
- You practice inaction in action.

**A few guidelines for turning karma into dharma:**

- Your work is not who you are. You are not an accountant, a doctor, a businessman, or a leader. It is about the evolution from tamas to rajas to sattva. Situate yourself as shown above and, no matter what you do, cultivate a sattvic attitude.
- Your sattvic motivation should be dharma and *moksha*.
- No matter what you do, dedicate it to the supreme and feel that you are an instrument for a higher will. Swami Sivananda says, "*Work is worship.*" Your work teaches you some skills, but the mind, the capacity, and the character are ultimately not you.

  Other people's minds are only mirrors on which you reflect for insight on how you think, feel, and respond to the various situations in which you find yourself.

  Life's circumstances help you to see your true Self, the immortal *Atman*, that resides in everyone as the non-doer, beyond all actions, and doer of all actions. This means you can do everything, while not identifying with any particular situation or position. Seeking name and fame is a pursuit of the ego, mistaking the name and fame to be yourself.

  Work is an excellent opportunity to purify yourself as you have to detach and move from karma to dharma.

- Each struggle in your work or your life is an opportunity to see yourself a little more clearly. Try this and that and, eventually, the struggle helps you to know yourself more clearly.
- The ultimate benefit of struggle in action is realizing that the energy and skills I utilize are not mine; I am only the instrument through which the *Atman* is manifesting in the world.
- The process of working through your karma can be viewed as a process of purification, a thinning of the ego, and removal of the egoistic notion of self. See it as learning to become more selfless as an expression of the Divine working through us.
- If you want to find your dharma, you should start through selflessness and Karma Yoga. Dharma has to stand with selflessness. If you want to find your mission in life, you need to answer the question: What is the purpose of my life? Practice Karma Yoga or the Yoga of selflessness in daily life. You will have to offer yourself to the service of something higher, larger than yourself, without condition, without expectation or attachment to the result. Be an instrument.

## WHAT IT MEANS TO BE SELFLESS

Ideally, you will act selflessly, doing your best to contribute to others or the community without thoughts of rewards or praise. Each situation is a perfect opportunity to work out some aspect of your karma. It might take a long time, but if you practice correctly, one day you will fulfill both your karma and dharma together.

You may think that selflessness means weakness and not fending for yourself. *"I will be taken advantage of if I'm selfless."* There is a subtle distinction between being selfless and losing control over your consciousness. Please understand that nobody can take advantage of you, unless you allow them to, because only you control your consciousness. Whether a person tries to take advantage or not, you are the one who decides whether or not you offer your energy, mind, and body to the service. In selflessness, you offer your being to the service in question; you do so without a sense of yourself or ego in the act. You do not do it saying, *"I am good, because I do this; look how well I do this; I will gain prestige, because I do this; the world or this person will praise me, because I do this."*

When you act selflessly, you do it solely as an act of service, truly and wholly for another person, for humanity, for the Divine. It is an act of service and, thus, all of the reward is for the other whom you serve. This is what is meant by selfless service. This is the main teaching in the *Bhagavad Gita*. You also find this teaching in the book *The Practice of Karma Yoga* by Swami Sivananda.

Whenever we consider the nature of selflessness, we are essentially considering the nature of the ego and egoism. Patanjali defined egoism as the association of the *Atman* with the instrument of seeing, the *antahkarana*. The *antahkarana* is the totality of the mental faculties; *Antah* means "inner" and *karana* means "instrument." The *antahkarana* is made up of the mind *(manas)*, intellect *(buddhi)*, subconscious *(chitta)*, and ego *(ahamkara)*. Thus, selflessness means detachment from or non-identification with the mind, the subconscious, the intellect, the ego, or the instrument of perceiving. When you are detached from the inside, you don't identify with your personality, with your ego, or with a separate sense of self.

If you want to find yourself, if you want to find your mission, your purpose, understand that it is a deep spiritual question about your highest purpose in life. To find an answer, you will need to stop acting with ego—which is at the whim of desire and emotions and the outside world—and stand firm in practicing selflessness. The more you are selfless, the more you thin out the ego, and the more your purpose will be revealed to you. Know that it will take time and significant effort and struggle, but your purpose will be revealed. Learn through the circumstances of your life: if you are a teacher, be a selfless teacher; if you are a mother, be a selfless mother; if you are an employee, be a selfless employee. Whatever you do, do it selflessly. Put your heart into your work. Do your best, aim for the best result you can, but do it without ego and detach from the result. Whether you succeed or fail, whether you are praised or criticized, promoted or fired, you know that you are sincere, dedicated, and selfless.

To repeat, when you work with a sense of selflessness, you will begin to reveal your dharma—and you will also begin to find peace. The ego and its desires and attachments, and thus its longings and pains, are reduced. Through selfless work, you work out your karma, you feel more deeply fulfilled; you struggle less with your ego. The key to remember, here, is that selflessness is detachment from the idea of doer-ship. As you practice, observe when ego creeps back in; observe when you long to be praised or seek the rewards of your actions. Do not get discouraged; merely recenter on your goal of selfless action. It is a practice, so it will take time.

## WHAT IS KARMA YOGA?

Karma Yoga can be practiced full-time or part-time. You can offer your time and energy in charity work or volunteering full-time or part-time, or selectively. Karma Yoga is, in itself, a spiritual practice that can lead to the highest realization of Self. *Sannyasins* are renunciates. They are renouncing not actions, but the desires and fruits of action. The *Bhagavad Gita* says, "*The sages understand Sannyasa to be the renunciation of action with desire; the wise declare the abandonment of the fruits of all actions as Tyaga*" (or renunciation) [XVIII:2].

Karma Yoga can help you turn your thinking and your actions around. Karma Yoga asks you to focus on whatever is in front of you to do and to do it with a good attitude. Work for work's sake. Use your duty, your *swadharma*, whatever it is, but turn it into selflessness; use it to practice becoming an instrument. Do the action, but without the ego.

Feel yourself as an instrument. When you become the instrument, when you act without acting, when you act without ego, you cancel out your karma. This powerful practice can help you sort out the strong attachment you have to your actions and their results. Again, Karma Yoga can help you learn to detach from what you do. The practice of Karma Yoga works to liberate you from this ego-self—this body and mind; this outward, separate life, with which you are very much identifying. All teachers of all religious paths regularly prescribe the practice of Karma Yoga, as a starting place.

Here are a few examples:

*S. is a carpenter. As a professional, he had a very good job with very good pay. But he decided to become a Karma Yogi at the ashram. By doing so, he converted all of his actions, all of his skilled actions as a carpenter, into* punya *(merits), or pluses in his karmic bank balance. He is a very good Karma Yogi, able to help with many projects and he is constantly obliging and doing. By his attitude, he is working through his karma.*

---

*This story is told on the internet: An Indian woman, when she was young, was abused physically and mentally by her family and was eventually thrown out to live on the street. She had a very hard time, working many menial jobs. She was later abused by her husband. But, she took her karma, her suffering, and turned it around by later opening an institution, a home for young girls, who were experiencing the same abuse and suffering she herself had undergone. Gradually, she adopted all these unfortunate women and gave them a home. The institution has since grown quite large. Through her suffering, she has become a powerful force in helping to relieve the suffering of other women. She turned her karma into dharma.*

---

*Another famous example is Mahatma Gandhi. He was a lawyer, trained in the legal system. He understood well how to formulate often-complex arguments to win his cases. He, eventually, took this skill as a lawyer and used it to help lead India to independence from British colonialism. He found his dharmic mission.*

---

*Imagine a woman desires to have a child but cannot. This is her karma. One way she might turn it into dharma would be to direct the love she felt for the children she wanted to have and channel it into caring for other children who may lack parents, like working for an orphanage.*

---

*Let's say that you grew up in extreme poverty. But through this poverty, you gained a wealth of experience and understanding of the challenges of being poor, the struggle to make ends meet that most people just don't understand. You can offer up this poverty by working for other poor people who don't have enough to eat and live in slums. By doing so, while you lacked material wealth, you found a richness of heart. You were able to convert your karma of struggling into an asset that you then shared with others.*

As you serve others, your mind will change and your soul will become richer. Karma doesn't have to be terrible, all pain and suffering; it can be the source of great spiritual wealth and goodness for the world and others. By letting go of the ego-identification and focusing on selfless acts for others, you can connect with your true love—with your true Self and the love that exists within you—and turn it into spiritual joy and happiness. This is the formula for how to turn your karma into dharma.

**Nine keys for Karma Yoga**

To make this idea more practical, let's talk briefly about the nine keys to finding success with Karma Yoga:

1. **Have the right attitude.** It's not what you do that counts, it is the fact that you do it selflessly that matters for spiritual growth. It is your attitude *while doing* that determines if the act will help you towards liberation or bind you into further karma. And as we have discussed, the attitude must be one of selflessness.
2. **Have the right motivation**. Your motive must be pure. Commonly, we work only for ourselves; we work for the reward or for recognition of our labors. Transform your motivation so that you are acting solely for the benefit of others.
3. **Do your duty.** Do action according to your nature, following your specific dharma and karma. This depends on your age, caste, and motivation; everyone has a duty, a role to play in this world.
4. **Do your best.** Whatever you do, do your best. Give yourself wholly to what it is that you do; do your duty the best you can.
5. **Give up the results of your actions.** As we discussed, feel that you are the instrument; act without ego or notion of future reward. It is the detachment from actions that will dissolve the karmic seeds inside the actions. So don't be attached to your job, or the praise or reward you think you will get as a result. Be ready to give it up.

6. **Serve the Divine.** When you serve others, humanity, or a higher power, you serve the Divine. The correct attitude here is to do unto others as you would have others do unto you. Love your neighbor as yourself. Adapt, adjust, accommodate, and bear insult, bear injury. See unity in diversity and remain ever aware that you are part of something larger than yourself. Practice humility in action. Beware of power, fame, name, praise, and censure.
7. **Whatever work you do, be mindful of the discipline, the experience, and the lesson it has to teach you.** Each job involves a different requirement in terms of time, concentration, skills, and emotional input. For example, if you do Karma Yoga at the reception desk, but you don't like to smile, you will need to work on that tendency. If you work in reception, your goal is to receive others, instilling a particular feeling of welcome in them. It is not about you, it is about them, so you must be selfless. Learn the lessons in doing things that the ego might not like.
8. **Cultivate virtues.** Swami Sivananda says you have to be qualified to be a Karma Yogi—free from lust, greed, anger, and egotism. Cultivate these virtues to support your actions in Karma Yoga.
9. **Combine Karma Yoga with other paths of Yoga.** Karma Yoga, when it is well-performed, needs to be done with devotion (Bhakti Yoga), concentration, meditation, and an attitude of self-control (Raja Yoga), and self-knowledge (Jnana Yoga). Performing Karma Yoga this way allows you to spiritualize all of your activities.

In the *Bhagavad Gita*, Sri Krishna says, *"Abandoning all duties, come to me alone for shelter. Sorrow not, grieve not, I will liberate you from all sins"* [XVIII:66]. This significant quote about Karma Yoga means whatever you do, detach and act selflessly and solely for the Supreme. Free yourself from all karma.

**Signs of the wrong Karma Yoga attitude:**

- You are concerned about how important you are.
- Your desire is followed by disappointment.
- You do not stick to your duty.
- You work hard, but never feel it's enough, never feel it is satisfactory and lasting.
- You become upset when your work is destroyed by someone else.

- You find yourself competing with other people.
- You feel joylessness derived from work. If you do Karma Yoga without joy, your ego has surely infiltrated your Karma Yoga. Your spirit is not embracing the selfless attitude of the Karma Yogi.
- Work without pay doesn't mean that it is necessarily Karma Yoga.
- Working, but with complaints, criticism, comparison, jealousy and envy is not the spirit of Karma Yoga.
- You say, *"I have come here to learn something, and I had to wash dishes all day long. I could do the dishes at home. So why come here to do dishes?"* You have lost the Karma Yoga attitude, looking around to find fault.
- You think that someone else benefits from your labor and you do not benefit from it.

To conclude, the *Bhagavad Gita* says that Yoga is "skill in action." Have the capacity to work out the karma, progressing and not accruing new karmic debt; that's a skill. Karma comes from desire, the past, and how you're living your life now. Your goal is paying off your karmic debts, while trying not to create new ones. This is where selfless action and Karma Yoga help to liberate you. *"Endowed with wisdom (evenness of mind), one casts off in this life both good and evil deeds; therefore, devote thyself to Yoga; Yoga is skill in action"* [*Bhagavad Gita* II:50].

## RENUNCIATION AND ACTION

It takes courage to face your karma and value yourself differently, not through your accomplishments or skills, but through your renunciation of ego. Attachments and desires are, in the end, obstacles to true happiness. Happiness does not come from your emotions or thoughts, or from work and success, or any karmic situation. Your True Nature is Bliss Absolute, the non-doer of all actions. Be detached from what you experience. The goal of life is not experiencing life; life is just a means, it is not the goal. Try to avoid entanglement by understanding that true freedom resides in non-attachment, and non-entanglement with the causes of suffering. True freedom is freedom from the ego-self and all that comes with it. You will have to take yourself and your desire for liberation very seriously and work steadily to disentangle yourself, step by step.

Become a wise person and live in the present; let go of the past and the future. Thinking about the past will bring regrets, reawaken unfulfilled desires, and prior injuries to the ego-self. Thinking about the future will reawaken the ego's desires and notions of what it needs to be fulfilled and complete. It will stir desires—and thus attachments by projections and expectations—which will, in the end, lead you back to suffering and future regrets.

Be in the present, truly present, without attachment and desire. There is peace. Think less. Immerse yourself in the present, using Karma Yoga to live a selfless life, detached from what you have to experience. Cultivate the undaunted spirit of selflessness; this will keep you on the path to true liberation.

Karma Yoga can lead to *moksha*. Albert Einstein declared, *"No problem can be solved from the same level of consciousness that created it."* In karmic terms, no karma can be undone within a mind that is not enlightened.

You will find your life's mission when you understand that you can only see your dharma, when you are free from your karma. When you learn to live selflessly, your dharma will reveal itself. Use the practice of Karma Yoga to live selflessly and, eventually, you will live your dharma selflessly for the rest of your life. Finding your life's mission will set you free.

Every karma is unique. Once you find your dharma, remain steadfast where you are. This is the sublime attitude to keep throughout life. Do not allow it to change according to your will; this is merely ego creeping back in. Happiness comes from peace of mind and peace of mind comes when we exist selflessly caring for others. It is then that we understand our dharma, and it is then that we find true peace of mind. In Yoga, we say it is the balance between self-effort and relaxation. Selflessness is a balance of acting in the world without being affected by the worldly mind.

In the *Bhagavad Gita*, Krishna advises us to become a perpetual *sannyasi* or renunciate. Krishna said you need to, *"live a life of action without acting, inaction in action."* If you achieve this, you are living a selfless life, without the ego, having renounced all attachments and desires in this life. In conclusion, in the *Bhagavad Gita*, Lord Krishna also says, *"The harmonized person, having abandoned the fruits of action, attains eternal peace. The non-harmonized person, impelled by desire and attached to the fruits of action will remain eternally bound"* [*Bhagavad Gita* V:12].

## *INSPIRED STORY*

**Awareness heals**

*A Christian monk, about 45 - 50 years old, has severe physical and mental weakness, many times hospitalized for depression, Parkinson's disease, and muscle tone, and has to take medicine every day. If he takes the medicine at the wrong time or when the medicine loses its effect, he will lose control of his muscles and may fall at any time.*

*After a gentle asana class followed by a counseling session with me for 90 minutes, a few hours later I heard from my family that this person could go for a normal walk this afternoon without taking medicine. After revisiting, I understood that it was the teachings of Karma Yoga that helped this person see his way.*

*This person is very fiery (pitta temperament), very well educated, a lawyer with high ambitions, but with a habit of non-stop work, with the intention that he wants to build a good community and a good church. He worked for many years and forgot about himself, that he is only a tool for the will of God to manifest, so he suffered from chronic stress to the point of weakness.*

*Even when he was in the hospital bed, his mind was still worried about work. It is the teaching of the Karma Yoga path that reminds him of detachment from action and makes him remember that everything is really in God's hands, not in our hands, that makes this person see his mistake in thinking that ruined his health. He remembers on that day that "illness is an opportunity to learn" and he remembers that for his spiritual development, he should stop complaining, be grateful, and be detached from doer-ship. It was the spiritual power and connection with His True Self that restored the mental and physical health of this person, instantly, miraculously, without drugs, and he was able to walk!*

**QUESTIONS**

1. *What are the criteria to determine your swadharma?*
2. *Summarise the 9 principles of Karma Yoga.*
3. *How do you find your purpose?*
4. *Give 3 examples of the conscious journey from Karma to Dharma.*

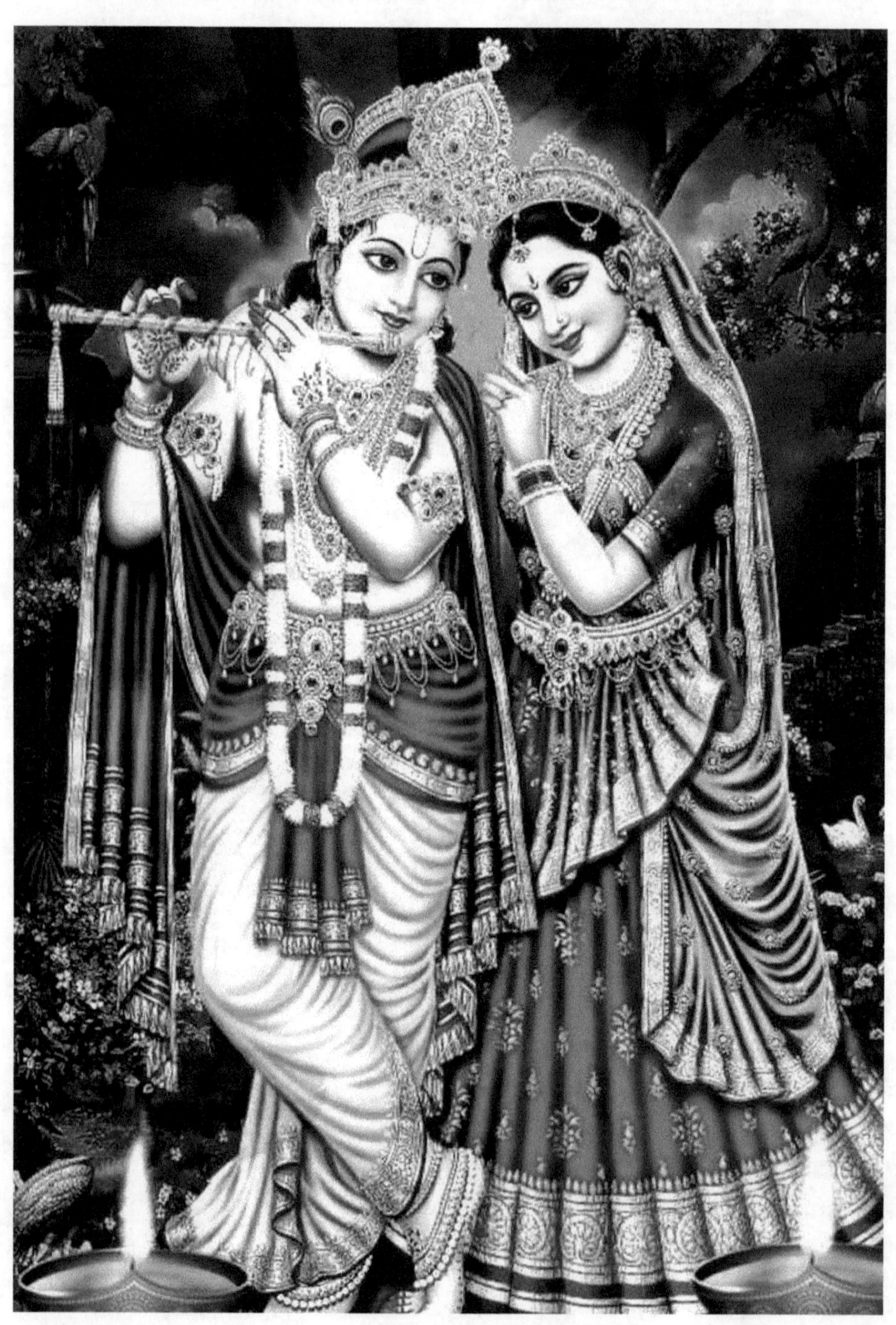

RADHA KRISHNA

CHAPTER 13

# Sublimating Desires

***"If one clearly understands the serious damage that comes through an impure life, and if he determines to attain the goal of life by leading a pure life, he must keep his mind busily engaged in divine thoughts, concentration, meditation, study of religious books and service of humanity."***

\- SWAMI SIVANANDA in *Practice of Brahmacharya*

We have been talking about Self-healing and Self-realization as a process of going inward and upward. Our journey in life is often outward and downward; we look for fulfillment out in the world of the senses and usually through our lower mind and desires. How can we convert the energy so it turns inwards and ascends upwards and helps our journey towards Self-realization?

## DESIRES & SUBLIMATION

Sublimation of desires or sexual energy is a process of redirecting the physical energy and desire towards higher, such as spiritual or creative, goals. In the context of sexual energy, sublimation involves channeling the energy generated by sexual desire into other areas, such as work, art, or spirituality. A conscious effort is required to redirect the energy, rather than to suppress or deny it.

Some of the common techniques for sublimation of sexual energy include:

1. **Transmutation of the energy:** This involves using the energy to create something productive, such as art or writing.

2. **Pranayama:** This is the practice of transforming and controlling the prana, balancing it, and channeling it upwards. It is very helpful for channeling sexual energy.
3. **Asana, mudra, and bandha of classical Hatha Yoga:** This practice uses asanas (postures), mudras (seals), and bandhas (energy locks) and helps to awaken and channel the dormant spiritual energy in the body.
4. **Meditation:** This allows us to focus the mind on the Divine and let go of physical desires
5. **Brahmacharya:** This is a celibate life, dedicated to realizing Brahman. When we set higher spiritual goals in life, it helps to divert our energy and attention from lower desires and channels it towards more meaningful pursuits.
6. **Cultivating a Yogic healthy lifestyle:** A healthy lifestyle that includes a nutritious diet, regular exercise, and adequate sleep can help to keep our physical and mental energies in balance.
7. **Engaging in activities that require physical effort:** Engaging your body in sports or exercise helps to channel the energy into productive outlets.

It is important to remember that sublimation does not mean suppressing or denying sexual desires, but rather transforming them positively and constructively in alignment with our higher consciousness. With regular practice and perseverance, sublimation can lead to profound changes in our consciousness and a greater awakening of our spiritual potential.

The *Chandogya Upanishad* says, "*The individual is made of desires. As is your desire, so will be your motivation. As is your motivation, so will be your actions. As are your actions, so you will eventually attain and become.*"

The important point here is that desire is at the root of the mind and is the source of motivation, and is thus the seed of other pursuits, such as spiritual and creative goals. Sublimation is a technique that has been practiced in multiple cultures for centuries. As the root of the mind, desire is also the root of willpower, imagination, effort, and seeking. We are all motivated by desire, which is the basis of all our actions, and determines our karma. Our karma is what keeps us trapped in the cycle of birth and death, in the ocean of samsara. Thus, if we wish to understand and transcend our karma, if we wish to be liberated from the ocean of samsara and our suffering, we must change the nature of our desires. On the path of Yoga, the way to transform our desires is through sadhana, spiritual practice, and the sublimation of the desires.

The *Bhagavad Gita* says that desire arises from spiritual ignorance, from not understanding our True Nature as *Satchitananda*, the state of absolute being-ness, absolute consciousness, and absolute bliss. In the state of spiritual ignorance, the rajasic mind will project its desire onto an object in the outside world. But, given the nature of the outside world, either we will not get this object of desire or we will get it, but eventually lose it. In either case, the result is anger, disappointment, and suffering from unfulfilled desires. With each outward desire, we move further from our true self, moving outward and downward into the realm of suffering and karma.

## WHAT IS DESIRE?

A desire, or vasana, at its core is just a thought wave, a mental modification, that arises through the forgetfulness of our *Satchitananda* nature. All four paths of Yoga, all Yoga philosophy and techniques, are designed to understand the root and nature of our desires and liberate us from them.

## FOUR KINDS OF DESIRE - FOUR PURUSHARTHA

In Vedanta, it says there are four kinds of desire, or four kinds of motivation, that we are born with; these are called the four *purushārthas*, out of which, two are sattvic and two are rajasic and tamasic *(see chapter 12)*.

1. **Moksha** is the desire to be free from karma and samsara, from spiritual ignorance that is the source of suffering.
2. **Dharma** manifests as the desire to grow, to understand, and to be in line with the rules of life; it is the desire to do and be good.
3. **Kama** is seeking pleasure and enjoyment of the senses. But with this desire, you might create problems for yourself. Too much enjoyment creates karmic debts and leads to the suffering that comes from attachment; it leads to imbalance and diseases of the body and spirit. The more you are aware of this motivation for pleasure, the more you will try to temper this seeking for pleasure, as you understand the cost.
4. **Artha** is the desire for wealth. You have to make a living and in some way support yourself in this life, so there must always be some desire for wealth. However, accumulation of wealth only leads to attachment to what is accumulated. Wealth can be wealth of virtues and good qualities. You can also donate a portion of your wealth to charity.

## THE FOLLOWING STORIES ILLUSTRATE THIS IDEA:

### Desire blinds: the story of a woman searching for a needle in the wrong place

*(also on p. 167, regarding attachment to objects)*

A woman lost her needle while sewing in her house, but because it was so dark in the house she went outside where the light was better, thinking this might help her find the needle. She was outside searching for a long time, until someone pointed out to her that it was impossible to find the needle outside, if she lost it inside.

The moral of this story is that the house is us, our inner awareness. But, because the mind and senses are so active, we cannot see much of anything, let alone the Atman at our core; it appears to be darkness. So, we turn outward to the world of noise and stimulation looking for our needle, our True Self. It does not occur to us that we will never find our True Self outside.

One of the central themes of Yoga is the practice of stilling the mind and senses such that we can turn inward and successfully find our True Self.

## 2 Desire robs you of your freedom: the story of the monkey and the cookie jar

A monkey put his hand in a cookie jar, trying to grab as many cookies as possible. But when he tried to remove the big handful of cookies, it would not fit through the mouth of the jar; he was stuck. He had the cookies, the object of his desire, in his hand, but he could not get them out of the jar. No matter how much he jumped around and banged his hand, it remained stuck in the jar.

The only way he could truly liberate his hand was to let go of the object of his desire. Likewise, our issue is that we remain attached to our habits, and our desires and, thus, can never liberate ourselves from our suffering.

We can never find the peace and true happiness—that we ultimately seek, but mistakenly look for outside—in our objects of desire.

### 3 Desire is an illusion: the story of a thirsty man walking in the desert

*(also on p. 168, regarding the illusion of pursuing happiness outside ourselves)*

In the heat of the day, a thirsty man in a desert found a tree and took shelter under it. The tree provided him some shade, but he saw an oasis about 15 minutes walk away. It did not take him long to decide that 15 minutes in the sun would be worth the effort to get some of that water. So, he left the shade and walked 15 minutes towards the water. He stopped, looked back, and saw the tree about 15 minutes behind him, but the water was still about 15 minutes ahead. He continued towards the water. But after 30 minutes, he could barely see the tree 30 minutes behind him and the water was still 15 minutes ahead. And so, he continued and the tree got further away and the water remained elusive, as it was a mirage.

If this man could see reality clearly, he would understand that where there are trees, there is water. The water is just below him, not in front of him. The oasis is his True Self, he just needed to turn inward and dig to find the satiation he was after. Instead, he looked outward and merely chased a mirage.

4

## Desire is insatiable: the story of King Yayati

King Yayati was a wise and powerful ruler of his kingdom. He was blessed by Indra, the king of the gods, with immortality. Yayati was pleased with this blessing. However, he soon realized that immortality alone could not guarantee him happiness. He felt a strong desire to experience the pleasures of youth and decided to use his boon to its full potential.

Yayati called his sons and asked them to exchange their youth for his old age. All of his sons, except the youngest, refused. The youngest, Puru, accepted his father's request, and Yayati enjoyed his youth once again.

However, Yayati soon became aware that his desires were insatiable, and he was never satisfied with what he had. He kept longing for more and more pleasure and his lustful desires took over him. He began to fall in love with other women, forgetting his loyal wife Devayani, who had stayed with him through thick and thin.

One day Devayani caught Yayati with another woman, and she was deeply hurt and angered by his lack of loyalty. She questioned his unquenchable desires, and Yayati realized that he had been foolish to think that he could satisfy his desire for pleasure and happiness. His insatiable desires had only brought him more misery and loneliness.

Finally, Yayati came to his senses and realized that his happiness could not be guaranteed by external things such as youth or wealth; it was within himself. He gave back the youth to his son Puru and requested forgiveness from Devayani. He realized the futility of materialistic desires and devoted himself to spiritual practices, which ultimately brought him inner peace and happiness. The story of King Yayati teaches us that insatiable desires can never bring us true happiness.

## 5 Our desires keep changing: Yama explains to Nachiketa

Yama explained that our desires are like droplets of water falling on a lotus leaf. They change their position constantly without affecting the leaf itself. Similarly, our desires change but our True Nature remains unchanged. Yama taught Nachiketa the importance of focusing on the True Self, which is eternal and unchanging.

Desires are multiple and never-ending. We keep chasing after them, but they only lead to temporary pleasure and eventually bring us pain and suffering. True happiness comes from within; we need to cultivate inner peace and contentment to lead a fulfilling life. The trick of desire is that it is always there; you cannot suppress desire, for it will merely shift to some other object or location. Desire has been compared to a balloon. If you press in one area to shrink the balloon, the air will merely shift, and the balloon bulges in a new location. So the question becomes, how do we successfully rid ourselves of desire, if removing it in one area will merely surface a new desire elsewhere?

**So the main question is how do we overcome and free ourselves from these desires?** We fulfill our desires through the mind, the senses, and their interaction with the outside world. Our senses connect us with the world by the organs of perception and the organs of action or *indriyas*. *Karma indriyas* are the organs of action.

To overcome our desires, consider how we might sublimate them. How could we channel the energy that would normally go into these desires—and the organs through which we interact with the world—into higher pursuits, like our sadhana practice and other more sattvic activities that elevate the spirit?

We could talk specifically about sensual sublimation and brahmacharya, which is what comes to mind when most people think of sublimating the senses and desires, however, sublimation of a whole range of desires is central to the various teachings of classical Yoga.

## CLASSICAL YOGA ON DESIRE

**In Raja Yoga,** the yamas and niyamas are fundamental qualifications for the practice of Yoga and aim at changing our core desires. Raja Yoga focuses on meditation and the mind seeking calmness and equanimity, free from the pendulum of attraction and repulsion.

**Bhakti Yoga** is essentially the practice of sublimation of emotion and relationships.

**Karma Yoga** is the sublimation of actions, the desire for results, and the egoistic desire to be somebody.

**Jnana Yoga** focuses on discrimination and *vairagya* or dispassion through self-inquiry, to liberate us from desires that come from incorrect thinking. In fact, in Jnana Yoga, the focus is on dispassion and renuniciation of worldliness. We realize that the object of desire is only a projection of our mind. The way to true peace is to renounce desires and the objects of their focus. Basically, it is renuniciation of the ego and the mind, the I-ness and my-ness.

As introduced on p. 174, the *Yoga Vasistha* presents seven stages of knowledge. In the first stage, it lists the *Satsampat* or six-fold virtues that must be acquired to become a sadhaka or practitioner of Yoga:

- **Sama** - serenity or the ability to be calm and control the vasanas, desires, of the mind
- **Dama** - the ability to control the senses and, therefore, reactions to external stimuli
- **Uparati** - satiation and renouncing anything that doesn't fit your dharma (duty)
- **Titiksha** - endurance or perseverance, despite suffering
- **Shraddha** - faith or trusting in the path of Jnana Yoga
- **Samadhana** - one-pointedness of mind or total concentration and focus on the goal

On top of these virtues, the aim of all the practices of Yoga is purification or thinning out of the mind. With fewer negative thought waves, the mind becomes calm. In essence, the four paths of Yoga speak about how to deal with desire by fostering detachment.

Swami Sivananda's last words were "Detach, attach," meaning detach from the thoughts of this world and attach with single-pointed focus to the Divine, the absolute, or higher power. All practices of Yoga—meditation, asana, pranayama, pratyahara—are training and building the health of body and mind in preparation for deeper self-inquiry and for complete awareness.

## PRATYAHARA & UNDERSTANDING THE SENSES

On a deeper level, Yoga helps with alleviating desires through the practice of pratyahara, or control of the senses. The senses are the interface between the mind and the outside world. It is important to understand the information we are receiving and the organs that deliver it.

Below is an excerpt from Dr. David Frawley, also known as Pandit Vamadeva Shastri, about *pratyahara*, the senses, and the importance of controlling them for our spiritual journey:

> *"The five senses' functions are outward going. They are our instruments for perceiving anything in this world. How we use our senses, the information they convey and the decisions we make with that information determine how we will live.*
>
> *Learning to use our senses correctly, then, is one of the main skills we need to master our existence and experience life optimally. It is important to understand that our experience of pleasure and pain, of happiness and sorrow, depends on our use of the senses. Our mind depends on the senses for all the information that we receive about the outside world and our bodies.*
>
> *In some respects, we can say that the senses give, and nourish, the impressions through which the mind is either calm or disturbed. We do not want our senses to deteriorate. That is, we do not want the quality or quantity of the information coming from the senses to go down, as this will be a loss of information, of wealth, about the world we live and navigate in. But at the same time, we do not have an innate knowledge of how best to manage, understand, or care for our senses, and we often end up abusing them or using them to satiate sensory desires.*
>
> *The senses play an important function on the spiritual path. Both Ayurvedic medicine and Yoga say one of the*

> *main causes of disease is the misuse of the senses, overusing them. They can be obstacles that make us more attached, or they can also play a positive role as we work to perceive higher consciousness. So, it is very important to understand, that at least initially, the practice of pratyahara is not to numb or destroy or shut down our senses. The senses are a tool that is neither good nor bad, the good or bad arises in how we use them.*

Dr. Frawley highlighted this point succinctly: If it were merely a matter of shutting down or numbing your senses, then all the people who have sensory handicaps—the deaf, the blind, the mute, and so on—would routinely be more enlightened as a result of that "advantage." It is very important to understand this correctly. We need to learn how to control and use our senses correctly to aid our practice toward liberation.

Pratyahara is the fifth of the eight limbs of Ashtanga Yoga. It is a practice, just as pranayama and asanas are optimizing the body and mind for the spiritual path toward liberation. We use pratyahara as a practice to purify our senses, learn to use them well, and make them stronger, in the same way that we use pranayama to improve the flow, increase the level, and gain control of prana.

So according to Dr. Frawley, "*When we practice pratyahara, on the one hand, we deepen our senses, improve sensory perception, adding more subtlety or increasing sensory resolution. And at the same time, we purify the senses by learning to filter what we allow to come through, what we allow our attention to be drawn to, and removing the patterned cognitive responses that create negativity in us as a default.*"

## SHIFTING OUR ATTITUDE TOWARDS THE SENSES: A LIST OF PRACTICES

A change of attitude toward our senses is needed. We must know them fully, and understand the ways they are received through the mind. When pure, or in moments of clarity, the senses reveal the sacredness of life through the beauty and divine energy we see in nature. Nature's magnificence can speak directly to our hearts, through the awe and interconnectedness we feel in its presence. In this way, the senses can be used as instruments of worship. Every time we stand in awe of the divine presence perceivable in this life, it is an act of honor and devotion. In ancient times, the rishis recognized this sacredness of life; they referred to the different elements they saw as divine presence, and they connected the elements to the senses through which they perceived them. For example, the sun god, Surya, and light are related to the eyes. The ears connect to the different directions in space, the nose relates to the cosmic air, and the mouth to fire. You can study these connections in greater detail as a way to contemplate on the Divine.

Below is a list of ways to use the senses in a positive manner. These practices lead to Self-healing, and help awaken our inner senses through the practice of pratyahara and contemplative meditation.

1. Use the tradition of **classical Tantra which teaches about the presence of gods and goddesses around us.** It teaches how to communicate with them through sacred worship. We can see them in the form of a *murti*, a symbol of the Divine, statue of a god.

   We also learn how to recognize the gods and goddesses in nature, which manifests as a feeling of bliss and unity. We connect with the *shakti*—the cosmic energy, the goddess, or divine power—that resides in all things; we connect with the essence—the *rasa* or *soma*, the divine nectar—that exists in the object of our perception. The *shakti* is behind everything we see; it is the energy or power of pure consciousness. It is this that gives us the sense of delight, the sense of happiness that we experience in nature.

   It happens when we turn away from our ego and towards the pure consciousness within. We must redirect and retrain our senses to focus on that inner light. Our senses have been tarnished and polluted by mundane external experiences, sensory pleasures, and the superabundance of sensory overload from modern-day social media and technology. As a result, we forget the divine presence that is possible to see and experience in everything—if only we turn our focus there.

2. Practice **Puja, a ceremonial worship or ritual.** Following the wisdom of tantra, we guide our senses to see the shakti all around us and learn to know it. We must honor this divine energy that brings life and being to all that is. We do so through three practices of remembrance: we visualize the gods and goddesses that are manifest in shakti; we perform actions to connect with them; and we repeat mantras to honor them, invoking them through divine energy in word. We can combine all three of these actions of remembrance through the ritual of Puja.

   Puja is a humbling celebration of spirit, where we enact the divine play. We use our senses to celebrate through chanting of mantra and kirtan to express our devotion to the divine energy. Puja is our celebration and connection to the world of nature, through our subtle senses; we still use the senses—still see, smell, and touch—but we connect to the divine or cosmic energy as the source, rather than the object itself. We connect consciousness to our heart of devotion.

Puja can be done elaborately or simply, but the essence and the sixteen steps are the same:

01. *Dhyana* – Meditating on the deity that is being invoked
02. *Aavaahana* – Inviting the deity to the altar
03. *Asana* – Giving the deity a seat
04. *Pandya* – Washing the deity's feet with clean water
05. *Arghya* – Offering the deity water to rinse hands and mouth
06. *Aachamana* – Offering the deity water to drink
07. *Snaana* – Bathing the deity with various auspicious items
08. *Vasthra* – Dressing the deity in clean clothes
09. *Yagnopaveetha* – Offering the deity a clean sacred thread
10. *Gandha* – Spreading fresh sandalwood paste on the deity
11. *Pushpa* – Offering fresh flowers while chanting the deity's names
12. *Dhoopa* – Spreading incense smoke throughout the altar
13. *Deep*a – Waving a lamp or offering the fire to illuminate the freshly decorated deity
14. *Naivedya* – Offering the deity some food
15. *Taambula* – Offering the deity a refreshing mix of betel nut and leaves
16. *Pradakshina & Namaskar*a – Circumambulating the altar and bidding farewell to the deity

After puja, we feel that we are bathing in the light. We wash outside, but we feel that we are immersed in the sacred water and sacred light.

3. **The *agnihotra*, or homa, a Vedic fire offering** can be performed at sunrise or sunset. First, create a sacred space with an altar, a space separate from all other activities in the home. Or it can be the meditation room. Purify and clean the energy in the room and air using incense of sandalwood, rose, jasmine, myrrh, champa, eucalyptus, mint, tulsi, or cinnamon. Place

an oil lamp on the altar to represent the fire or divine light. The space can be made more sacred and can be honored through decoration with *murti*, sacred stones, flowers on or around the altar, and with yantra and paintings or pictures of deities. Every deity has a sacred environment, with its associated energy of mountains, forests, water, flowers, and animals. In front of this home altar, perform mental puja. It does not have to include all the steps listed above, but rather it is imagined in detail, bringing the divine scene within through the senses, perceiving the shakti, the divine energy, in all things. This will spiritually nourish you.

4. **See the sacredness in nature.** Use your senses, tune them to see and focus on the sacredness when walking, hiking, or just spending time in nature. This activity has been called forest bathing or *shinrin-yoku* in Japan, where the concept originated. Forest bathing is walking or being in nature consciously, and mindfully connecting with what is around you—appreciating the wind, a tiny flower in the grass, the diversity of plants and trees and animals, the sky, rivers, ocean and so on. When you are in tune with nature and tuned into its essence, or *rasa*, you are in tune with the Divine.

5. Similar to forest bathing is **the practice of pilgrimage**. On a pilgrimage, you also walk, hike, and travel—often on a path well-traveled by many other pilgrims over many lifetimes, visiting places that are beautiful and sacred. The practice, again, requires you to be mindful and fully present, tuning into the essence of the sacred energy residing in the pilgrimage site. This is a good method of sublimating our desire for movement or change in landscape, in lieu of taking a tourist vacation. On pilgrimage, we adopt the attitude of seeing the Divine in all things. We surrender to the journey as we visit beautiful temples, pagodas, churches, and other sacred places where saints have lived, visited, or died and have left their bodies. Uplifting sacred places like this exist in many countries.

6. **Attend spiritual festivals**. In these events, you take part in or witness sacred celebrations, experience chants and rituals, hear storytelling or theater, and hear the subtle sounds of spiritually-elevated people.

7. **Gardening** is a very good sublimation method. Gardening is a very rich sensory experience—we touch the ground, dig in the soil, and smell the earth and the watch the different plants grow. Gardening is an ongoing sensory tuning with the earth, plants, and seasons; it can become part of our regular practice to keep our mind in tune with nature and the divine essence that can be experienced there.

8. A form of **sensory meditation,** we focus our attention on some aspect of nature like a landscape—or the universe—that helps us contemplate the fact that we are a part of something much larger than we generally realize. Lie back and meditate upon a sky full of planets and stars and distant galaxies. Gaze at the distant horizon during the day—sitting before the ocean, a lake, or a faraway mountain range. These sights are often so grand and magnificent that just looking at them will elevate you.
9. Meditate, using the mind to **visualize and comprehend the boundless space.** As we visualize, we try to see the whole, rather than focusing attention on any particular spot or aspect—shifting the mind from perception to proprioception. For example, we can visualize a sphere of golden light circulating around us. Along with this, we can chant mantras. Or we can see a dark blue light around us, visualize the expanse of space and chant Om Namah Shivaya. Similarly, we can meditate on the sounds and light that we can hear or experience within.
10. **Practice Yoga nidra,** deep relaxation, or Yogic sleep. Cultivate deep sleep, allowing the mind to be renewed in deep awareness. Use mantra and meditation to facilitate this deep relaxation.
11. **Practice abhyanga,** the Ayurvedic practice of herbal oil massage. In this massage, we use the sensation of touch on the skin in the moment, but also the deeper muscle sensations and the relaxation of tension and release of prana that results.
12. **Practice mindful hydration.** Throughout the day, drink warm water infused with herbs, such as tulsi, sage, mint, ginger, turmeric, or green tea. Sip from the cup while mindfully sensing the taste of the different herbs used. You can also drink golden milk (warm milk with turmeric) before you sleep at night. This practice helps to reconnect us with our senses.
13. **Karma Yoga** is a very good way to sublimate all our desires and senses. Service involves many of our senses. Karma Yoga is the skill of inaction in action through which we purify and uplift ourselves. In Karma Yoga, we have the inner motivation to be selfless, to do good for others, and we harness our senses to perform these acts of devotion.

## BRAHMACHARYA - SUBLIMATION OF ENERGY & DESIRE

Another important topic in the sublimation of energies and desires is *brahmacharya.* We have spoken of *pratyahara,* the practice of withdrawing our senses, turning our senses inward and shifting our attitude towards the senses as a means of sublimating sensory input.

At its simplest, *Brahmacharya* is control of the reproductive *indriya*, or sexual continence or complete abstinence. But *brahmacharya* is much larger than this and applies inwardly, as well as outwardly. It is control of all senses and, thus, all desires in thought, word, and deed.

**What is *brahmacharya* practice?**

The word *brahmacharya* is composed of two Sanskrit words: *Brahman* and *charya. Charya* means "occupation with, engaging, or following" and is connected to the idea of *acharya*, or teacher. So, in this instance, it means "a follower of Brahman" or "Brahman is the teacher." This powerful statement suggests that the *brahmachari* is one whose whole life is focused on moving inward and upward towards Brahman.

*Brahmacharya* is a life of self-restraint and sublimation of sexual energy—of all energy—into *ojas shakti. Ojas shakti* is the power and sustenance of life. *Ojas shakti* gives you contentment, perseverance, and happiness in living this life. You could say it is your spiritual immune system; it prevents disease. Put another way, *ojas shakti* gives you rest, relaxation, energy to overcome stress, and the endurance to move through life in a peaceful, happy, contented manner. Through the practice, you gain tremendous energy to keep your brain clear and increase your power of concentration, inquiry, perception, understanding, and memory. In this way, it is the foundation of a Yogic life, a divine life. It is the secret of health and longevity, and necessary for Self-healing.

Swami Sivananda wrote a book called *The Practice of Brahmacharya*. In it, he said that this world is nothing but sex and ego. *"Passion is the instinctive urge for external normalization through self-preservation and self-multiplication."* He said that diversifying energy makes you distracted and fragmented. We know that the force of Yoga, the focus of Yoga, is to come back to One. In this light, the force or instinct to procreate is opposed to the focus of Yoga and the force towards unity and the integration of opposites in being. Thus, if you control your passions, sublimate and focus your energies on Yoga, rather than procreation or other opposing desires, you will more successfully pursue the path of finding the Truth. Thus, *brahmacharya*, the path of self-control, is controlling the instinctive urge. The practice is applied to men and women in all places and at all times.

To practice *brahmacharya* successfully, you must understand *samskaras. Samskaras* are mental impressions, the deep patterning in our brains that form our default patterns of behavior. One very deep *samskara* in the mind, aimed at finding happiness through the senses, is the desire for sexual satisfaction. *Samskaras,* however, can be a large source of unhappiness and suffering. A *brahmachari* needs to be aware of these *samskaras;* we follow them out of habit and then they obstruct the Self-healing process, both physically and mentally.

## BRAHMACHARYA PRACTICES

These practices will assist you in pursuing the path of *brahmacharya.* Keep in mind that there are two parts here: practices for the renunciate or full celibate initiate and practices for the "householder."

### PART 1 – Brahmacharya practices for the renunciate

- **Choose your place of living.** To pursue dedicated practice, chant mantras, and practice sadhana, you need to have a space to live that is elevating, healthy, peaceful, and joyful. It is best to live in nature—or even better, in an ashram in nature surrounded by a satsang, or community of like-minded people also on the spiritual path. Sivananda said, "You should not live by yourself; you should not live with friends; you should not live with acquaintances; you should not live with relatives." Consequently, you need to live in spiritual company with people who have the same aspirations and motivations. You should not just go and live in the middle of the city, say, next to a movie theater or next to bars and clubs or other non-sattvic environments; the negative energy will make your struggle harder, rather than supporting your spiritual practice.
- Be careful of the **company you keep**, and who and what energy you surround yourself with. As mentioned above, you need to live with spiritually-advanced people, but "company" is also the people and ideas you expose yourself to through various media. Beware of reading books and consuming all forms of media content, except those that are directly spiritual. For example, the newsstand has hundreds of magazines, but they are all about fashion and how to be sexy and beautiful, what kind of car or motorcycle makes you look good in society's eyes; all are focused on vanity and ego. Stay away from this type of content. "Company" also includes movies. Resist the habit of watching movies with romantic, sexual content that will only excite your lower instincts. Beware of people or media content from those channels that are eager to present negative news and scandals that will merely disturb your mental peace.

- **Practice spiritual sadhana.** Swami Sivananda said that lack of spiritual sadhana is the main cause of all sexual attraction. Consider that you are sexually active when you have no practice, but if you practice spiritual sadhana, you will not find any ideas of sexual attraction in your mind; it is focused on spiritual practice. You cannot easily abstain directly without practice; you need Yoga and spiritual sadhana to transform and sublimate that energy.
- **Cut the formalities of social life.** By formality, Swami Sivananda means to remove yourself from the influence of peer pressure and the expected social behaviors that go with it. For example, if you don't want to go to a party, but your friends go and keep calling and telling you to come, you will feel inclined to oblige, just to be friendly. Or you don't want to drink, but people around you drink, so you give in, saying that one drink won't hurt. A similar idea applies to smoking, fashion, fitting in, and all kinds of social events. Swami Sivananda says to cut this obligation from your life. If you are sincere in your quest to pursue the sublime life of spirituality, then cut this formality and lead a devotional life free from the business of bodily existence. Don't focus your life on the needs of the body, focus it on the spiritual quest.
- **Study sacred scriptures.** You will need to study a lot and endeavor to acquire knowledge. Always be reading the sacred scriptures, studying the *Bhagavad Gita* and similar texts.
- **Do daily devotional practice.** For example, you can practice sun salutations with the feeling of mantra and devotion to the sun. Consider doing the practices during the time of sunrise and sunset. You can do a fire ceremony practice yourself, alone at sunrise and sunset. You should also do japa, repetition of mantra, any elevating practice. You can repeat the Gayatri Mantra daily and also your personal mantra. The point is to have a daily devotional practice to keep your mind focused inward and upward.
- **Do service to the guru,** according to Swami Sivananda, for twelve years. When you live in service of the guru, the teacher of wisdom, you are exposed to the highest teaching and spiritual energy.
- **Abstain from the company of the opposite sex.** Be more strict with your choice of company. When you are in the company of people you are attracted to, or even just seeing them, it automatcally creates desire, because of the deep *samskara* in your mind. This *samskara* is said to be intergenerational.

- **Go to sleep early and get up early,** and sleep alone in your own bed.
- **Do not overeat.** *Mitahara* means "to eat half" or "half full." One of the many aspects of *brahmacharya* is proper diet. The sattvic diet must be simple, spiceless, calming, and non-stimulating. It can also include the practice of fasting at times, which is a great help in the path .
- **Do tapas,** austerities for purification. Swami Sivananda liked taking cold baths. Every day, he would go down to the river Ganga and take a cold plunge. It is considered a nervine tonic; it helps calm the nerves of the genitourinary system.
- **Practice purity.** Abstain from body decoration, beautifying the body, wearing nice and fashionable clothing, using perfumes, etc.
- **Have good conduct.** Spiritualize all of your relationships. Behave with respect toward teachers, elders, and your classmates. Do not have connections with people of the world, even on social media. Do not cause injury to anybody; do not gossip or indulge in scandals. Practice ahimsa.
- **Cultivate a pure heart and pure knowledge**: Swami Sivananda said the senses should not be suppressed, but to cultivate a pure heart and pure knowledge, as discussed above in the discussion of *pratyahara*. Understand that desire cannot be extinguished through enjoyment, and suppression of the senses will only increase desire, blazing up like a fire fed with ghee. The practice of sense control and shifting the attitude towards the senses should be pursued.
- **Respect your teacher's wisdom.** According to Swami Sivananda, it should be considered superior to that of parents. The parents gave birth through lustful meetings and the physical body, while the wisdom of the teacher gives birth to your real immortal Self.
- **Cultivate humility.** Avoid the fetters of name, fame, and worldliness. Humility is very important, because when you cultivate external power, you empower the ego and cannot control yourself.
- Practice regularly the **Hatha Yoga methods** of asana to help check the sexual impulse, especially the inverted postures of *sirsasana* (headstand) and *sarvangasana* (shoulderstand), and the meditative posture *siddhasana*. These asanas draw the mind inwards and help control the senses.
- **Pranayama** helps to gradually transform the mind from gross to subtle. Regular daily practice of alternate nostril breathing, *anuloma viloma*, helps balance the mind. During your practice, you should feel joy and not too much exertion.

- ***Mula bandha*** is a Yogic *kriya* that takes the downward-flowing energy or sexual energy called *apana* and, through long practice, controls and transforms it into *ojas shakti*, the spiritual energy discussed above. Advanced Hatha Yoga practices, such as this, should be done under the supervision of a teacher.

- **Do *kriya* practice.** You can practice *uddiyana bandha*, which is done by exhaling completely and drawing the abdomen in for a few seconds. Then release the abdomen and inhale. Then you can do *nauli*, which is done by churning the abdominal muscles from side to side. These practices draw the prana upwards and reduce the flow of apana.

- **Practice mudras.** The purpose of Maha Mudra is to improve control over sexual energy. In Yoga, *mudra* means "seal of energy."

- Practice the nine methods of **Bhakti Yoga.**

- Practice the **yamas and niyamas** of Ashtanga (Raja) Yoga.

- **Practice *vichara*, self-inquiry, and the aspirant's qualifications (above).** Strengthen your will, eradicating *raga-dvesa*. Once you cultivate a strong will—will is a powerful enemy of passion—passion will die.

**PART 2 - Brahmacharya practices for the householder**

Householders can learn to see their relationship not as mere sexual coupling, but rather as a sacred union.

Even within marriage, there is *brahmacharya* for the householder. Without taking the vow of abstention, the married couple would be encouraged to spiritualize their relationship. They needn't abstain from sexual relations, but are advised to keep the vow of moderation and to transmute sexual energy into spiritual energy, as much as possible.

- Spiritualizing the relationship involves both partners engaging in daily meditation, japa, and spiritual practices.

- Try to develop pure love beyond lust. Live a life of spiritual partnership, supporting each other on the path.

- Think of God and the Devi, or the goddess, to spiritualize your relationship. A husband can consider his wife as a sister, as a goddess, or as the *Atman*. Likewise, a wife can consider her husband as a brother, as a god, or as the *Atman*.

- Know that continence is not harmful. It conserves your energy on all levels and it gives immense strength and peace. It is the sublimation and spiritualization of sexual energy, offering it in humble dedication to the service of God and humanity.

- Beware of social environments that promote intoxication and sensual indulgence. Include being in sattvic environments as a goal in life.

**Here are some ways that sublimation can be practiced in marriage:**

1. **Nurture emotional intimacy.** Connect with your partner on a deeper level by openly sharing thoughts, feelings, and vulnerabilities. This creates a strong bond between partners, which can help to sublimate sexual energy into a deeper emotional connection.
2. **Cultivating shared interests** or hobbies can help to channel sexual energy into more productive and meaningful pursuits. Engaging in activities together strengthens the bond between partners and allows for more dynamic ways to connect.
3. **Serve others.** When couples engage in service, it helps to create a sense of purpose. It generates joy and fulfillment, which can contribute to a sense of spiritual connection.
4. **Building strong communication skills** helps to create and maintain a strong bond between partners. It encourages empathy, understanding, and compromise, which leads to a deeper understanding of one another and strengthens the relationship.

Sublimation in marriage involves using sexual energy as a foundation for deeper connection and spiritual growth. By channeling the energy in more meaningful ways and building a strong emotional bond, couples can achieve a sense of fulfillment and joy in their relationship.

## HEALING FROM ADDICTIVE BEHAVIORS

Ingrained habits or addictive behaviors stem from the subconscious mind and can be challenging to change or overcome. *Raga-dvesa*, like and dislike or attraction and aversion, are the two main mind currents that drive behavior. *Raga-dvesa* are deep tendencies carried from lifetime to lifetime. They are the two currents of the mind that bind us to the wheel of samsara. They are the driving forces behind deep habits and addiction.

Working with addiction requires a special understanding and special attention. To understand the root cause of an addiction, we must identify and understand the root cause of the imbalance that is causing it. *(See the book "Yoga of Recovery" by Durga Leela, who has been teaching this program for many years at Sivananda Yoga Vedanta Centers.)*

**Five senses therapy**

Ayurveda uses five senses therapy to work with hard-to-change habits and addiction. We use our senses and their respective organs to heal ourselves. Everything in this world is composed of the five elements: earth, water, fire, air and ether. We must be familiar with the five elements and how the senses connect with them to understand and apply sense therapy.

- Smell is the sense connected to earth. Earth gives a sense of groundedness, solidity, stability, and presence.
- Taste is connected to water. Water is the sense of flow, of fluidity, which can be translated as compassion and feeling for both self and others.
- Sight connects to fire. Fire, the sense of light, relates to heat and digestion and hormonal transformation. The virtue of fire is clarity and decisiveness.
- Touch connects to air. Air is the idea of movement, circulation, coordination, and the nervous system. The virtue is adaptability and creativity.
- Hearing connects to ether. Ether is the sense of space and proprioception, the peripheral sense of the body in space. You need to develop openness if you want to connect to others, but also time have good personal boundaries.

The five senses are connected to the five elements and the five elements are connected to the motor organs, or organs of action, called the *karma indriyas* in Sanskrit.

- The anus is related to the earth.
- The reproductive organs are related to water.
- The feet are related to fire.
- The hands are related to air.
- The tongue and speech are related to ether.

If there is a misuse of the reproductive organs, relating to the water element, which is damaging to our prana, to our health and peace, then we can determine an appropriate therapy to self-soothe, recover, and heal, without feeling deprived. For example, it could be that you were eating only fast food, drinking artificial forms of water like soda, and not attending to your emotional needs; you have a negative emotional imprint. The remedy would be hydration, bathing with herbal water, adding ghee to the diet to replenish the brain, and implementing nourishing self-care like self-abhyanga (self-massage using warm sesame oil), and extra care for our relationships.

What we want is to find and develop healthy and useful self-practice—a practice we can apply on our own that brings a feeling of satiation, satisfaction, and pleasure. Seek gratification that is creative, constructive, and healing.

## CONCLUSION

There is a lot to do to ward off the many obstacles to sublimating the senses in our attempt to bring the energy inward and upward. We must exert to counteract the powerful force of desire that pulls us outward and downward in sensual and sexual energy expenditure. We now have a sense of what we can do to begin to understand and counter that tendency. We can now appreciate the importance of mindfulness and dedication, how everything is connected in small, subtle ways in daily life. The more we are aware, the better the chance of improving our life, applying the Self-healing therapies that can guide us.

**Be who you are**

*N., a 19-year-old male, is a law student living with his parents. He is gay, but his parents do not accept his sexual orientation. Both of his parents are lawyers and judges, and exhibit strict and demanding behavior towards him.*

*His mother is emotionally attached to her children. His parents encouraged him to study law; he pursued it, despite not genuinely enjoying the field.*

*He enjoys composing music and singing in his free time, achieving success in writing songs for singers on YouTube.*

*Outwardly, he appears cheerful and outgoing, but he struggles with insomnia and anxiety and is always hesitant to express his thoughts, as he fears not being accepted. He was advised to use positive affirmations regarding self-love and to establish a deeper connection with his mother to feel stronger.*

*He then associated his deep love of the pine forest with the idea of his mother and began to consider her as a sacred forest. He was also encouraged to write a journal to understand his thoughts.*

*After practicing these techniques for a month, he underwent a complete transformation and felt happy and fulfilled by being able to share his thoughts with his parents. He realized that he is constantly loved and protected by his dedicated mother. His insomnia and anxiety disappeared, and he stopped placing excessive importance on others' opinions of him.*

**QUESTIONS**

1. *Where does desire come from and what is its main characteristic?*
2. *What is pratyahara? Name five practices of positive use of the senses that will help in sublimation of the senses.*
3. *What is brahmacharya? Name five practices for celibate renunciates that will help the process.*
4. *Name five practices for householders that will help regulate sexual energy.*

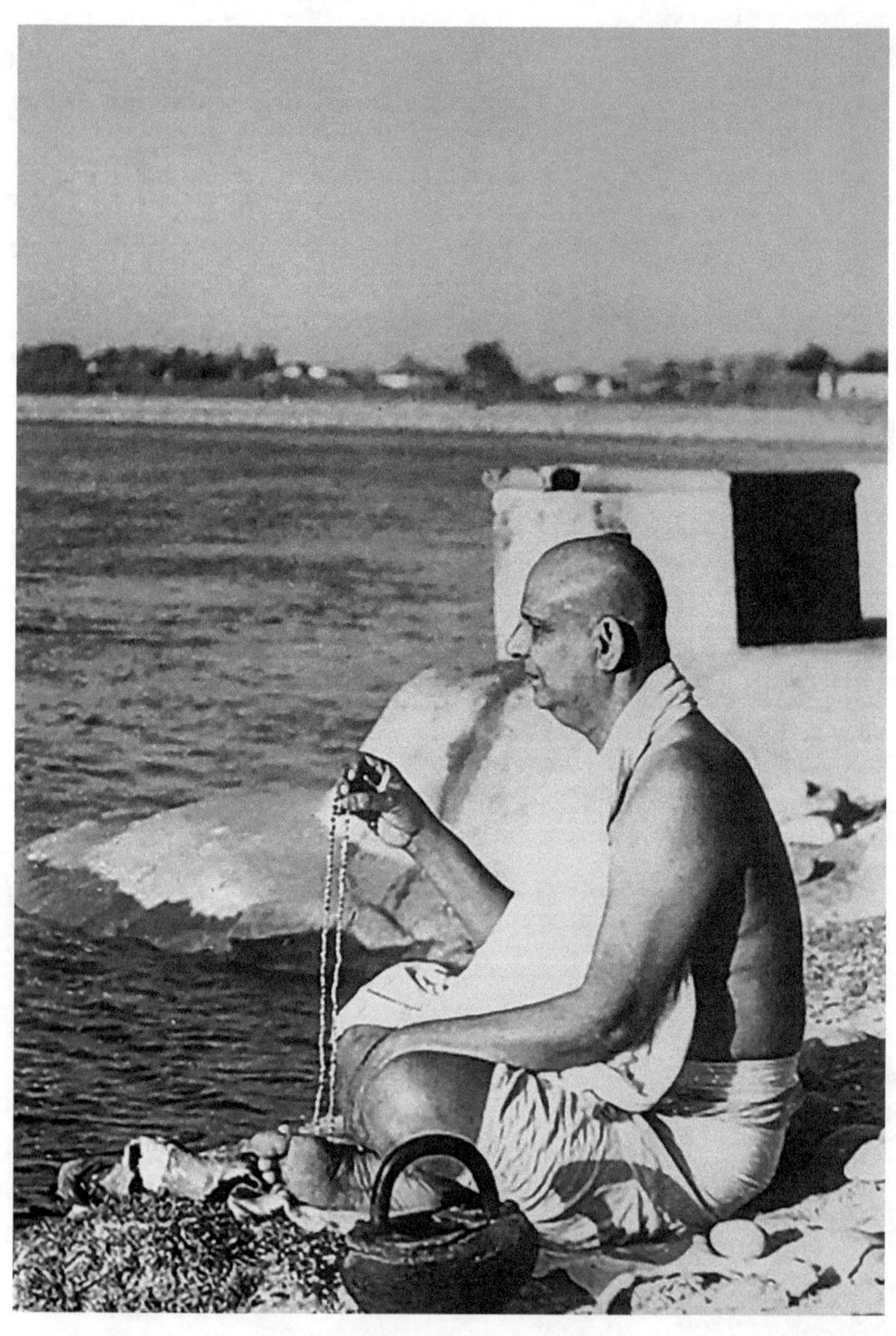

SWAMI SIVANANDA DOING JAPA BY THE GANGA

CHAPTER 14

# Protecting & Strengthening the Mind with Mantras

***"Mantras are Sanskrit invocations of the Supreme Being. Reinforced and propelled by japa meditation, they pass from the verbal level through the mental and telepathic states, and on to pure thought energy. It is the most direct way to approach the transcendental state."***

*- SWAMI VISHNU-DEVANANDA in "Meditation and Mantras"*

Swami Sivananda wrote in his book *Bliss Divine*, *"Meditation is the only royal road to the attainment of freedom. It is a mysterious ladder, which reaches from Earth to Heaven, from error to truth, from darkness to light, from pain to Bliss, from restlessness to abiding peace, from ignorance to knowledge, and from mortality to immortality."*

Spiritual aspirants need to meditate. The mind is an instrument for Self-healing and Self-realization; protect it from negative influences and keep it focused on the highest thoughts. Understand the mechanics of the mind and know that Japa Yoga is the most powerful way to turn the mind around, destroy the *vasanas*, or habitual thoughts, and protect the mind from new harmful impressions. The word *sankalpa* refers to thoughts, memories, old negative patterns, old mistakes, fancies and fantasies, depressing moods, innumerable desires, and different *samskaras* or impressions in the mind.

## MECHANICS OF THE MIND

Here is a summary of how the mind works and the importance of repeating a mantra and doing Japa Yoga.

1. The mind is always restless and moving. Our lives are constantly unstable; the mind projects different ideas externally and we run after them. We can compare the **ripples on the surface of a lake,** to the mind, constantly having thought waves. We need to endeavor to keep the mind calm at all times.

2. The mind is not only restless, but constantly jumps around in a disorganized manner, like **a drunken monkey.** To counteract this restless mind, we need to concentrate it on one point, one object of focus.

3. The mind is unruly. It has certain habits and doesn't like to be told what to do. We feel confused by the mind, with its favorite thoughts and secrets. It's like **a wild horse** that resists being tamed. When we know to stay away from certain harmful habits, we are sometimes at a loss to know what to do instead. In the same manner as training a wild horse, we need to be patient, gentle and consistent, showing the mind that we are the master.

4. The mind has deep secrets. It is like **a shy lady** who does not want to be seen, so she hides herself and, when we are not looking, she sneaks out. The subconscious mind is very strong and has endless thoughts, patterns, habits, and desires. For an untrained mind, it is said that 95% of the mind is unknown and belongs to the past. When we function out of our subconscious, we know very little of what is in our mind.

   We cannot trust the mind; we must train it. If we use the mind without awareness, we will do things that lead us away from our ultimate goal, which is to grow and to become enlightened. We need to start to be aware and maintain our awareness at a high level. We need to be very serious in working with the mind.

5. The mind is like **an old music record,** functioning out of grooves or habits, patterns, *samskaras*. The mind is just a bundle of habits. We need to replace negative habits with positive ones. For example, if we have the bad habit of waking up late and, first thing, turning on the news, now we replace the news with self-affirmations and the practice of counting our blessings. We can change thought patterns to positive ones.

6. The mind is extremely fast, **like a ceiling fan**. It is so fast that it escapes our awareness. We need to slow it down, to be able to understand a few of the main thoughts that are causing disturbance and need to be dealt

with. Asana and pranayama help to calm and refocus the mind. Mantra repetition keeps the mind one-pointed and simple.

7. **The mind is connected to the body**. There is an intimate connection between what we feel in our mind and in our body. Moving through an asana sequence moves the prana and directly affects the mind. That's why we do asana, to control the mind.

8. **The mind is connected to the breath**. Pranayama controls the breath and controls the mind. When we do japa, we repeat mantra, coordinating it with our breath. the mind is connected to the breath. For example, when an artist has stage fright, by controlling the breath, the emotions calm down. Pranayama helps to balance the flow of energies in the mind.

9. **The mind is connected with the senses.** There are many effective techniques to withdraw the senses from their myriad objects of fascination. This is part of *pratyahara* practice (see chapter 13).

10. Although the mind is very fast, it can only think **one thought at a time,** like a computer. Thus, focusing on mantra repetition brings the mind easily to a concentrated state.

11. **The mind works with names and forms.** It thinks via words and images. This world is projected by the mind. If you want to see the Truth of your Self, you will need to transcend the limiting names and forms of this world into the Divine. Mantra science uses sacred sounds and sacred images to attract the mind and then changes its workings through high vibrations.

12. The mind **works through association.** One thought leads to another, and you can find yourself lost in thoughts. The mind is easily influenced. Use of mantra will help the mind to keep good association and stay on a positive track.

## BENEFITS OF JAPA YOGA

Japa Yoga, systematic repetition of a mantra, is like soap for the mind. It intensifies spiritual *samskaras*. Not only does it clean up past negative *samskaras,* but it installs new positive, spiritual *samskaras*. The practice of Japa Yoga fosters concentration, which leads to meditation. Often, spiritual aspirants do not understand the true benefits of mantra repetition. Occasional repetition will not create grooves deep enough to change consciousness.

Swami Sivananda says, "*Every name or mantra is filled with countless shaktis or powers.*" Mantra repetition is the most direct way to cleanse the mind. It gives the mind new kinds of powers and connects us with the Divine. The glory of the mantra can be realized, but only through constant repetition of the name.

The mind can be our best friend or our worst enemy; it depends on how we use it. Master the mind; don't let it pursue power and divert us away from our goal.

## THOUGHT POWER

Thoughts, when deep enough, have the power of influence. Thoughts of the same nature attract each other. Thoughts have wavelengths and different levels of vibration. Thoughts have prana. Consider the relationship between thoughts and prana. High-prana thoughts have higher wavelengths. They are powerful and impactful and bring us closer to the Truth. Low-wavelength thoughts involve less prana and yield less impact, less power of influence; they lead us to pain and suffering.

## THOUGHT INFLUENCE

We are constantly swimming in an ocean of thoughts. If the the "water" is clear, we feel light, clean, and refreshed. But, if we swim in a muddy lake with smelly, stagnant water—meaning the thought environment is made up of tamasic thoughts—then we come out feeling polluted, heavy, and dirty.

Therefore, if you want to strengthen and protect your mind, you must learn to purify your thoughts and consciously choose a clean thought environment. Guard yourself from the inside and from the outside. When you keep your thought vibrations high, low-level thoughts cannot enter; they cannot affect you. Or you might choose to consciously "tune down" to lift others up.

## WHAT IS MANTRA YOGA?

Swami Sivananda wrote in his book *Japa Yoga*, the most comprehensive and authoritative treatise on mantra scriptures, *"Mantra Yoga is an exact science; by constant thinking of mantra, one is protected and released from the rounds of birth and death."* Your thoughts will all be positive; you will no longer have negative thoughts. You will be free from karma, the realm of birth and death.

Japa Yoga is achieved by a mental process. In the word *mantra*, there are two words: *man* is "to think," as it comes from *manas* meaning "mind," and *Tra* comes from the word *trai*, which means "to protect or to free." The mantra frees you from what? It frees you from the bondage of the phenomenal world—the world projected by our minds and our thoughts.

*"A mantra, when constantly repeated, awakens consciousness,"* wrote Swami Vishnudevanandaji in his beautiful book *Meditation and Mantras*. He says, *"A mantra is a mystical energy encased in a sound structure. Upon repetition of the mantra, the energy is released; mantras are Sanskrit invocations of the Divine."*

**How does a mantra work?**

When you repeat a mantra, a certain energy, a certain power, is released. The "mystical energy" hidden in the formula of sound—not any sound, but a Sanskrit sound—is elicited. Why Sanskrit? Sanskrit is called Devanagari or the language of the gods. It is not a foreign Indian language, it is an ancient universal language. The fifty letters of the Sanskrit alphabet are based on the pure vibrations of our chakras, our inner energy centers. When we repeat a Sanskrit mantra, it strikes directly on our inner energy system. Using the mantra, we create a certain pure vibration in our astral body and mind and rid ourselves of all our impurities and negativities.

A mantra cannot be created or tailored for an individual. It is a sound formula given to us by the Rishis, the sages or the seers of ancient times. The Rishis have used the mantra and attained the highest realization. There are six conditions of being a mantra: it has a seed, a *shakti*, a specific energy, a presiding deity, a specific meter, a specific wavelength, and a plug or lock. Use of mantra is an exact science and needs to be studied properly under the guidance of a teacher.

Japa Yoga uses the sound vibration of the mantra. It is the most effective method of meditating and clears out negativities. It helps make our minds strong by increasing our concentration. Remaining focused on a pure vibration, helps us counteract the constant jumping and restlessness of the distracted mind. We can repeat the mantra verbally or mentally, at a specific time or all day long when we can remember; there are many ways to use a mantra.

We need to be thoroughly convinced of these profound benefits, so we will be motivated to practice. When a mantra is repeated consistently enough, it moves consciousness from a low level to a very high level of thought.

**The four stages of sound:**

- *Vaikhari* is dense, audible sound at its maximum differentiation, gross audible sound.
- *Madhyama* is a subtle, more internal state; sounds are inaudible to the physical ear, but higher in wavelength and more powerful.
- *Pashyanti* is even higher, a telepathic and universal vibratory level. It's beyond the mind, beyond the specifics of the mind.

- *Para* is sound that is not expressed, a potential state of sound, undifferentiated. It's the unchanging, primal substratum of all languages. It is the source of the universe. It links directly to *Para Brahman*. In the undifferentiated, *Ishwara* and *shakti* are one. *Shakti*—the power of sound, the power of thought—and consciousness become one.
- A mantra awakens supernatural powers or consciousness, which we call *chaitanya. Chaitanya* means "spiritual consciousness" or "the knowledge of the Divine."
- A mantra generates creative forces and has the power to release the cosmic and the super-cosmic consciousness.
- Mantra repetition works by changing the vibratory wavelength of the thought. Thought and prana go from the gross manifestation of nature that you see, into higher wavelengths, and even higher wavelengths, and finally to the highest wavelength. Remember the *Para* stage of sound; at the highest level, thought goes beyond different languages. It is beyond language itself.
- There is a relationship between sound and image, we can "see sound." The science of Cymatics studies how a sound frequency creates a specific design in space. If you change the sound, it creates a different beautifully intricate design. If you destroy the image and play the same music or make the same sound, then exactly the same image will appear again. The mind works with sound or name and image. It is the mind that prevents us from seeing the Absolute. It prevents us from realizing ourselves because of its cacophony of thoughts. Our manifested world is also very confusing. A simple sound will create a certain form in the invisible world and affect our astral body. If you have an oscillator, you can capture the image on a metal plate. Sounds produce shapes, and particular notes will give rise to particular forms. A combination of sounds creates very complicated shapes. If you want to generate a particular form, you must produce a definite note in a particular pitch. This was taught by the Rishis, but now, slowly, research has started to figure out the science behind it.
- Repeated recitation of a mantra will produce in the mind the form of the devata or the deity, or the cosmic energy that is connected with the mantra. Repetition of the mantra *Om Namah Shivaya* will produce the form of Shiva. Repetition of *Om Namo Narayanaya* will produce the form of Vishnu. Every sound corresponds to the sound and form of the Divine. When it is on a high level, it reaches the Divine, the *chaitanya*—the spiritual

consciousness, a world we are unfamiliar with as it is beyond our physical world. There are so many worlds with different kinds of cosmic energy.

- The mantra of the devata is the devata himself. Mantra is the means of invoking the devata, the cosmic energy or being.

Swami Sivananda says, *"Japa purifies the heart."* This suggests that we will directly open to pure love.

*"Japa steadies the mind. Japa destroys birth and death. Japa burns sins. Japa scorches samskaras. Japa annihilates attachment. Japa induces vairagya, which means detachment. Japa roots out all desires. Japa makes one fearless. Japa removes delusion. Japa gives supreme peace. Japa develops prem or devotion. Japa unites the devotee with the Lord. Japa gives health, wealth, strength, and long life. Japa brings God-consciousness. Japa awakens the Kundalini. Kundalini is a spiritual power. Japa bestows eternal bliss. Japa washes the subtle body and the astral body."*

**Four types of mantras**

1. *Saguna mantra:* mantra accompanied by the form of a deity
2. *Nirguna mantra:* mantra without form
3. *Abstract mantra:* the *Pranava* or "OM" mantra, or Vedantic mantra
4. *Bija mantra:* the mono-syllable seed sound hidden in all mantras

With consistent repetition of the mantra, the sadhaka, or the person who meditates, will develop the virtues and the powers of the deity that presides over the mantra. The person inherits the power hidden in the mantra. A different mantra manifests a different *shakti*.

**How to choose a mantra**

- You can choose a mantra according to the sound vibration you find attractive.
- You can choose a mantra based on the image of the deity that is meaningful and attractive.
- You can choose a mantra according to the meaning of the mantra, for example: love, peace or prosperity.

**How many times should you repeat the mantra?**

Repeating a mantra three times is the minimum invocation, but that is not enough. We then say it three times three or nine times. Then we increase to 27 times, 54 times, 108 times, or 1,080 times. If we are very sincere, we may take a vow to do, for example, 108 repetitions (one mala) of a particular mantra three times a day.

**The different mantras**

- Mantra of Shiva: *Om Namah Shivaya. Om Namah Shivaya. Om Namah Shivaya.*
- Mantra of Vishnu. *Om Namo Narayanaya. Om Namo Narayanaya. Om Namo Narayanaya.*
- Mantra of Krishna, who is an incarnation of Vishnu. *Om Namo Bhagavate Vasudevaya. Om Namo Bhagavate Vasudevaya. Om Namo Bhagavate Vasudevaya*

Here are the mantra of the three forms of Shakti/Goddess.

- Mantra of Goddess Durga: *Om Sri Durgayai Namah. Om Sri Durgayai Namah. Om Sri Durgayai Namah.*
- Mantra of Goddess Lakshmi: *Om Sri Maha Lakshmiyai Namah. Om Sri Maha Lakshmiyai Namah. Om Sri Maha Lakshmiyai Namah.*
- Mantra of Goddess Saraswati: *Om Aim Saraswatyai Namah. Om Aim Saraswatyai Namah. Om Aim Saraswatyai Namah.*

There are many more mantras:

- The mantra OM is composed of A-U-M. It's as if there are three sounds, when there is only one sound: OM…OM…OM.
- A bija mantra is a seed sound mantra. It is not used for Japa.

**How do you get a personal mantra?**

A mantra cannot be created. The energy of the mantra in the form of mystical knowledge is passed on to the ripe individual. The best way to receive a mantra is to study or learn from a guru or a guru lineage. *Guru* means "the removal of darkness." The Sivananda organization has evolved from a lineage of teachers. Our two most contemporary gurus are Swami Sivananda and Swami Vishnudevananda. The current *acharyas* initiate students into mantras on behalf of the lineage of gurus. It is important to choose and stick to one lineage of teachers.

The guru/disciple relationship is an age-old tradition where spiritual energy is transmitted from one person to another through mantra *diksha*, or mantra initiation. The mantra, once initiated during the ceremony, creates a link between you and the spiritual teacher. This psychic and spiritual relationship should then be kept alive by daily mantra repetition. The longer and more consistently you work with the mantra faithfully, the faster the purification will be. Faith is important in mantra repetition. It's not blind faith. It's scientific. You become what you think about most. In Japa Yoga, faith is essential, superceding the intellect and the ego.

What was the trick used to control the mind of this giant servant? He represents our mind. What is our mind always doing? It is full of desires. We satisfy a desire and another one comes. Truly, this unending allure is killing us. What can we do to control the mind? What does the tree in the courtyard represent? Think of a string of mala beads or a rosary. The mala beads are the tree and the giant servant/the mind is climbing. Om Namo Narayanaya, Om Namo Narayanaya, Om Namo Narayanaya, one step at a time, one bead and one mantra at a time. When we arrive at the end of 108 beads, and meet the Meru bead, we flip it around and roll it again one step at a time. The bead rolling with mantra helps the mind to slow down and become one-pointed and calm. At that time, we can feel who we are. This is the beauty of Japa Yoga.

**Practical advice for doing japa**

- The best time for japa is dawn or dusk—early morning, sunrise, or sunset.
- Sit in a dedicated space, facing north or east.
- Keep a steady pose, a cross-legged sitting posture.
- Sit on a wool or cotton blanket or keep the vibration using a certain type of skin or grass mat for insulation.
- Prepare for the Japa Yoga session with some prayers and some intention.
- Repeat correctly with good articulation. The mind needs to be kept alert.
- Mantra repetition can be done by repeating verbally, murmuring, or repeating silently. Mental japa is more powerful than verbal.
- Do not change the mantra; always keep the same mantra.
- Learn how to use a japa mala (rosary) properly. This of great help in the beginning.

- Optionally, place a picture of the deity of the mantra in front of you while doing japa.
- Endeavor to complete a fixed number of japa malas or follow a fixed amount of time.
- After meditation, sit quietly for ten minutes to absorb the vibration of the mantra.

**Additional guidelines for doing japa**

### The story of a buffalo farmer

*Govinda wanted to be initiated by his teacher. He asked for a mantra and the teacher gave him one. Whatever the teacher gave, he forgot; he could not remember. Then finally the teacher asked him, "So, what do you like the most?" He said, "Oh, I don't know, I just have my buffalo. Every day I go out with my buffalo, so I love my buffalo the most." So the teacher said, "Okay, I will give you the mantra. Your mantra is "Om buffalo." You keep repeating the "Om buffalo" mantra and then you meet me again and I will give you further instructions.*

*Some time passed—weeks, months—and the teacher hadn't seen Govinda. The teacher went to the village and asked where Govinda was. Nobody had seen Govinda. So he went to Govinda's hut. The hut was a small cabin made out of mud with a wood frame. The teacher called his name, "Govinda, Govinda, I know you're there, come out!" Then he waited and then called again. Then he heard some sounds and asked, "Are you there? Can you please come out?" Then came Govinda's answer, "Oh teacher. I'm so happy that you have come. I wanted to come and see you, but I cannot come out through the door." The teacher asked, "Why can you not come out through the door?" He said, "Oh, my horns are too big. I can't come out through the door."*

*What does this story illustrate? Govinda repeated, "Om buffalo," and after some time, he became a buffalo. Thus, the teacher knew that Govinda was ready and initiated him into a mantra and he was able to attain a high level of consciousness.*

**The story of a woodcutter**

*A woodcutter is cutting wood to make a living. He is getting old. He's afraid he won't be able to chop wood much longer, so he prays. His guru appears in his dream and says, "Okay, I will send you a servant, but on one condition: You have to keep him busy, otherwise, he will kill you." The woodcutter agrees, saying, "No problem, I have plenty of work to keep him busy. Please send him fast!"*

*The servant arrives—a big, tall, and powerful guy who says, "Master, give me work." The woodcutter replies, "Okay, cut the wood, bring it to the market, sell it, come back." He does that. "Okay, build a fence around the property." He does. Dig a well, he does. Build a bigger house, he does. Whatever the woodcutter could think of, this guy did incredibly fast. The servant asked, "More work, master. Next?" The woodcutter was starting to become afraid, as he was running out of ideas.*

*Again he prays and, again, the guru appears and says, "I'll give you a trick to control the mind of this servant: Tell him to go to the forest and find a straight tree. Cut off all the branches, cut the tree down, and bring it to the courtyard. Dig a big hole and secure the tree. Then tell him his job is to climb from bottom to top. When he arrives at the top, tell him his new job is to go from top down to bottom—bottom to top and top to bottom, bottom to top and top to bottom. The wood cutter did as instructed.*

*So, after some time, guess what happened? The giant servant could do any kind of work very fast, always wanting more, but he could not do this job. He begged the woodcutter, "Please release me from this job; I promise I won't kill you; I cannot do this anymore!" Thus, he was subdued.*

- Use the right hand, not the left.
- Avoid using the index finger.
- Hold the japa mala high, close to the body, and not down near the level of the navel or below. Hold it nearer to your chest or face.
- When you use the japa mala, cover your hand with a cloth or shawl, as it is a private, sacred activity.
- When you roll the beads of your japa mala, you can turn the beads towards you or push them away from you, one at a time.
- Repeat the mantra at a medium speed. Don't hurry, or go too slowly.
- Before sitting, decide on a fixed number of rounds you will complete—for instance, three or six malas every time you sit. Or go by time— fifteen minutes or half an hour or more.
- You can also do likhita japa, continuous writing of a mantra with concentration in a notebook.
- Do not change your mantra. Keep the same connection to the source, to the lineage, that gave you the mantra. Stick to repeating the one mantra alone, don't switch from mantras to mantra. Never change your mantra.
- Remember the mantra with every incoming and outgoing breath. Then, it becomes part of your breath. You can do mantra sadhana while working or at any time when you do not have to be focused on an external task—for example, when you're driving or doing Karma Yoga. Repeat the mantra as often as you can and gain the benefits. The effect is cumulative, as you gain power. There will come a time when the energy is built up enough and you will experience a shift in energy. You'll feel it.
- Keep the mantra to yourself. Do not disclose it to people who don't understand.
- There are different types of mala beads. Choose one that's easy to roll. Generally, a rudraksha mala is for Lord Shiva. Tulsi and sandalwood malas are for Lord Vishnu. There are many types of crystal beads for the Devi.
- Keep your mala around your neck, under your shirt, or in a pouch, or you can keep it on your altar.
- Keep a daily record of your japa. Count how many rounds you do per day and write it down. It's like money to deposit in the bank.
- Do not overload the stomach before you sit for japa.

- You can do three sittings a day: 4–6am, 4–5pm and 6–8pm.
- Establish a clear concentration point, which you use all the time—the point between your eyebrows or the point in the middle of your chest.
- It is said that the practices which are most helpful for everyone in Kali Yuga are Mantra Yoga, Japa Yoga, and kirtan.

## WHAT IS KIRTAN?

### How kirtan can help us elevate our mind, open our heart, and protect our mind

Kirtan is singing of the divine names. Kirtan is done using Sanskrit mantras, it is singing with faith, love, and devotion. People sit together and sing. *Kirt* in the word *kirtan* means "praise." In the singing of kirtan, we are glorifying the Divine, so we need to bring a positive attitude when we do it.

Even though we may not understand the mantra, the feeling is important. It is not a religious practice. It is invoking the pure energy of the universe that resides in our hearts. It does not contradict any kind of religious belief. It will help us to be healthy physically and mentally. It supports the prana flow. It calms the nerves and helps transform emotions toward the positive.

While chanting kirtan, we feel the presence of the divinity in our hearts. This gives us a lot of strength to face life's difficulties. It is a powerful mental tonic. It melts the heart. Often our thinking blocks our feelings, so when we chant kirtan, it needs to be out loud. Then we ultimately enter the superconscious state, we transcend all of our mental limitations. Our mind is elevated, uplifted. Kirtan melts the stone-hearted person. Kirtans are made of Sanskrit mantras, which correspond to the vibrations of our chakras, thus making it easier to awaken the spiritual energy.

Any kirtan is good to learn. Start with chanting the kirtan of your chosen *Ishtadevatā*. In the Sivananda organization, kirtan sessions in Satsang begin with our Daily Chants. We pray to Ganesha to remove obstacles and then honor all forms of wisdom and the teachers of the highest Knowledge. We then choose from different songs in our Kirtan Book—organized mostly by deity—according to the energy of the day of the week.

- Monday - *Shiva*
- Tuesday - *Subramanya or the strong form of Devi*
- Wednesday - *Krishna*
- Thursday - *Guru*
- Friday - *Devi*
- Saturday - *Shiva or Hanuman*
- Sunday - *Rama and special Sunday prayers*

**Other mantras for protection:**

- *Maha Mrityunjaya mantra,* also called the *Om Tryambakam* mantra, is used daily for protection. It can be used before we step onto an airplane, when the airplane takes off, when we get into a car, and when the car pulls out. When someone is sick, you can send them this prayer, this mantra. When someone celebrates a birthday, we can chant this mantra for health, long life, liberation and prosperity. When someone transits out of this world, when they die, we can repeat this mantra. On any occasion, we can repeat the *Om Tryambakam* mantra.
- There are additional peace mantras that come with the *Om Tryambakam* mantra.
- The *Dhyana Slokas* are mantras used before we start any kind of endeavor, especially a spiritual learning class.
- Sing *kirtan daily* to invoke all the different energies of the universe.
- There are special Vedic *Shanti mantras* to be chanted the Vedic way, to foster peace.
- The *Guru mantras,* also a Vedic chant, have a very beautiful meaning.
- *Arati* is the ceremony of light. This is also a very good mantra to use for cleansing and protecting a space, such as your meditation room or your room where you sleep. Do *arati* to your altar and follow the *arati* mantras with the dedication song, with the intention of offering your actions to the Divine.
- Chant a mantra before eating. Dedicating your food helps with nourishment and digestion.
- Always pray for the world. The *Lokah Samasta* chant is one such prayer: "*May the world attain peace and harmony*" (see last page of this chapter).

**Kirtan for different deities**

Kirtan is to be sung out loud with feeling from your heart, visualizing the deity and some of their features. It can be sung in groups or solo and can be accompanied by harmonium, cymbals, or tambourine. Clap your hands to keep rhythm; it is said that when you clap your hands, you are chasing away your karma! There is a corresponding quality of the day associated with the planets:

- Monday - *Moon*
- Tuesday - *Mars*
- Wednesday - *Mercury*
- Thursday - *Jupiter*
- Friday – *Venus*
- Saturday – *Saturn*
- Sunday - *Sun*

## SHIVA SONGS

*Shambo* means "the quiet auspicious Shiva, the quiet auspicious presence of the Divine in our hearts." Lord Shiva is detached and austere and sits on the high mountaintop, near the snowy peak. From his hair flows the River Ganga. The sacred Ganga River represents the nectar of immortality. Lord Shiva represents the Supreme Consciousness, as well as the aspect of the cyclical transformation of Nature and the cleansing of negativities. Shiva will give us this power to purify. Lord Shiva taught austerity, simplicity, and detachment in meditation. Here are a couple of examples of Shiva bhajans:

**Shiva Shiva Shiva Shambho**
*Shiva Shiva Shiva Shambho* (x2)
*Mahadeva Shambho Mahadeva Shambho* (x2)

**Shambho Mahadeva**
*Shambho Mahadeva Chandra Chuda*
*Shankara Samba Sadashiva*
*Gangadhara Hara Kailasa Vasa*
*Pahi mam Parvati Ramana*
*Shivaya Shivaya Shivaya Namah Om*
*Om Namah Shivaya Om Namah Shivaya*

## SONG OF SUBRAHMANYA/DEVI

Subrahmanya is a powerful son of Shiva. He has the same energy as Shiva, but he is the God of righteous action, the leader of the army of Gods, the warrior who will help us gain victory over negativities. This song is sung at a fast tempo, because he's a strong warrior.

*Subrahmanya Subrahmanya*
*Shanmukhanatha Subrahmanya*
*Subrahmanya Subrahmanya*
*Kartikeya Subrahmanyam*
*Hara Hara Hara Hara Subrahmanyam*
*Shiva Shiva Shiva Shiva Subrahmanyam*

On Tuesdays, we can also sing a song of the Devi, honoring her strength. Tuesday is the day governed by the planet Mars, known for its very strong energy. The Devi kills all the demons. In the following bhajan, we find the demon Chamunda. Ambika Devi is the name of the strong form of the *shakti* of the universe that removes all nonsense.

*Devi Devi Devi Jagatmohini*
*Chandika Devi Chandamundaharini*
*Chamundesvari Ambika Devi*

## KRISHNA SONGS

These can be chanted or hummed all the time, but, specifically, we chant the kirtan of Sri Krishna on Wednesdays. Krishna has very sweet energy and represents divine love. He also gives us knowledge, guides us, and reminds us of the Divine in the *Bhagavad Gita*. There are many songs praising the glories of Sri Krishna. Krishna is an incarnation of Lord Vishnu, the aspect of the Divine that brings peace, sustenance, and harmony. Krishna exemplifies divine love. Often, Krishna songs include Radha, his favorite devotee.

**Hari Hari Bol**

*Hari Hari Bol Hari Hari Hari Bol*
*Keshava Madhava Govinda Bol*
*Sri Krishna Govinda Hare Murare*
*He Natha Narayana Vasudeva*

**He Radhe**

*He Radhe Radhe Radhe Shyam*
*Govinda Radhe Sri Radhe*
*Govinda Radhe Radhe Shyam*
*Gopala Radhe Rahde Shyam*

## GURU SONGS

On Thursdays, we chant songs for the Guru. We pray for Knowledge. We praise our connection to the Guru to receive knowledge. The Guru is close to us, guides us, teaches us and shows us the way.

**Gurudeva**

*Gurudeva Gurudeva Jaya Gurudev*
*Sivananda Gurudeva Jaya Gurudev*
*...Vishnu Swami Gurudeva...*
*If you want to be like Him*
*You must follow Him*
*Not my will, but Thy will my Lord*
*Not my will, but Thy will*

## DEVI SONGS

Devi is *shakti* or force of nature. We refer to her with love and affection, like our Divine Mother.

**Namo'stu Te**
*Namo'stu Te Namo'stu Te Jaya Sri Durge Namo'stu Te*
*Namo'stu Te Namo'stu Te Jaya Sri Shakti Namo'stu Te*
*Namo'stu Te Namo'stu Te Jaya Sri Kali Namo'stu Te*
*Namo'stu Te Namo'stu Te Jaya Sri Laksmi Namo'stu Te*

## RAMA SONG

Sunday chanting is dedicated to Lord Rama, along with Sita and Hanuman. Hanuman represents the power of devotion and selfless service.

*Rama bolo Rama bolo bolo bolo Ram* (x2)
*Sita bolo Sita bolo bolo Sita Ram* (x2)
*Hanuman bolo Hanuman bolo bolo Hanuman* (x2)
*Shiva bolo Shiva bolo bolo Shiva Ram* (x2)

## DAILY CHANTS, SUNDAY PRAYERS, DEDICATION PRAYERS, SPECIAL MANTRAS

We chant a special group of prayers on Sundays, dedicated to Lord Rama, the Devi and Lord Shiva. They are very beautiful. Unlike kirtan, they are sung in unison, as opposed to call-and-response.

## MAHAMRITYUNJAYA MANTRA

This mantra is used for protection on different occasions. It is recommended to repeat it daily three times.

*Om tryambhakam yajamahe*
*Sugandhim pusti vardhanam*
*Urvarukamiva bandhanan*
*Mrytyor Mukshiya ma'mrtat*

## PEACE MANTRAS

*Om Sarvesham Svastir Bhavatu*
*Sarvesham Shantir Bhavatu*
*Sarvesham Purnam Bhavatu*
*Sarvesham Mangalam Bhavatu*

May auspiciousness be unto all.
May peace be unto all.
May fullness be unto all.
May prosperity be unto all.

*Sarve Bhavantu Sukhinah*
*Sarve Santu Niramayah*
*Sarve Bhadrani Pashyantu*
*Ma Kaschid Dukha-Bhag Bhavet*

May all be happy.
May all be free from disabilities.
May all look to the good of others.
May none suffer from sorrow.

*Asato Ma Sat Gamaya*
*Tamaso Ma Jyotir Gamaya*
*Mrityor Ma Amritam Gamaya*

Lead me from the unreal to the real.
From darkness to light.
From mortality to immortality.

*Om Purnamadah Purnamidam*
*Purnat Purnamudachyate*
*Purnasya Purnamadaya*
*Purnameva Vashishyate*

Om that is whole (complete, perfect).
This is whole.
From the whole the whole becomes manifest.
From the whole when the whole is negated what remains is again the whole.

**This chant means that, at all the times, everything is perfect.**

*Om shanti, shanti, shanti*
*Om peace, peace, peace*

## ARATI (short version)

| | |
|---|---|
| *Om Na Tatra Suryo Bhati*<br>*Na Chandra Tarakam*<br>*Nema Vidyuto Bhanti*<br>*Kuto Yamagnihi*<br>*Tameva Bhanta Manubhati Sarvam*<br>*Tasya Bhasa Sarvamidam Vibhati* | The sun does not shine there, nor do the moon and the stars, nor this lightning and much less this fire. When He shines, everything shines after Him. By His Light, all this is illuminated. |
| *Om Gange Cha Yamuna Chaiva*<br>*Godavari Saraswati*<br>*Narmade Sindhu Kaveri*<br>*Namastubhyam Namo Namah* | Our salutations to you holy rivers: Ganga, Yamuna, Godavari, Saraswati, Narmada, Sindhu, and Kaveri. Salutations to you again. |

## DEDICATION SONG

*Twameva* means that, every day, we dedicate all our actions. It's good to chant this at the end of each day. We offer every action and have no residue; we have no karma.

| | |
|---|---|
| *Twameva Mata Cha Pita Twameva*<br>*Twameva Bandhuscha Sakha Twameva*<br>*Twameva Vidya Dravinam Twameva*<br>*Twameva Sarvam Mama Deva Deva* | O God of Gods, Thou alone art my Mother, Father, Relative, Friend, Learning, Wealth, and Everything. |
| *Kayena Vacha Manasendriyairva*<br>*Buddhyatmana Va Prakrite Svabhavat*<br>*Karomi Yad Yat Sakalam Parasmai*<br>*Narayana Yeti Samarpayami* | Whatever actions I perform with my body, speech, mind, senses, intellect, nature, or emotions, all these I dedicate to the Supreme Lord. |
| *Sarva Dharman Parityajya*<br>*Mam Ekam Sharanam Vraja*<br>*Aham Tva Sarva Papebhyo*<br>*Mokshayishyami Ma Shucah* | Abandoning all duties, take refuge in Me (the Lord) alone. I will liberate thee from all sins, grieve not (Bhagavad Gita XVIII – 66) |

## MEAL PRAYER (*Bhagavad Gita* IV:24)

*Om Brahmarpanam Brahmahavih*
*Brahmagnau Brahmana Hutam*
*Brahmaiva Tena Gantavyam*
*Brahmakarma Samadhina*

Before you eat, say this prayer to protect you, so you don't get a disease from the food, but also to give gratitude to all those responsible in the process of giving you the food.

## PRAYERS FOR THE WORLD

*Loka samastha sukhino bhavantu* (3x)
"May the whole world attain peace and harmony."

*OM Shanti, Shanti, Shanti!*
*Om Peace, peace, peace*
"Peace to me and all my thoughts
Peace to my family and connections
Peace to the whole world."

**Testimony of a Sivananda Yoga Health Educator**

*"I understand other people better. I realize more clearly for this person with this problem, which sadhana to practice, which Yoga tool is appropriate for them. The more I learn, the more my own karma is solved, especially relationship karma. My whole family became my students. I see that when a relationship becomes 'spiritual teacher and student,' it becomes pure and all karma is released.*

*Although my students do not have serious illnesses, they live normal healthy lives, they still suffer spiritually, because they don't know selflessness or pure love in life. As a teacher, I must show them that I am the embodiment of that selflessness, so that they will have faith. I realized that we have to get closer to our true inner self first, then we can help others."*

*V.*

**Testimony about Self-healing and healing others**

*"Thank you to everyone who supported me during this two-year course. The course is about the process of self-purification. I had to deal with my own problems and needed to heal myself. I want to thank my mentor, who patiently guided me to love my students, so I had more motivation to learn and develop more love for myself.*

*During the practice, I realized that faith is very important, faith in the Yoga students who have problems—mental or physical, this or the other—faith that they will heal themselves. Also, you need to develop faith in yourself; from that faith, you develop patience and pure love. And more importantly, you, yourself, can be a serious sadhana practitioner. Thank you all for allowing me to serve and grow myself."*

*M.*

## QUESTIONS

1. *Explain the mechanics of the mind and how mantra repetition helps to control the mind.*
2. *What is a mantra? How does mantra work?*
3. *What is kirtan?*

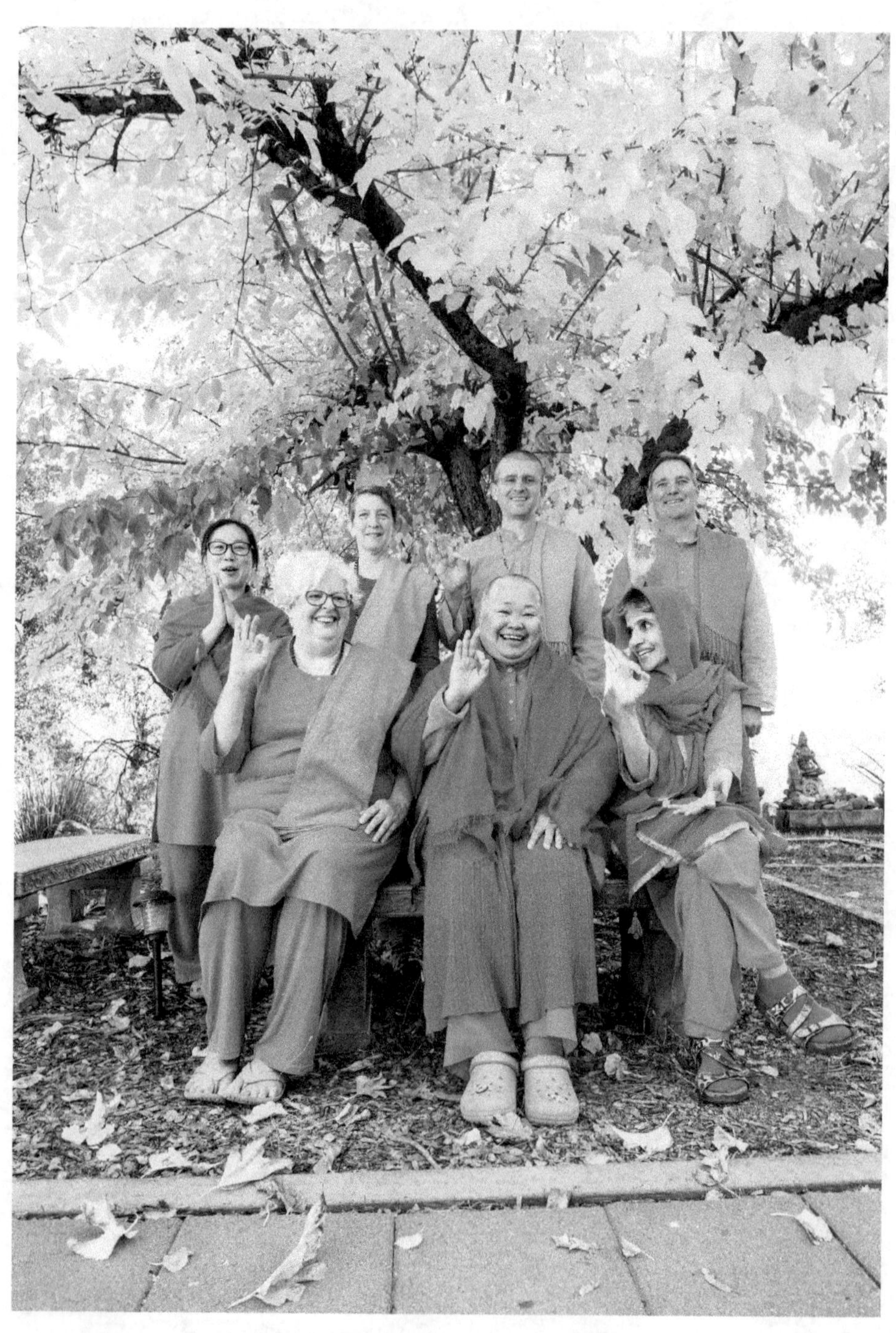

SWAMIS IN HAPPY MOODS TOGETHER

## CHAPTER 15

# Positive Thinking in Daily Life

***"Cheerfulness is the state or quality of being joyful, lively and of good spirits... A cheerful man is like a sunny day. He radiates brightness all around. Be cheerful, sweet, happy, and smiling. You will become very healthy and you will radiate health in every direction."***

- SWAMI SIVANANDA in *How to Cultivate Virtues and Eradicate Vices*

**Regarding thoughts, we need to know:**

1. how thoughts work. What is the best thought to think?
2. how to transform from lower-mind thoughts to higher-mind thoughts.
3. how to convert thoughts through the thought techniques toolbox.
4. how to cultivate virtues and good thoughts.
5. how to eradicate or remove negative thoughts.

## WHAT IS THOUGHT?

In *Thought Power*, Swami Sivananda tells us that, *"Thought is a vital, living force, the most vital, subtle and irresistible force that exists in the universe. The thought-world is more real relatively than this physical universe. Thoughts are living things."* Swami Vishnudevananda, who was always very positive, said *"There is a power and energy which each person can tap into if he knows that it is available. This force inspires, encourages, enforces, and gives strength to those who seek to grow in a positive direction."*

So, what is positive thinking? Positive thinking is moving from the lower mind to the higher mind through conscious thought. It is understanding that everything is an opportunity for growth and self-development.

Swami Sivananda says, *"Life is a great opportunity provided by the Lord for His children to evolve into Himself. The great central aim of life is the conscious realization of our oneness with all."*

To turn around a negative thought or feeling, we need to consciously see things from the point of view of our oneness with all, with the Divine, and not from our separate individual points of view. Life is a great opportunity for us to transform our tendency of negative thinking into the positivity that already exists in nature. So, we need to let go of our individual point of view to embrace positivity.

We live in a multi-dimensional universe. , While we find ourselves physically here, at the same time, there is another world that is not physical, called the astral world. It's more subtle and we are not usually aware of its existence; we are only aware of our familiar physical reality.

If there are 20–30 people in the same room, there will be countless thoughts, although we cannot perceive them. If we put a radio in the room and tune it, we may have the Chinese Opera and BBC News. All kinds of people from everywhere will be talking right here and now. In reality, we live in that multi-dimensional universe, but we forget that. We think that our world is just what our senses perceive.

Thought is a very subtle force and is very powerful; thought can build and destroy, like an atomic bomb. Thought can destroy many things and kill many people. Please be aware that, when you are thinking, you are interacting in and manipulating the subtle, invisible force. If your thinking is negative, it can be very destructive and bring about depression, stress, illness, and friction—for you and others.

**Thought is energy; thought is prana.** Not all thoughts are of the same value in terms of energy. Some thoughts are higher frequency and higher vibration, and some are lower vibration and lower energy.

Yoga teaches methods to **increase your vibratory wavelength**. Our duty, when living this life, is to increase our vibratory wavelength to the maximum. We accomplish this by purifying our minds through appropriate methods of Yoga. The aim is to increase your energy. If your energy is high, your thoughts will automatically be of higher frequency.

Thought is not only subtle, but it is all-pervasive, it is everywhere. If you swim in the ocean and there are strong currents, there will be struggle and the currents might sweep you away—no different than the thought currents in your mind.

Similarly, we need to be aware of the thought atmosphere we bathe in. We mistakenly think that wherever we go, the energy is the same. Here at the ashram, we are in a beautiful area with mountains and lakes, but the thought energy is very different than at the resort next door, although it, too, has mountains and lakes. In the ashram, people do meditation, chant, do asanas, and work on their thoughts. In the resort, even though they are in the same kind of landscape, people are free to think whatever thoughts they like. The thought energy at the ashram is of a higher wavelength due to all the daily practices. The ashram's high positive energy is very noticeable; we can actually feel it. A newcomer arriving feels instantly how positive, peaceful and energetic life is here. Our bodies, mind and spirit benefit from bathing in the thought atmosphere of the ashram.

## THOUGHT POWER AND THOUGHT INFLUENCES

Be aware of the thought atmosphere when you make choices in life. Try to choose, not only the physical surroundings but also, the thought atmosphere. The astral world is real; our mind bathes in the subtle astral world and will be affected by the dominant indwelling thoughts.

A dominant thought has been repeated for a long time. In a casino, the thought is "winning, winning." In an ashram, the thought is "sharing, loving, giving." If people have a tendency to think certain thoughts, then those thoughts will collect and remain in the atmosphere. Then when other people come there, they feel it. The financial district in a big city, with its collection of banks and financial institutions, will resound with the thought of "profit, profit, money, money."

And what is the main, pervasive thought in a person's mind as they walk around a shopping mall? "Buy, buy, buy!" You don't need anything, but when you go there, you will most likely buy something, because the dominant thought is about consuming. Take the example of a window dresser displaying a dress in a department store. The designer has spent three hours setting up the eye-catching display. How many thoughts are in the dress now? There are a lot of thoughts, yes—how the light shines on the display, the placement just by the elevator, etc. Hours of deliberation have been invested by the designer in that winning display. As a result, when people pass by, they will be fascinated by the dress; they respond to the thought and energy involved. This is how thought power works.

It also could happen that a person takes a walk in town and, inadvertently, visits the red-light neighborhood, which is full of sexual movies and topless dancing clubs. All of a sudden, lustful thoughts enter the person's mind. Their mind was concentrated and chaste before, but now has imbibed these desirous thoughts from the atmosphere.

*"I have a student who moved into an apartment near the financial district of San Francisco. Then she told me: "I realize all of a sudden that I have changed; now I always calculate, even how much money the meal cost me that I served to my friend, who came to visit me..."*

*So she realized: "Oh my God, I have changed!" and she moved out of the financial district realizing that she had been influenced by the energy that is there.*

We need to understand how thoughts can influence without words. Knowing that, it behooves us to keep our minds in a healthy environment, and choose our company wisely. Even when we are in someone's company without conversing, we are being influenced by the strong dominant thoughts of that person's mind.

**Remember that we are like a radio transmitter and receiver**

We tune to different wavelengths. We transmit our thoughts without even talking, and we attract and receive thoughts of the same nature as our own. Our body and mind are like this radio, constantly broadcasting and receiving thoughts. Therefore, if we have a positive goal in life, it is essential for us to strictly choose our company.

Yoga practice keeps the body and mind strong and allows us to receive and transmit powerful vibrations. In this way, we can contribute to the world—just by working on ourselves and elevating our thoughts to a high, powerful, positive thought wavelength. Yogis can help the world, even at a distance, just by meditating and transmitting positive thoughts.

**Helping others by holding positive thoughts**

A student in a Positive Thinking class said, *"Before, when my husband was down and I felt good, I would lower my vibration and happiness to be on the same wavelength as he was."* After the Positive Thinking class, she said, *"Now when I'm happy and he's not happy, I maintain being happy and he also becomes happy like me!"*

This is what we can do. Avoid sinking to the level of people who are negative and unhappy. Remain positive. We lift people up just by our thoughts.

Positive thoughts have a higher vibration than negative thoughts. Positive thoughts have more energy than negative thoughts. But positive thoughts are more difficult to come by. Why? Why it is easier for us to be negative than positive? Positive thoughts require more prana. Usually, people don't have enough prana to be positive; they spend a lot of prana on useless activities. Negative thoughts are easier to produce; they require no effort.

Your body and mind are like a thought factory. If you don't have enough energy, the thoughts produced will be negative. Whatever the situation, your reaction will be negative. But, if you have enough energy, the thoughts you generate will always be positive. Therefore, relax and work on your positive thinking, instead of complaining.

**"What you think is what you will become,"** according to Swami Sivananda. Hence, you must tend your thoughts, like you would care for your children, all the time. *"You create your destiny through your thoughts. You always attract to you thoughts of the same nature and you repel other thoughts. If you think that you're strong, then you become strong. If you think that you are weak, then you become weak."*

But in reality, you are not your thoughts. Yes, thoughts are very powerful, but Yoga philosophy clearly states that we are not our thoughts. We simply need to take responsibility for our thoughts. Thoughts and the mind are just our instruments. A thought is just energy or force, a modification of the mind, a *vritti*, a disturbance in a peaceful lake of consciousness.

## HOW THOUGHT WORKS

Imagine a very calm lake of thought. In an ideal situation, when a thought wave arises in the mind, if we do not feed it, the wave will fall back into the ocean of consciousness. A thought manifests like a wave; it rises and falls. The wave does not have a reality in itself. It only has a reality insofar as we name the wave and give it meaning.

We start to think about this wave, *"I'm not happy because of this and that."* Then we start to identify with it. If we feel it and think about it, the thoughts become more solid and they gain more power and seem real.

We then have a choice. We can make these thoughts a reality or we can make blissful thoughts the reality. The Yogis look at the thoughts to understand them. They don't feed into the thoughts. They don't give the thoughts energy, they let them go. They also can transform the thoughts from darkness to light.

**The mind is made of thoughts. The mind is constantly changing. The mind has different levels and functions.** But the mind is not who we are. Our thoughts and feelings are not ours, even though they might feel familiar. We tend to repeat familiar thoughts and feelings—and then lose ourselves in them. Learn to navigate your thoughts and emotions. If you know how to develop your mind, you will know how to accelerate a process of spiritual evolution and Self-healing.

For example, we can exercise contemplating the highest kind of thought—the nature of the *Atman*. This thought comes from enlightened beings and scriptures. These thoughts are for us to contemplate and think about deeply.

*"The Atman, which is your true Self, is beyond all thoughts."*

It is your Self. You need to think of your Self, your Truth. It is pure Consciousness. It is *Sat-Chit-Ananda*.

It is Existence Absolute; it has never been born, and will never die.

It is Knowledge Absolute, it is the source of our intelligence.

It is *ananda*, the source of bliss.

**Here's an example of highest thinking:**

*"My true nature is Sat-Chit-Ananda, beyond birth and death, beyond the understanding of my mind, and beyond this temporary happiness that I have in daily life. My Atman, my Self, is Bliss Absolute, beyond conditions."*

We are not educated to think like this. But we can exercise our thinking and train our mind to think such high thoughts.

*"The Atman, my Self, is neither inside nor outside; it is dwelling within, and it can be perceived through the subtle and pure mind.*

*It is everywhere. It is beyond time and space.*

*It is not material. It's eternally present.*

*It is the Truth that is always there.*

*It is Truth. It is pure and perfect. It is beyond duality, beyond any kind of split.*

*Sometimes you might feel, "I'm here but I want to be there." You always feel split. "I love this person, but I love that person, too." Again, you feel split. But if you go to the true Self, then your Self is everywhere. There is no duality.*

*The Self is not white, the Self is not black, the Self is not male, the Self is not female.*

*It is eternal. It has no equal, it cannot be compared to anything else.*

*It's transcendent and it is fully illuminated by itself, fully enlightened.*

*It exists by itself, like the sun. The moon needs the sun to be enlightened, but the sun is the source of light.*

*My Self, my Atman, is without names and forms and yet there is a long list of words attempting to describe it.*

*If you think incorrect thoughts about it, sooner or later it will bring you pain.*

**Positive thinking means moving from the lower mind to higher mind.**How do we train the lower mind and awaken the higher mind? The lower mind is the vast subconscious mind, of which we are unaware. It is made of past thoughts, carried from lifetime to lifetime; instinctive thoughts; emotional thoughts; impulses; past habits; programming; memories; and *samskaras*, or thought imprints. To think more positively, we must replace thoughts from the lower mind with thoughts of the higher mind.

Yoga philosophy teaches that we store in our subconscious thoughts not only of this lifetime, but also of previous lifetimes. These thoughts create karmic patterns called *samskaras*, or habits, which occupy 95% of our mind. That means most of the time we function on autopilot (see chapter 11).

The subconscious mind governs not only the automatic functions of the body, like breathing and heartbeat, but also stores our learned experiences. Even though we might seem to have forgotten, past impressions will still condition our behaviors and feelings. For example, driving lessons are tedious in the beginning, as we have to consider everything—our speed, others' speed and distance from us, obstacles, and possible hazards. But after programming all these factors into the subconscious mind, we can simply drive without thinking.

**Positive thinking means being more conscious and aware.** The more we become aware of our thoughts, the more we can transform our thoughts from negative to positive. Begin to recognize thoughts of an instinctive nature: selfish thoughts, habitual thoughts, survival thoughts, learned thoughts, needy thoughts, desirous thoughts, and sensual thoughts. Replace them with fearless thoughts, spiritual thoughts, truthful thoughts, self-affirming thoughts, open and all-inclusive thoughts and, finally, intuitive thoughts and insightful thoughts.

**Develop the higher mind and intellect to think positively.** The lower, subconscious mind consists of powerful hidden and submerged thoughts of the past. The subconscious mind is instinctive; it is the seat of our animal instincts. The instincts are fast, powerful, and irresistible. We have the instinct of survival, the instinct of procreation, the herd instinct—following the group, following the leader—and the territorial instinct. We act according to our ever-present instincts. For example, if a person goes where they know there is little food, they take food with them, due to the survival instinct. If there ends up being food left over, they will give it to family members before giving it to a starving stranger standing nearby. This is also due to the survival instinct.

The subconscious mind is largely emotional. We suffer considerably from our emotions—anger, fear, greed, hatred, jealousy, envy, and lust. These emotions are very strong and they lead us onto a roller coaster. Emotional impulses are imperative and very difficult to resist.

The higher mind is the conscious mind. The function of the conscious mind is to regulate emotions, control our instincts, and resist our unhelpful habits, so that we can make better choices in the present, replacing negative habits with positive ones.

The subconscious mind, if well-trained, will work for us like 100 helpers. It follows orders and listens to our auto-suggestions. It is our best, most trustworthy friend when well-trained and can be our worst enemy when not.

Once well-trained, we can trust our subconscious mind. It's like a personal assistant who obeys our clear orders: wakes us up on time, reminds us of our appointments, etc. The subconscious mind is related to the past, memories, habits, and imprints. We feel confirmed by identifying with the past, but then when the past projects itself in the future, we feel worried. We are always in the past and future, missing out on the present.

**The conscious mind is the higher mind and is the seat of the intellect.** It functions in the present and needs to be developed and purified, as well. The conscious mind and our power of reasoning, when well-developed, can help us make wise and intelligent choices for our progress. It can compute, compare, and reason about pros and cons and will not be usurped by the subconscious mind. It is, therefore, not subject to manipulation and justifications. The high end of the conscious mind is the discriminative intellect, which is the faculty to know the difference between the Self and the not-self, the permanent and the impermanent. The more we function out of our higher mind, the closer we move to a place of freedom and well-being.

For a person who is on the journey of Self-healing, or self-development, the conscious mind needs to be exercised more. Note that the intellect is also limited by time, space, and causation, and can make mistakes; it cannot see past the mind to see the Truth, unless it switches to the realm of the superconscious mind or intuition.

With the intellect, we also develop the capacity for self-awareness, knowing ourselves as Sat-Chit-Ananda and not as the limited ego. We feel this deep within as the Truth within our heart.

The conscious mind helps us to remain in the present, which is to be alive and well. We feel that we *are* life. Otherwise, we feel that we are missing out on life, living mostly in the past or the future.

**The third level of the mind is called the superconscious mind,** the seat of intuition. This higher mind is not developed in the majority of people. Intuition allows us to know in a flash and does not make mistakes. Intuition comes from a pure mind; it is not impulsive. It's very different from the emotional, instinctive mind. Intuition and instinct are both very fast and strong. Due to this, they can sometimes appear to be the same, which causes confusion. The superconscious mind is warm, wise, insightful, and closer to the truth of pure love and unity.

The journey of positive thinking is the navigation of these three levels of mind. We must:

- Overcome the unconscious and the animal instinct.
- Exercise reason and discrimination, and consciously practice sadhana to accelerate the process of moving from darkness to light.
- Surrender personal will to the higher will.

During meditation, we clean the subconscious mind's impressions; we activate the conscious mind, which becomes clear, and intuition develops.

**Nurture positive thinking by the five points of Yoga Life.** Equip your thought toolbox with well-rehearsed positive thinking techniques. Almost everyone entertains some negative thoughts. Become your own doctor. Know how long these negative thoughts have been there, how persistent they are and what their nature is. How strong are they? How serious are they? How often do they occur? How many times a day does the thought arise? What is the nature of the thought? Be as precise as possible.

Imagine that you have a thought toolbox. A carpenter has a toolbox; a nurse or a paramedic, who responds to emergency calls, also has a toolbox. Equip your thought toolbox with techniques to deal with negative thoughts. Use these techniques together or separately. The more you use them, the more familiar with them you become and they will be readily available for you to make use of when needed. Here is a list of the techniques to deal with negative thoughts.

**Techniques to switch negative thoughts to positive thoughts, according to Raja Yoga:**

- **Replace negative thought with the opposite.** (See exercise below.)
- **Be indifferent** to the thoughts when they arise.
- Through **sublimation,** channel and transform the power of a thought into something positive. (See exercise below.)
- Through **positive visualization,** develop a mental picture of what you want to become. For example, if you have thoughts of freedom and imagine yourself walking toward the sunrise, envision yourself very relaxed and smiling. If you want to be very peaceful, then visualize the ocean or a lake, without any waves, so clear. For beauty, you can visualize a beautiful flower, a lotus flower that has opened in the sunshine. Use the power of imagination, as long as it is positive.
- A **positive affirmation** is asserted as a positive fact. We create a positive sentence and repeat it to reinforce a helpful belief, idea or thought about ourselves or our life situation. Take the negative—whether a tendency, an insecurity or a problem of any sort—and rewrite it into a positive. Then, repeat it many times a day, looking at yourself in the mirror, affirming it. This makes the thought very strong. For example, if you have the recurring thought that, "Nobody loves me, I'm not good enough," the counter suggestion and positive affirmation would be, "I am love itself; I love everyone and everyone loves me; God loves me and I am lovable." Repeat the affirmation to retrain the mind to something that serves you better.
- Practice **concentration.** Keep your mind very concentrated and reduce distractions. Live a simple life. As a result, the mind will become positive. Conversely, if you have a very complicated life, then, most likely, the mind will be very busy, distracted, and it will be more difficult to stay positive. Making the mind more concentrated is like building the muscles of the mind. Make the mind strong by repeatedly coming back to concentration, such as on a sacred mantra.
- Cultivate **cheerfulness.** Keep a cheerful, smiling disposition. Always look at things with optimism and a sense of humor.
- **Think of one thought at a time.** To avoid confusion, focus on only one thought at a time. Concentrate on it and be very clear.
- Notice **thought associations.** Be aware that negative thoughts never come alone. One negative thought will be followed by another negative thought,

one after the other. For example, if you think, *"People don't love me,"* then you will also think, *"My father and mother, do not love me,"* and next, *"My father doesn't love my mother,"* and then, *"My grandmother also doesn't love my mother,"* and then, *"The neighbor of my grandmother doesn't love my grandmother."* Thought is like a chain. We think of something negative and ten negative thoughts come with it, invade our consciousness and we lose ourselves in negativity. The opposite can also be true: invite one positive thought in, and then the positive thought will bring its ten associates and friends and, all of a sudden, you feel good.

- **Kirtan or chanting mantra** is a very powerful, easy way to switch your mood. Sing or listen to kirtan. It is positive, joyous and uplifting.
- **Asana**, Yoga postures, if performed daily, will help move the prana, clear mental blockages, and restore positivity. The proper sequence of the asana needs to be observed. Also, when we practice asanas we need to have proper concentration, with relaxation in between postures and a deep, final relaxation. Practicing a balancing posture every day will also help keep the mind balanced.
- **Pranayama** will recharge our batteries with vital energy to restore positive thinking. Practice regular abdominal breathing exercises using the diaphragm to recharge. Practice alternate nostril breathing to balance the two hemispheres of the brain. These simple breathing techniques can be done anytime and are very effective in bringing back balance to the emotions and the mind. Imbalanced energy, too much logic or too much emotion, will make us lose our center and well-being. When both nostrils flow, we immediately become balanced.
- **Relaxation** of the body and mind brings back a positive state of mind.
- **Eat a balanced diet.** Avoid eating too much sugar and a diet that will aggravate the mind. Avoid eating junk food, especially when the mood is negative.
- **Meditate** and find calm to refresh the mind.
- **Cultivate** virtues and eradicate vices (see exercises below).

**From the other three paths of Yoga, add more affirmations to the thought toolbox.**

- From the **Karma Yoga** path, techniques affirm that, *"I'm just the instrument."* Let's say you do some work, but you don't feel that you're good enough and you fail; you become very negative. At that moment, you need to switch to the idea, "I'm doing the best I can," and "I'm just the instrument. I'm doing my duty. I give up and I offer the results. I do the best I can."

- From the **Bhakti Yoga** path, it's believed that everything always happens for the best. God knows best. We affirm, "It's not my will. It's God's will. I surrender to God's will."
- From the **Jnana Yoga** path, affirm that:

> *"I am the silent witness. Life is just a play. I'm just an actor in the play of life."*
>
> *"This too shall pass."* In the world where everything changes, even pain will not last forever; it will change, it too shall pass.
>
> *"I am not this, I am not that."* Jnana Yoga also uses affirmation in this *Neti Neti* formula. It ensures that we don't get attached to the false idea of ourselves. *"I am not this emotion. I'm not this idea. I'm not this name, I'm not the fame."*
>
> *"This is only my illusion. It is my wrong perception. It is a superimposition, a projection of my mind."*
>
> *"We are one; there's nobody out there; there is no other; everybody is myself."*
>
> *"I see myself in You; I am your Self. The paths are many, but the Truth is one."*

## LIST OF VIRTUES FOR SELF-AFFIRMATION

- **Adaptable:** flexible, not stubborn or rigid, flowing with life
- **Ahimsa:** nonviolent, respectful; anger comes from desire unfulfilled
- **Austere:** conscious restriction of senses and mind, in order to bring them inward, not indulgent
- **Balanced:** not too rational, not too emotional; being centered
- **Beautiful:** see beauty, feel beautiful
- **Blissful:** happy mood of the soul
- **Bright:** Feeling light, knowledgeable
- **Calm:** the emotional thought waves are under control, not up and down

- **Charitable:** giving heart, generous
- **Cheerfulness:** always express the joy of the spirit, smiling disposition
- **Clear mind:** clear intellect, knows what is bad and good
- **Compassion**: Selfless love, feeling empathy, love, and concern for others' suffering
- **Concentrated:** the mind is fixed on one goal, the pre-meditative state, equated to being mindful
- **Connected:** connected to Self, to the universe, connected to others to feel strong
- **Conscious:** comes from a higher mind, not subconscious habits
- **Considerate:** considering others' needs
- **Consistency:** continuous, regular practice; not changing, not intermittent
- **Contentment:** desireless; not restless; lack of jealousy, envy; comes from surrendering to God's will
- **Courage:** strength of mind, counteracting fear; a very important quality, which allows you to change
- **Creative:** new and positive, soulful and resourceful thinking
- **Decisiveness:** opposed to indecisiveness and procrastination; coming from strong faith and higher mind determination that all is good and is divine play
- **Detached:** not attached, anchored in the Self; be witness to all external happenings involving body-mind-emotions/senses
- **Devotion:** love for the highest in your heart
- **Disciplined:** in a positive manner, i.e. do the right things at the right time
- **Discrimination:** knowing intuitively the difference between real and unreal, Self and not-Self, permanent and changing
- **Dispassion:** detached while being fulfilled; does not mean being bored; based on discrimination, not falling to the illusion of senses, emotions or past impressions
- **Dutiful:** the way to *dharma* and *moksha* is to fulfill our duty (*swadharma*)

- **Empathy:** understanding other people's conditions and sufferings
- **Endurance (forbearance):** to be able to bear the difficulties of karma without complaining, having faith that this too shall pass
- **Equanimity:** even-mindedness in success or failure, in likes or dislikes, in between waves of *raga* and *dvesha*, not up and down and high and low
- **Even mind:** calm, same as equanimity
- **Expanded:** feeling of being big and great
- **Faith:** it will make you peaceful and secure, the opposite of doubt
- **Flexible:** adaptable
- **Flowing:** floating with life, instead of being stagnant
- **Focused:** it helps you to be present
- **Forbearing**: be able to bear, persevere, and keep calm in difficulties
- **Forgiveness:** going forward in life, accepting responsibility, and letting go, not to say that the wrong action was right, but forgiveness is necessary to move on, not holding any grudge towards anybody
- **Forward:** feeling of moving forward
- **Gratitude:** open heart practice, to be thankful for all things
- **Growing**: going upwards
- **Happy:** not permanent happiness, but the general disposition of the mind
- **Harmonious:** sharing energy of oneness and joy with all around
- **Healthy:** think about health, rather than disease
- **Honest:** be sincere about where you are
- **Humble:** recognizing the supremacy of spirit over personality and the habitual sense of a separate self
- **Independent:** self-reliant
- **Intuition:** from the superconscious, not to be confused with instincts or impulses that come from the lower mind; intuition is higher than emotion and intellect and does not make mistakes
- **Japa Yoga:** focused on mantra, sacred sound
- **Joyful:** a general disposition to be joyful will give you more prana

- **Knowledgeable:** follow scriptural guidance to find truth, not just intellectual information or belief
- **Knowledge:** to learn, to become curious about knowledge to get out of ignorance
- **Letting go:** detached, non-attached, not identifying with changing phenomena of body-mind-circumstances
- **Light:** instead of heavy
- **Loving:** toward everybody, this is a quality of heart and soul, different than being emotional
- **Moderate:** not extreme
- **Moderation:** balanced between pairs of opposites, avoiding extremes
- **Non-violent:** ahimsa; no anger, impatience or willfulness
- **One-pointedness:** elevated and concentrated state of mind at the exclusion of other distractions
- **Patience:** all happens in God's time, not in your time
- **Peace:** a quality of the soul; not temporary peace stemming from the satisfaction of desires, but a deep quality of heart; a mixture of contentment, self-surrendering attitude, wisdom, acceptance, and self-control; emotional thought waves are calm
- **Productive:** being able to flow with the energy of beneficial work for the good of all
- **Relaxed:** not stressed
- **Renunciation:** detachment does not mean not to have; it is the highest stage of life, when convinced that only Truth will set you free
- **Respectful:** see others and self as honorable and divine
- **Self-analysis:** to understand our mind
- **Self-confidence:** strength stemming from a sattvic mind, that had a glimpse of the Truth of the Self
- **Self-control:** control of senses
- **Self-discipline:** not following our lower mind or impulses
- **Self-reliance:** not depending on others, relying on our own self-effort
- **Self-sacrifice:** letting go of the mind's cherished attachment to ideas, objects, comforts in search of Truth

- **Self-surrendered:** acceptance of everything as from divine will, no ego
- **Selfless:** not egoistic
- **Sensitive:** understanding other people's needs, not only your own
- **Serene:** calm, content
- **Soft-spoken:** do say things, but nicely
- **Steadfastness:** carry on practicing; control of mind, no matter the circumstances
- **Strong:** just being yourself; not abusive, but anchored in your Self
- **Surrendered:** having faith, relaxed, no need to control everything
- **Thoughtful:** instead of being indifferent and insensitive
- **Tranquil:** calm, content
- **Truthful:** quality of heart, be close to heart for self-expression
- **United:** feeling connected and one with all, not separated
- **Uplifted:** feeling light
- **Upwards:** feeling of moving upwards; advancing
- **Vigilant:** be careful not to be indulgent and fall back in bad habits
- **Wholesome:** feeling together, feeling oneness
- **Wise:** choosing the right response, when faced with challenges

## ERADICATE VICES BY THINKING OF THE OPPOSITE

| | | |
|---|---|---|
| Abusive | › | respectful |
| Addictive | › | disciplined |
| Egoistic | › | humble |
| Angry | › | being content, letting go of expectation |
| Anxious | › | having faith |
| Arrogant | › | humble |
| Attached | › | detached |
| Blaming | › | taking responsibility, no victim attitude |
| Brooding | › | let go of the past |
| Careless | › | caring |

| | | |
|---|---|---|
| Chaotic | ➤ | harmonious |
| Complaining | ➤ | content, taking responsibility |
| Contempt | ➤ | respectful, humble |
| Crazy | ➤ | in order, grounded |
| Depressed | ➤ | joyful, energetic, endowed with faith, hope |
| Desirous | ➤ | contented |
| Dishonest | ➤ | honest |
| Distracted | ➤ | focused, mindful |
| Doubtful | ➤ | having faith |
| Dreaming | ➤ | grounded, logical, practical |
| Dull (tamasic) | ➤ | concentrated, sharp |
| Envious | ➤ | content; be more realistic about who you are |
| Exaggerating | ➤ | being truthful |
| Exhausted, tired | ➤ | energized, enthusiastic, capable |
| Fanaticism | ➤ | tolerance |
| Fault-finding self | ➤ | habit of seeing good qualities in people/ |
| Fearful | ➤ | courageous |
| Feeling down | ➤ | feeling "up" |
| Feeling empty | ➤ | feeling fulfilled |
| Feeling lack | ➤ | feeling fulfilled |
| Feeling limited | ➤ | feeling expansive, unlimited |
| Frustrated | ➤ | accepting |
| Greedy | ➤ | generous |
| Hatred | ➤ | loving |
| Illusion | ➤ | clear thinking, truthful, courageous |
| Imaginative | ➤ | factual, conscious |
| Imbalanced | ➤ | balanced |
| Inconsiderate | ➤ | considerate |
| Inconsistent | ➤ | consistent |

| | | |
|---|---|---|
| Indecisiveness | ➤ | unafraid of making mistakes, making decisions with confidence and offering actions to God |
| Indulgent | ➤ | disciplined |
| Inferior | ➤ | oneness; in truth, no one is inferior or superior; we are one |
| Irresponsible | ➤ | responsible |
| Irritable | ➤ | patient |
| Jealous | ➤ | accepting own karma, accepting self |
| Judgmental | ➤ | accepting, tolerant |
| Lazy | ➤ | enthusiastic |
| Lustful | ➤ | pure |
| Manipulative | ➤ | straightforward |
| Mean | ➤ | generous |
| Naive | ➤ | realistic |
| Obstinate | ➤ | flexible |
| Perverted | ➤ | pure, good |
| Pessimistic | ➤ | optimistic |
| Possessive | ➤ | generous, sharing |
| Procrastinating | ➤ | do it and surrender results; overcome fear and confusion |
| Proud | ➤ | humble |
| Resentful | ➤ | grateful, forgiving, content |
| Restless | ➤ | peaceful, calm, poised, turning inward |
| Revengeful | ➤ | forgiving |
| Rigid | ➤ | being flowing, flexible, adaptable |
| Self-doubt | ➤ | Having faith in Self |
| Self-hatred | ➤ | self-love |
| Self-justification | ➤ | honesty (lower mind always tries not to admit to our faults) |
| Self-righteous | ➤ | self-surrendered |

| | | |
|---|---|---|
| Selfishness | › | selflessness, switch to "we" and "ours" or (egoistic; "Thee" and "Thine" based on "I" and "mine") |
| Sensual | › | austere, turning inwards, ascetic, passionless |
| Shy | › | self-confident, bold |
| Sinful | › | dharmic, virtuous, innocent |
| Skeptical | › | having faith, certain, convinced |
| Slothful | › | caring, active, energetic |
| Spiteful | › | forgiving, benevolent, kind, friendly |
| Stagnant | › | flowing, progressing |
| Stingy | › | generous |
| Stuck | › | flowing, inspired |
| Undisciplined | › | disciplined |
| Unhappy | › | happy |
| Unhealthy | › | healthy, aware |
| Unrighteous | › | righteous |
| Unstable | › | stable, steady |
| Vicious | › | considerate, ethical |
| Wasteful | › | conserving |
| Weak | › | strong |
| Worldly | › | turning inwards |
| Worried | › | having faith |

***Om Tryambhakam*** is a powerful prayer for health, peace, and protection. In this prayer, there is a promise that, in due time, when everything is right, liberation will happen, dropping like a ripe fruit. So don't worry. Don't be impatient. Don't be fearful. Just do your practice and everything will happen as it should.

**Healing through Satsanga**

*John came to the ashram for the weekend. He was suffering from an auto-immune disorder, but the doctors had yet to identify it. John had been practicing Hatha Yoga for 25 years, very physical in his practice. Now his body was emaciated from the disease and his sense of who he was as a physically-active person was causing great distress and fear. Nonetheless, he took the Yoga class and did all the postures as best he could, but was in tears at his current condition. He was ready to go home.*

*But then, he decided to attend the satsang meditation and kirtan and spend time with the ashram residents. Everyone was supportive and encouraging. The next day we had a conversation about Yoga life and remembering the greater purpose of life. We talked about the karma of the physical body and I reminded him that his real nature was not the body and that his True Nature (Atman) was healthy and alive.*

*By the end of the weekend, shared with positive company, eating nourishing food, and practicing meditation, prayers, and sacred chanting, John had rediscovered his joy, rediscovered his Self. Even though the physical body was suffering, he was able to detach from the perceived limitations of the body and identify more strongly with his blissful Self.*

**QUESTIONS**

1. *What is thought? How does it work?*

2. *Give an example of higher thinking about the Atman.*

3. *Positive thinking is moving from the lower mind to the higher mind through conscious thought. Give five techniques to switch negative thought to positive thought.*

4. *Give two positive affirmations from each of the Four Paths of Yoga (Karma Yoga, Bhakti Yoga, Raja Yoga, Jnana Yoga).*

5. *Name five vices and their opposites. Name five virtues for contemplation and self-affirmation.*

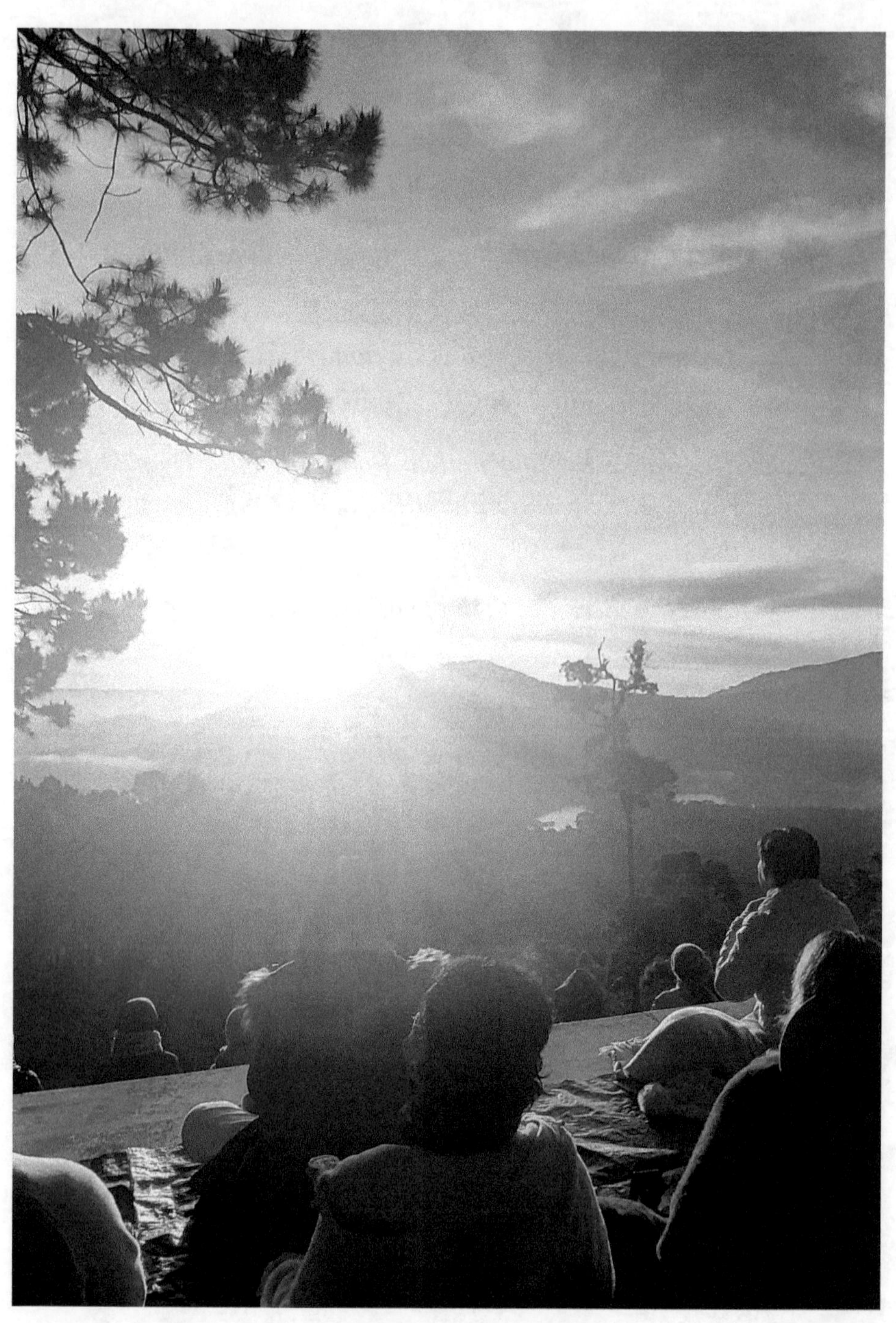

SUNRISE MEDITATION

CHAPTER 16

# Meditation in Daily Life

***"Fear not. The mind is no doubt extremely turbulent. Through repeated attempts, you can perfectly subdue it. You are the master of the mind. By abhyasa (practice) and by vairagya (detachment), assert your mastery. Feel the power, bliss, and splendor that results in perfect self-conquest."***

- SWAMI SIVANANDA in *Sivananda Upanishads*

Regular meditation practice is based on a fundamental understanding that the practice of quieting the mind and turning it inward is necessary to become physically, mentally, and spiritually healthy. You must be convinced that this is the reason you meditate.

## TECHNIQUE OF MEDITATION

This is a simplified version of the fifteen points of meditation according to *Meditation and Mantras* by Swami Vishnudevananda. Some of the steps are combined here.

1. **Be regular in time, place, and practice.** The space needs to be private, clean, ventilated, and reserved only for meditation. The first priority is to create your sacred space and set a specific time for daily meditation. The best times are from 4:00–6:00am and 6:00–8:00pm, with the minimum sitting being 20 minutes. Practice 20 minutes at dawn and again 20 minutes at dusk. Regularity of practice is very important. Ideally, meditate at the same place and time.

2. **Condition your mind to turn inwards.** Give instructions to the mind to be here and now, to let go of the past, the present, and the future, and to let go of the ideas of who you are and what you are doing.
3. **Prepare for your meditation posture.** You can try it now. Sit cross-legged with the spine erect, stretched upwards. The posture needs to be comfortable. If there is tension, there is blockage in the flow of energy. It is very important in meditation to be aware of the flow of energy.
4. **Prepare for the meditative breath,** conducive to meditation. First, take three long, deep breaths to bring oxygen to the brain. Bring prana to the mind, releasing tension and fatigue when you are exhaling. The deep breaths are followed by a rhythmical breath. When your breath is rhythmical, then the thought waves will calm down. So, inhale for three counts. Inhale 1-2-3, exhale 1-2-3. Inhale 1-2-3, exhale 1-2-3. Allow the breath to calm itself down even further to an imperceptible rhythm; the breath follows an imperceptible rhythm, a very quiet rhythm. At this time, the mind starts to turn inward.
5. **Next, prepare to focus.** To do so, choose a point of focus, one of the high-energy centers—either the point in the middle of your chest or the point between the eyebrows. Choose only one point, and always use the same point. Choose the point that is most comfortable and familiar to you.
6. **Turn inwards** and upwards by consciously **repeating the universal mantra OM.** Repeat this mentally. Or use any sacred sound formula that you have been initiated into—with which you have a special connection and have developed a devotional feeling towards. Take time to understand what a mantra is. It is important to tune your mantra repetition with your breath. Inhale mantra and exhale mantra. Meditation is getting back to your True Nature. It must be very natural.

   You can repeat the mantra accompanied by rolling mala beads. This helps you focus on one mantra at a time. You repeat verbally or mentally, with mala beads or not (see chapter 14 on Japa Yoga).

   Concentration on a sacred mantra should become a habitual practice, even outside the formal sitting meditation time. It can support you in daily life, while driving, working, or doing repetitive tasks. The more you practice, the better, as there is a cumulative effect of mantra repetition. After some time, it is no longer a struggle. Mantra repetition becomes very peaceful. The mantra stays in the mind and becomes the background of your thoughts.

7. If the mind drifts into any usual concern or thought, **withdraw it like a witness.** Just step back... let the thought come... and let the thought go. Do not fight with the mind, saying things like, "Oh, I'm not supposed to think about this," or "I'm not a good meditator." Just observe and let go.
8. At first, the mind wanders. Be gentle and relaxed. Do not struggle. Learn to step back and be the observer, **detach from the play of the mind, and return to focus**—to the breath or to the mantra.
9. Bring the mind to rest at the energy center, your point of focus. Allow yourself to sink deeply into the silence and the peace. **Relax, let go.** Do not be afraid.
10. Apply the chosen technique and **hold the sacred mantra**, the concentration object, throughout the meditation session.
11. As you progress, the meditator, the object of meditation, and the act of meditation **become one, as the thoughts become pure**. Eventually, it becomes effortless; you're not aware that you are doing anything. The process becomes very natural and you can just sit quietly for a long time. It is said that at that time, you have reached the state of pure thought.
12. After long-time practice, duality disappears and **Samadhi, the superconscious state** is attained. In your journey of meditation, if you encounter stagnation, then review your steps, find the obstacles, and readjust.

## BENEFITS OF MEDITATION

1. **1. Spiritual benefits:**
    - Meditation will bring us in touch with the true, the perfect, and the secure Self, which is the consciousness within each of us.
    - We need to remember that happiness is our True Nature. But then why are we sometimes unhappy? One of the very important ways to find happiness is to tune in. The idea of "tuning in" indicates the adjustment of our thought vibration towards our inner soul.
    - Meditation develops our self-awareness, our consciousness, and our discriminative intelligence. With this intelligence, we can distinguish what is truth and what is the mind's illusion. So, when meditation dawns, we will be able to know this.

- Meditation develops our intuitive capacities and faculties—which we have, but are not necessarily using—our inner knowing, the inner sensing of what is right and wrong.
- Meditation helps bring us to the here and now. Only when we live in the present do we feel peaceful, centered, and together. When we feel "together," we are strong and capable of facing any challenge. Living in the past brings regrets; living in the future brings anxiety. Consequently, we function in this life with our limited beliefs about who we are and what is the reality surrounding us.
- Meditation helps us understand who we are. We can find answers to such questions as: Who am I? What is the deeper meaning of my life, what is the purpose of my life? Why do I always feel that I'm lacking something? Meditation helps us connect with ourselves in daily life. It keeps us on track with ourselves, allowing us to go inward and deeper to rediscover who we are.
- Life becomes a repetition of the patterns in the mind, a series of projections of preconceived ideas. We, thus, become victims of our karma, our past impressions, or thoughts of the past. We are drowning in the ocean of samsara, the cycle of birth and death.

2. **Mental benefits:**

- Meditation helps to alleviate the subconscious from its load of impressions of past *samskaras*, addictions and habits.
- The mind is not trustworthy to show us the purpose of life, because it is constantly changing and being influenced by others. So, our experience is unstable peace and temporary happiness, as the mind constantly projects various ideas. The mind is constantly busy running in the different grooves; habits or *samskaras* often keeping us stuck in a loop as we struggle to find lasting peace and to overcome our repeated patterns. We often lose control of our minds; then the mind keeps moving on its own accord. When we lose control of our minds, we lose control of our lives. Meditation will, therefore, release stress and anxieties and recharge us with new faith and love.
- Meditation brings clarity to the mind, calms emotions, and opens the heart to forgiveness and love.

- Meditation heals relationships. Meditation is connected wholeheartedly with secure and fulfilled Divine love.
- Meditation is like a tonic to the mind. It gives peace of mind and eases the restlessness and the search for answers. It allows the mind to slow down. It helps us to tune ourselves to the spirit within. It cleans or purifies the mind.
- Three things happen during meditation: 1) cleaning the subconscious, 2) becoming more aware and conscious, and 3) developing our intuition.
- Patanjali Maharishi said, "*Yogas chitta vrtti nirodhah.*" The more we can calm the mind and the fewer thoughts there are in the mind, the more peace we have. If we are not able to control the thought waves, then we are lost, as we identify with the thoughts in the mind. We will be restless, projecting different ideas and running after them.
- Einstein said, "*No solution to a problem can be found by using the same level of consciousness that created it.*" To find the solution to a problem we need to go deeper and higher. We have to turn inward and upward and change our vibrations or thoughts, our patterns of thinking. The scripture of Yoga declares that future suffering should be avoided. If we know that when the mind functions in a certain way, it will bring us some kind of foreseen suffering, then we need to solve the situation first from the mind, so this tendency doesn't have a chance to manifest itself. Meditation helps us do this.
- During meditation, the old thought waves calm down and the mind becomes very clear and pure, and we can see the true reflection of ourselves in it. Thus, we come closer and closer to the source of wisdom within us.
- We will become stronger and we will come up with solutions, rather than just reacting to situations and blaming. We will be able to find creative solutions for our lives.
- Meditation will also lead us to self-inquiry; it will make the mind clear and give rise to the inner voice. We will recover quickly from grief—we all suffer from attachment so, therefore, will suffer from grief. Meditation is a remedy for this sense of loss, as we find our internal connection and the oneness of Spirit.

- The spirit or Self is One; we go deep within ourselves and find peace beyond expectations. We renew ourselves and become more flexible, tolerant, and open. This is akin to the concept of neuroplasticity; the brain is reshaping itself, renewing itself, and renewing the connections. This is good news; we don't have to be stuck in the same way of thinking; we can renew our thinking.
- We can also be free from anxiety, which is a very big problem nowadays. Stress and tension have become an epidemic. With meditation, we will find strength and solutions from within and become free from the fear of death, as we dis-identify with the body. The more we are able to detach from the body—because we understand that the body is our instrument and not us—the more we will not be afraid of death; much of the fear in life will disappear. We will become more grateful and appreciative of life.
- Meditation helps us to forgive and forget more easily. We become more enthusiastic and positive, as opposed to depressed or resentful. We quickly overcome anger and disappointment. We become more content and less desirous. We radiate peace and harmony, thus automatically influencing the world positively.
- It is said in the *Bhagavad Gita* that, "*A person who does not disturb the world and who cannot be disturbed by the world, who is free from exultation, jealousy, apprehension, and worry, he too is dear to me.*" (XII:15). People who meditate will become leaders of this world in their own right. They will become self-reliant, not be dependent on others and will not be driven by desires.
- Meditation comes with self-discipline. People who meditate will no longer suffer from loneliness, because they are deeply in connection with their true Self and they are in harmony with other people. They will have better relationships with themselves and with others. They will increase their capacity to love themselves and others. Their love will become more selfless. They can keep the heart open. Negative emotions like hatred, anger, envy, jealousy, lust, and desire vanish when we meditate.
- Meditation helps us to restore our faith and overcome self-doubt. Faith is of three kinds—faith in the Supreme Being, faith in the teaching, and faith in our own capacity to find happiness. Without faith, we are alone and our ego is the only reference. Then we can become very easily challenged and depressed, because we have

nothing to fall back upon. The ego all we have, when we do not have faith. With regular, successful meditation and the resulting faith, we eventually free ourselves from the conditioning of the past.

- Meditation helps us to keep life simple, reducing the complications in daily life. We plan incessantly—in a very complicated way. When we meditate, we can say, "It is okay; I don't need this, simple!" Otherwise, we waste a lot of time with these complications, created by the mind.
- Meditation is frees us from the swinging of the mind between attraction and repulsion, *raga-dvesha*. We cease both running away from the pain of the experiences of our past and running toward our attachments.
- Meditation is being aware of our inner guidance. We become strong, as we know that the source of wisdom is within.

3. **Physical benefits:**
    - **Reduced stress and anxiety:** Meditation activates the relaxation response, which helps decrease the body's stress response. This can lower blood pressure, reduce cortisol (a stress hormone) levels, and decrease overall stress symptoms.
    - **Improved sleep:** Regular meditation practice has been linked to improved sleep quality and duration. It can help calm the mind, reduce anxiety, and promote relaxation, leading to better sleep patterns.
    - **Boosted immune system:** Studies suggest that meditation can positively affect the immune system. It may increase the activity of natural killer cells, which are responsible for fighting off viruses and tumors, and it may also increase antibody production.
    - **Pain relief:** Research suggests that meditation can help alleviate pain by modulating the way the brain perceives and responds to danger signals. It can also help individuals develop a higher pain tolerance.
    - **Lower inflammation:** Chronic inflammation is associated with a variety of health conditions, including heart disease, diabetes, and certain types of cancer. Some studies have shown that regular

meditation practice can lower inflammation markers in the body, helping to protect against inflammation-related diseases.

- **Improved cardiovascular health:** Meditation has been linked to improved heart health. It can reduce blood pressure, lower the resting heart rate, and decrease the risk of heart disease and stroke.
- **Increased energy and vitality:** Meditation can help increase energy levels and improve overall vitality. By reducing stress and promoting relaxation, it allows the body to recharge and restore energy levels.
- **Improved focus and concentration:** Meditation enhances attention and cognitive control, helping to improve focus and concentration. Regular practice can lead to improved productivity and cognitive performance.
- **Slowed aging:** Meditation practices, like mindfulness, have been associated with increased telomere length, which is a protective factor against cellular aging. This suggests that meditation may have anti-aging effects at the cellular level.

## MEDITATION: FOLLOWING THE EIGHT STEPS OF RAJA YOGA AND THE FOUR PATHS OF YOGA

Over 2,000 years ago, Patanjali Maharishi, talked about the mistake we make when we identify ourselves with our instruments of seeing—the body and mind. The body and mind are precious, but they are not who we are; they are our instruments of perception. To realize this, we need to follow the eight steps of Raja Yoga.

**The steps to meditation are as follows:**

1. Yama – abstention; refraining from doing certain things that disturb the mind
2. Niyama – observance; doing certain things that will help calm and uplift the mind
3. Asana – steady pose
4. Pranayama – controlling the prana
5. Pratyahara – withdrawing of the senses
6. Dharana – concentration

7. Dhyana – meditation
8. Samadhi – the experience of superconscious meditation

**Meditation and the Four Paths of Yoga**

- In daily life, meditation can be done in action by observing the Karma Yoga attitude: letting go of results, and doing selfless service for others as a way to purify the ego and bring back balance and purity to the mind.
- Meditation comes easier with Bhakti Yoga, the Yoga of devotion and pure love. Either we cultivate devotion to God or humanity. Meditation needs to come with a harmonious relationship with others, including forgiveness, love, and compassion. Meditation comes with successful cleansing of the emotional baggage. When the baggage stays in the mind, it keeps projecting the idea of duality. We become stuck in that thought—everything is split; everything is imperfect and painful.
- Meditation is contemplation in Jnana Yoga. It is oneness, seeing unity in diversity. Meditation is self-observation and self-awareness. A regular habit of observing our thoughts is a stepping stone in the process of meditation. We have to be aware of our thoughts, be "mindful." You cannot meditate if you are not attempting to separate yourself from the mind.
- Meditation is also doing self-inquiry, which means inquiring about the true nature of reality and of the self. Meditation is asking the question, "*Who am I?*" and detaching—or attempting to detach—from false identification. It is a more advanced way of meditating; we dive deeper into the question, "*Who am I?*" and detach from the ideas: "*I am a man, I'm a woman. I'm 30 years old. I'm 50 years old. I'm intelligent. I'm rich, I'm poor. I'm Vietnamese, I'm Chinese,*" and so on.
- Meditation is self-affirmation: "*I am the Immortal Spirit, I am Satchitananda Atman.*" This is advanced meditation, the meditator rejects the unreal, not because they don't like it, but because they seek something deeper. They affirm the real, not because they are egoistic, but because they realize its value. The meditator goes on affirming the real, the permanent, and the unchanging.
- Another advanced method of meditation is meditation on the Self, a method by which the practitioner contemplates the meaning of the scriptural declarations, for example, *Tat Twam Asi* (That you are) or *Aham Brahman Asmi* (I am Brahman). After exhausting the intellectual process, the divine thought is also discarded.

## WHAT MEDITATION IS AND WHAT MEDITATION IS NOT

Meditation is a slow process, resulting from a successful turning inwards of the mind, with a conviction that there is a truth higher and more satisfying than what the mind and our intelligence can conjure up. Classical Raja Yoga meditation is called *dhyana*, the seventh of eight steps—which means it is an advanced step. We should not belittle ourselves if we are unable to meditate right away, if we first need to follow the steps and change our lifestyle to be more meditative.

To meditate, follow the eight steps and four paths of Yoga as outlined above, but also the five points of an integral Yoga lifestyle: 1. exercise (asana), 2. breathing (pranayama), 3. relaxation (savasana), 4. vegetarianism, and 5. positive thinking and meditation. These five points are part of the meditation life.

**What meditation is not:**

- Meditation is not escaping into an inner world, disconnecting from others, and isolating yourself.
- Meditation is not relinquishing your intelligence. It is consciously using your intelligence to distinguish between illusions and reality and, eventually, going beyond limited intelligence to tap into the intuitive source of knowing.
- Meditation cannot come with fear and desire. Replace them with courage and faith to face the experience of the unknown and tread new territories of the mind.
- Meditation is not separate from life. It's not saying, "I meditate and then go live my life." Meditation is integrated with life.
- Meditation is not ungrounded imagination, flying up in the air, astral traveling, or reading people's thoughts.
- Meditation is not relaxation. It is concentration; it is hard work!
- Meditation is not seeking experiences or fantastic psychic phenomena.
- Meditation is not a quick fix.
- Meditation is not wandering in the psychic world.
- Meditation is not dreaming, building castles in the air.
- Meditation cannot come to a weak, disturbed, neurotic, or fearful mind. It is better to do asanas and pranayama and go to therapeutic counseling to overcome the negative tendencies of the mind before attempting serious meditation. Regularly sitting quietly in an effort to calm the mind is already very helpful.

- Meditation is not seeking extra-sensory experiences, isolating oneself, or escaping into an inner world out of fear; meditation is not escaping from reality.
- Meditation is not shunning your responsibility.
- Meditation is not spiritual bypassing—pretending to be holy, but not recognizing the hurts, the fears, the hang-ups, the conditioning of the mind.
- Meditation is not to achieve a self-made goal; meditation is not a selfish endeavor.
- Meditation is not technical and dry, but includes a deep, sacred feeling.
- Meditation is not religious, even though one might have spiritual experiences.
- Meditation is not seeking spiritual experiences.
- Meditation is not free-roaming but, rather, a disciplined venture that follows step-by-step guidance.

## GUIDELINES FOR MEDITATION IN DAILY LIFE

- Imagine meditation as pouring a stream of oil from one vessel to another, continuously flowing. Therefore, we train the mind to be immersed in a meditative mood throughout the day, keeping the mind turned inwards and inspired.
- Start your day with meditation and end your day with meditation. Sit quietly, turning inward, for at least half an hour morning and evening.
- Integrate meditation into your daily routine little by little, starting with 20 minutes in the morning, and 20 minutes in the evening. It's possible. The next day 20 minutes, 20 minutes, and then maybe increase to 30 minutes—regularly. That's all that's required, don't miss a day.
- After waking up early in the morning, do self-affirmation. Create the affirmations yourself, or have somebody help you come up with an appropriate self-affirmation; the situation is always changing.

> *For example, a lady is always making plans to do this and that and then she feels nobody cares about her. Nobody asks her this and that, then she feels lonely and let down, like nobody loves her. I said, "You are always planning your*

*life so tightly that nobody can say anything to you. And now you blame people for not caring for you. They have no room to care for you."*

This is a mental pattern. It needs self-affirmation, such as, "I am love and I am loved. I am being taken care of by the Universe, even when I am not aware of it. I am relaxed in the support, which might be different than I expected."

- We have a tendency to fight, to compare, to be competitive. Make a self-affirmation that nobody is better or worse than anyone else; it is just my mind caught up in comparing. Repeat this affirmation throughout the day.
- Remember the abstentions, things that you should not do. Don't be angry. Don't steal; don't lie; don't accumulate, etc.
- Do purification practice for at least one hour daily with asana, pranayama, and japa.
- Practice gratitude and count your blessings.
- During the day, when planning what to do, where to go, choose well the surroundings where you will spend your time. If you find you must spend time in a negative environment, keep the mind at a high level of thought by repeating your mantra as much as you can.
- Spend less time chit-chatting, wasting time. Relax the mind with positive entertainment, like going for a walk in nature, observing the blue sky, contemplating flowers, sunrise, sunset, and moonlight. These are good, positive entertainments.
- Keep the mind concentrated at all times. Refrain from indulging in imagination. The moment the mind is not focused, it will jump to stories of the past or the future. In the past, we indulge in regrets and feeling bad, the future brings anxiety and fear. Always keep the mind centered in the present, focusing on selfless services and actions and repeat your mantra.
- Work mindfully with dedication. Do not sit idle: *"An idle mind is the devil's workshop."*
- When eating, do so with awareness, with a feeling of gratitude.
- Rest before sleep. Give instructions to the mind. Turn off all the screens one hour before retiring.
- Pay attention to the quality of your dreams. They are indicators of your subconscious mind.

- Chart a daily routine and follow a certain rhythm. Resist changing it. Have a very calm life, enjoy following the rhythm.
- Avoid unnecessary movement. Exercise is fine, but avoid finding excuses to move and do this and that. Conserve prana for meditation. Keep the mind positive and hopeful that you are advancing. We all need encouragement, "I'm progressing toward my goal, which is Self-knowledge."
- Be alert for obstacles in mind; always watch the mind. For example, check the wandering habit of the mind. Notice the effect of cessation of practice, ill health, improper diet, a diet that is disturbing to the mind, laziness, sleepiness, undesirable company, waste of vital energy in sensual pleasures, lack of spiritual preceptor and egoism.

***INSPIRED STORY***

**A Cushion For Your Head**
***Poem by Hafiz***

*Just sit there right now*
*Don't do a thing*
*Just rest*

*For your separation from God*
*Is the hardest work*
*In the world*

*Let me bring you a tray of food*
*And something*
*That you like to drink*

*You can use my soft words*
*As a cushion*
*For your*
*Head.*

**QUESTIONS**

1. *Summarize the technique of meditation.*
2. *List ten spiritual benefits, mental benefits and physical benefits of meditation.*
3. *Explain what meditation is not.*
4. *Describe meditation in the Four Paths of Yoga.*
5. *Give a few examples of how to practice a meditative lifestyle.*

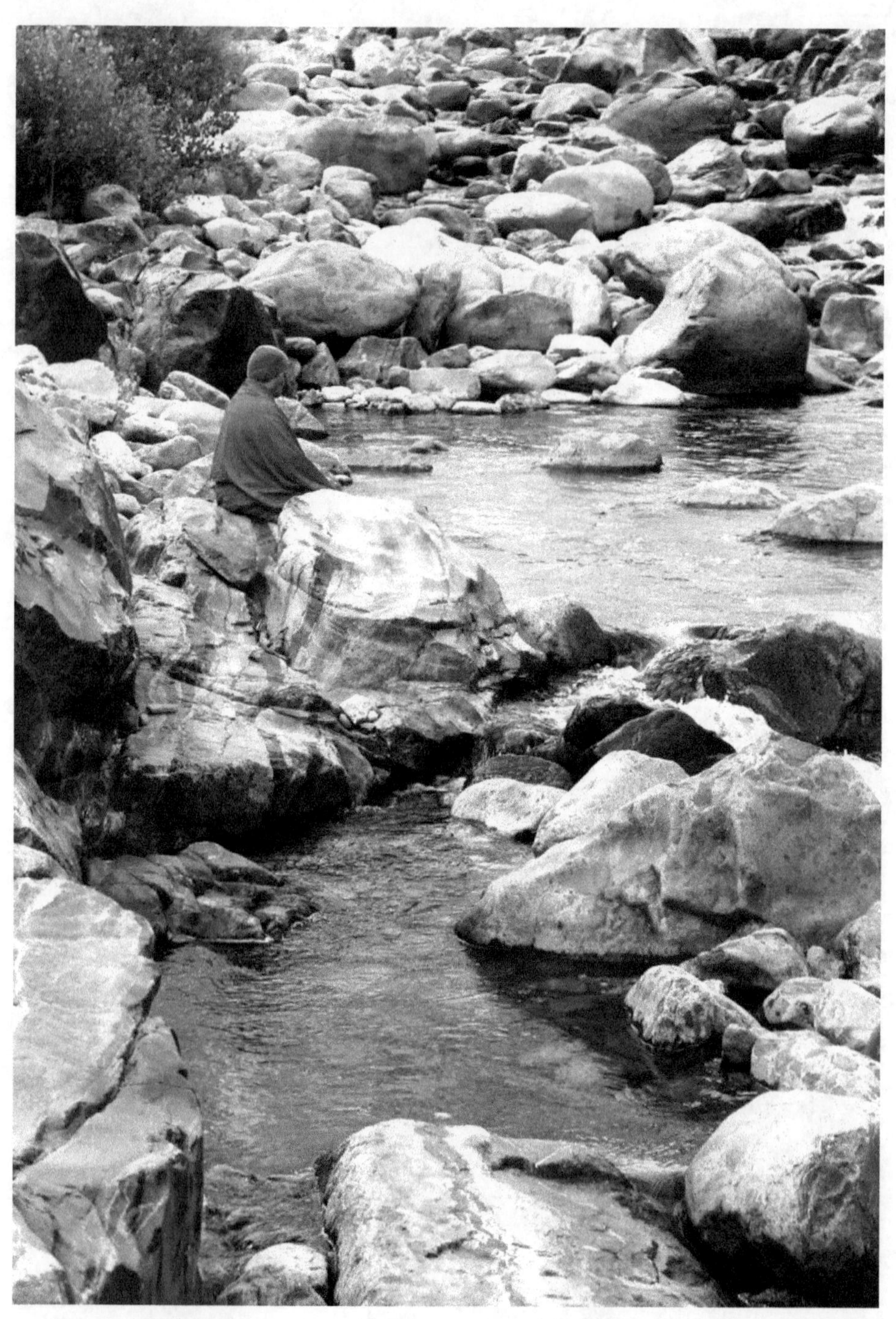

SELF-ENQUIRY BY THE YUBA RIVER

CHAPTER 17

# Self-Inquiry to Be Free from Karma

***"To break through the cycle of cause and effect in this phenomenal world, we must look for an existence which does not change and, likewise, is the cause or the causeless cause of these changeable existences... it is the Light of lights, Life of all lives, Mind of all minds, and Soul of all Souls. It is the hidden Life, vibrant in every atom. It is the hidden Light that shines in every creature. It is the hidden Love that embraces all in Oneness. It is the Silent Witness (Sakshi) of all activities in all minds. It is the Brahman of the Upanishads."***

—SWAMI SIVANANDA, *Practice of Vedanta*

## WHAT IS SELF-INQUIRY?

Self-inquiry is a meditation method to help us remember our True Nature as *Atman* and thus make us feel stronger in times of need. The practice has three aspects: self-awareness, self-surrender, and self-love.

This new way of thinking will help you feel strong at all times, particularly in times of fear, anxiety, and confusion when you feel lost or that your health and well-being are being threatened.

We are faced with uncertainty. Existential questions that haven't been dealt with, may come to the surface. This is a great opportunity to think deeply and find peace and strength through a new understanding of ourselves and our environment.

**The practice of Self-inquiry is the practice of asking the question "Who am I?" and breaking the habit of being yourself.**

Vedanta philosophy is a powerful philosophy coming from the ancient Vedas. It gives us new insights and solutions to our problems.

- It says that we need to solve our problems from a different level of consciousness than the one we are familiar with.

- It is about seeing ourselves and our environment differently.
- To do so, we need to think deeply and endeavor to distinguish between what is unchanging and what is changing.
- Something unchanging is real. Something changing is illusory.
- To get to the unchanging, we need to question what we believe to be true about ourselves and our perception of the universe we see around us.
- The whole meditation exercise is about asking ourselves "Who am I?" and breaking the false identifications. We do not know who we are, but we know who we are not. What remains is the "I."
- By this query, we recover the Self and feel stronger and happier. We free ourselves from suffering and fear resulting from our attachment to the false self. We realize it is a habit that we have harbored for a long time. Therefore, the meditation needs to continue over time.
- We become more and more detached.
- It takes strength and sharp intellect to do this.

**Our habitual mind keeps reproducing past illusions.**

Things are not the way we imagine them to be. The reality we see is the reality of our mind's projections. The classic story of "The Snake and the Rope" illustrates our situation well (see chapter 1). In the darkness, a person sees a snake and jumps in fright. Someone unafraid of snakes brings a light to shine upon the snake. Under the light, it turns out to be only a rope. A rope looks like a snake, but is not a snake. The rope did not become a snake, and the snake did not become a rope. All of these apparent changes happen only in the mind. The mind, already fearful of snakes, projects "snake." Our thoughts and memory are superimposed upon the truth. Similarly, in the darkness of our spiritual ignorance, we keep seeing scary and stressful things and react in fear. When we dare to inquire, knowledge sets us free. Then we can see things as they are and not as we imagine them to be.

**Why do we keep seeing the same thing?**

To be free, we must revisit the personal and collective past illusions. To wake up, we revisit our fears and see them for what they are—not real, and only in our minds. We become familiar with our mind's patterns and it is easier for us to recognize them; we catch ourselves when we are seeing the "snake" and not the rope. We thus become stronger, over time, as the memory of the rope becomes more and more established. Only then can we transcend the vision of the "snake." Our fears resulting from our weaknesses become more and more known and we become stronger and stronger. Self-inquiry helps us to do this.

**How to unveil the Self and be free of the habit of being ourselves?**

*First, you are not the body.*
*Upon asking the first question, "Who am I?"*
*The first answer is, "I am the body."*
*The body is made of the five gross elements:*
*Earth, water, fire, air, and ether.*
*It is made of food.*
*We are born with our constitution. There are three types of body constitution in Ayurveda, the ancient science of medicine. They are called doshas.*
*You can be solid, earthy, supportive, and steady, made of earth and water.*
*You can be fiery, sharp, active, inquisitive, made of fire.*
*You can be quick, sensitive, and moving like air in space.*
*The body constitution gives the predisposition*
*to think and be this way or that.*
*We are not seeing the same thing, as our constitution veils us.*
*Whatever constitution or body type we are,*
*The body is born, grows, decays, and dies, in due time. It is not meant to be forever,*
*It is not us; it keeps changing.*
*If we line up photos of ourselves at different times of our lives—from being a baby, a toddler, an adolescent, an adult, in our 30s, 40s, and 60s—the body looks different in size, shape, and weight and, yet, we point to each photo and recognize the same "me" exclaiming, "This is me, this is me!"*
*Think about this, there is a "me" that is not the body.*
*The body is our instrument on our journey, not the self.*
*Mistaken identity with the body creates fear and anxiety, especially the fear of death.*
*The body journey is a chapter in the book of our lives, not the whole story.*

*Apply the neti-neti method (Vedantic refutation method: not this/not that) to the body.*
*Affirm "I am not my gender, neither male nor female."*
*"I am not my race, black, white, yellow."*
*"I am not my age, young, old, older."*
*"I am not my physical beauty or appearance."*
*"I am the driver of this body vehicle."*
*"I am not the color or shape of the vehicle."*
*"I am not my muscles, bones, lungs, heart, nor hair."*
*"Nor my arms nor legs."*
*"Nor my nose, tongue, eyes, skin, nor ears."*

*"I am the driver of this body vehicle*
*and these organs and limbs are my instruments."*
*"I am the subject and these are the objects."*
*"I am consciousness and not the sum of my body parts."*

*Detach from the body.*
*Do not overly worry about it as yourself.*
*Being the caretaker of the instrument,*
*gives you strength and health,*
*frees you from the fear of death,*
*which is paralyzing in this time of virus threat.*

**The second identification is with the prana/life force.**

*The prana energizes the body and gives it life.*
*Prana is changing, sometimes low, sometimes high,*
*balanced and unbalanced.*
*Prana comes with the air we breathe,*
*the earth, water, fire, and etheric space.*
*We can identify with what we feel,*
*energetic or tired,*
*strong or sick,*
*blocked or flowing,*
*acting and enjoying,*
*moving here and there,*
*or staying still and sheltered in place.*
*But we are not our prana, life force.*
*So be aware, and take care of your prana.*
*Do pranayama to purify and regulate*
*your prana and emotions;*
*but we are not the prana.*
*Therefore, stay detached from it.*

**The third identification is with our mind and emotions.**

*Who am I?*
*I am worried, angry, fearful, joyful, sad, grieving.*
*Our states of mind and emotions*
*kidnap our identity.*
*We lose ourselves in our emotions*
*and become what we feel.*

*The senses are connected to what we feel*
*and keep us alternating between pleasure and pain.*
*They set the stage for the mind and emotions to play*
*its comedies or dramas.*
*But comedy turns to drama and drama turns to comedy.*
*Snake turns to rope and rope turns to snake.*
*Nevertheless, the sense of "I" is lost, drowned in the emotions*
*Of all our relationships,*
*Which makes us feel ups and downs,*
*Happy and unhappy,*
*Loved and separated.*
*Stay still, turn within,*
*Happiness is within.*
*Love is already there,*
*Calm down, detach.*
*I am not the mind and emotions.*

**Fourth, I am not my ego and intellect:**

*I can tell the story of my life,*
*Over and over again.*
*To one person, hundreds of people, thousands,*
*To my children, grandchildren,*
*Yet I am not my story,*
*Even though I might be attached to it.*
*My story even well-rehearsed*
*From lifetime to lifetime,*
*Generation to generation*
*Keeps changing*
*As my lessons keep changing.*
*I keep acting out what I think myself to be,*
*My level of consciousness,*
*My level of self-awareness,*
*My level of being the silent witness*
*To myself.*
*My understanding of who am I,*
*Separated or connected,*
*Isolated or together,*
*Alone or involved,*
*Unstable or stable,*

*Worthy or unworthy,*
*Proud of accomplishments,*
*Better or worse,*
*Achiever, intelligent or a failure,*
*My level of self-knowledge is changing.*
*Therefore it is not me, the unchanging.*
*Truly, there is something beyond the ego stories*
*That cannot be described.*
*This is who I am, the background of things,*
*The movie screen*
*On which the movies, stories play*
*And yet unaffected,*
*Detached Witness I am.*

*The calming of the mind and the ego,*
*The realization of the silent witness,*
*Becoming the observer of my thoughts,*
*Becoming the conscious awareness itself*
*makes me feel strong.*
*I find myself and do not lose myself*
*When I detach myself from my stories*
*And stop justifying myself.*
*I am not my ego.*

**The fifth level of identification is more subtle.**

*As it speaks about my purpose,*
*As my question becomes deeper,*
*I realize that I have been there, done that*
*For a long, long time.*
*The purpose of this birth and its lessons*
*is revealed.*
*As long as the "I" is conditioned, attached,*
*My sense of purpose is distorted.*

*Now I realize the purpose of this birth.*
*My journey is from karma to dharma.*
*And I am blissful and happy.*
*No more fear,*
*No more separation,*

*No more doubt,*
*No more agenda.*
*I am consciousness and bliss.*
*I am free.*

**Self-inquiry meditation is thinning out the veils.**

*See through the illusions of self and others.*
*Turn within and solve your problems from*
*A different level of consciousness.*
*It can only get better.*
*We are not losing anything.*
*Only gaining in strength and courage*
*To face our lives*
*By being ourselves.*
*This meditation and Self-inquiry are forced upon us*
*In this time of crisis when all established habits are being questioned,*
*And reinvented.*
*The more the veils are thin,*
*The happier and steadier we become.*
*The more this world will come to peace*
*As we understand that my self and your self are one.*
*Perceive unity in diversity.*
*Celebrate our interdependence*
*And let go of fear,*
*Clinging to the past,*
*Projecting in the future.*

**There is only one Truth**

*There is not your truth and my truth*
*Because both are only reflections.*
*There is only one sun*
*Reflected on many surfaces.*
*Reflected on a rock surface, the light shines a little.*
*Reflected on water, it becomes distorted with the waves.*
*Reflected on a wood surface, the light is dim and stable.*
*Reflected on a shiny mirror, the light is bright and the image sharp.*
*There is only one consciousness,*
*The same in all beings,*
*Whether mineral, animal, human, or superhuman.*

*We are one.*
*The differences are external*
*But the essence is one.*

**We do not know the truth and act out of ignorance**

*Forgetting the big picture,*
*Forgetting to do self-inquiry,*
*Forgetting the search for the truth,*
*Forgetting our purpose,*
*We become greedy, senseless, and abusive towards animals and nature,*
*Not thinking, not respecting,*
*Constantly creating pain for others*
*For our pleasures.*
*This is the time*
*We need to wake up and turn inward,*
*Question our ways,*
*Cease to blame,*
*But taking responsibility.*
*Stop the killing*
*Of innocent animals,*
*Their abuse and torture.*
*Become vegetarian.*
*Stop the wasting of resources*
*And the appropriation*
*Of planet Earth.*
*Stay still and Meditate.*
*Everything you want is right*
*Here and now.*

## HOW TO FOSTER SELF-AWARENESS

- **Self-awareness is intuitive, beyond mind and intellect.** When we talk about self-awareness, we talk about the spiritual insights beyond the workings of the mind and intellect.

  We are using the inner instrument (*chitta, manas, ahamkara, buddhi,* subconscious mind, conscious mind) to comprehend our experience. But the intuitive insights come from the superconscious mind, the seat of intuition. It is the moment of clarity that gives answers and it is undeniable.

Allow yourself to think about the problem and let it be. The answer comes in a flash.

- **Self-awareness comes with sattva.** The function of self-awareness is fundamental for healing, but it is not easy to access. People who are sick are generally in tamas and rajas, while self-awareness requires sattva. All of the therapeutic interventions of a Yoga Therapist or Yoga Health Educator are geared towards increasing sattva and fostering self-awareness. They do this by bringing people to awareness of the slow and smooth breath—without effort—and by bringing awareness to the present moment, which is perfect in itself.
- **Self-awareness is spiritual healing.** It implies healing on a deep level. The individual no longer sees themselves as a separate individual, identifying and struggling with body and mind (the *jiva*), but has glimpses of the *Atman*, the indweller.

  **How to apply?**

  - Diminish the ego, that feels separate and alone in the experience of a larger reality or group consciousness.
  - Use the word "we" instead of "I."
  - Refer to each other as a "soul," "spirit," "God," "the universe," or "Mother Nature," as it is something obvious and not hidden or marginal.
  - Ask yourself how you feel, not referring to the emotions, but to something deeper.
  - Know that all happens for the best, even if we do not understand.
  - Teach whomever you come into contact with to stop and turn within and feel their heart/soul intelligence and start to trust it.

- **Self-awareness and God-awareness are the same.** In other words, it would also be correct to say that the individual realizes their connection with the Divine. The individual becomes grateful and realizes God's grace and mercy, knowing that all is perfect. No more blame, guilt, anger, resentment, despair, rejection, self-pity, or self-victimization.

**How to apply?**

- Match the belief system to your individual religious background, knowing that all paths lead to the same truth. God can be defined as "not I," so awareness of the "not I" is self-awareness.
- Do exercises on gratitude for the "not I."
- Affirm "God loves us," "We are not alone."
- Understand the positivity, the synchronicity, as glimpsing the presence of God.
- When we feel most alone, God is actually carrying us or caring about us, transporting us beyond our pain and sorrow.

*There is a beautiful poem by Mary Stevenson entitled "Footprints in the Sand." In the poem, in a dream, someone sees two sets of footprints in the sand, one set of their own and one belonging to God. In the dream, looking back on life, at the saddest and most difficult times, there is only one set of footprints. Troubled by this, the dreamer asks God why, at the hardest times of life, when needed the most, was he not there. God replied, "My precious child, I love you and will never leave you, never, ever, during your trials and testings. When you saw only one set of footprints, it was then that I was carrying you."*

- **Self-awareness is self-acceptance and self-surrender.** Accept your non-acceptance of the imperfect self, the ego, the idea of who we are. Accept, on another level, that you are perfect and untouched by all that is happening. Often, we reject some aspects of ourselves (rajas), or *everything* about ourselves and the universe (tamas). Acceptance is an important step towards healing. There are no more preferences; you accept everything and love everything. There is peace and contentment. This can happen only when you get out of your self and are relaxing internally in the love inherent in their own deeper Self.

**How to apply?**

- Do not reject anything, do not think that something is better.
- Limit the running towards and away from anything.
- Breathe into the pain, physical or mental. Dissolve the pain in acceptance.
- No effort, no fight. Stay calm in all conditions. Everything is perfect as it is.
- Do Restorative Yoga, savasana, and relaxation in all aspects.

- **Self-acceptance is Self-love.** Usually, there is self-rejection, lack of self-confidence, and lack of self-care when we are tamasic and rajasic. Self-love turns the love that is addressed to others into the love of our true Self. The patterns of attachment and disillusion are fundamentally changed, as we can live and let live and find our place in life and destiny. There is perfect contentment.

  **How to apply?**

  - Detect patterns of attachments. Excessive attachment to something external shows a lack of self-love.
  - Remember to self-love. Take time for self-care. For example, do asana, pranayama, take a walk, etc.
  - Take care of the body as a temple, take time to eat well, and enjoy life.
  - Give words of appreciation to your own self and also learn to appreciate others.
  - Avoid comparing yourself with others.
  - Avoid wasting energy on something you cannot change. Be ready to change something that needs to be changed. Know the difference.

- **Self-acceptance is self-surrender to God's will.** You become like a co-partner with the Divine. You become relaxed and accept all life's happenings and outcomes as a gift, instead of resisting and fighting, trying so hard to make a life, instead of simply being.

**How to apply?**

- Adopt a policy of no complaints.
- Have a smiling attitude, cooperate, and be flexible.
- Adopt the idea that, "There is no other, everything is our own self."
- Remember the Self in others to let go of control.
- Remember the Self in others to let go of fears (from attachment).
- Let go of anxiety.
- Share stories of grace.

• **Self-surrender is relying on Mother Nature to heal and to do what She wants.** Your connection to Nature is restored. You becomes wise in your choices, as you become like a child in the mother's lap. The forces of Nature will then do their recuperative work.

**How to apply?**

- Trust that the body has intelligence and knows how to heal itself.
- Trust that Nature has intelligence and knows.

• **Self-awareness, self-love, and self-surrender imply increased faith and courage.** Have faith in your capacity for healing, faith in God or Nature the healer, and faith in the doctor or therapist.

**How to apply?**

- Increase trust in yourself and others. Avoid excessive suspicion and anxiety.
- Eat with faith and confidence that your food is nourishing. Pray before eating. Bless the food and the cooks.
- Keep an object/image as a reminder of the Indweller. Bring it with you to places where there are inner distractions, such as a hotel, when you are traveling.
- Repeat the mantra with faith.
- Read scriptures and have faith in the teaching and the teachers.

- Dare to do things beyond your comfort zone. Try a new posture, a new endeavor and have faith that it will work out.

- **Self-awareness brings in self-responsibility.** I do my duty. I take the necessary steps, either by taking medicine, doing exercises, eating properly, meditating... but with the idea that I am performing a duty to the body as a temple, and not with an idea of the outcome. For example, avoid thinking, "May I be cured, so that I can continue life as before."
- **Self-awareness goes beyond death and diseases.** The immortal Self, the *Atman,* is diseaseless, deathless, birthless. It is only the karmas that are playing out in your life. Once the karmas are understood, you become ready for anything and find peace.
- **Self-awareness leads to intuition.** Emotions and desires almost totally govern most people's lives. Developing self-awareness means understanding that the spirit is the most important thing, because it comes before everything else. The mind comes from the spirit and the body comes from the mind. The subconscious mind, or lower mind, makes up a huge part of the total mind, so most people are helpless and at the mercy of their subconscious mind. The first step on the path to self-awareness is to be aware of our reactive tendency and our instincts and our habitual thoughts and feelings.
- **Slow down and change gears.** Without self-awareness, you are like a car going 100 miles per hour in one direction, and even though it might be heading towards a cliff, you cannot do anything about it.

That's why there are so many Yoga techniques—such as asanas and pranayama—to help you develop your awareness, so you can slow the car down the, change gears, steer our vehicle in a different direction, and ultimately change the course of your life.

Spiritual growth means becoming aware of the subconscious mind and being able to put the mind into a different gear. Awareness means examining yourself. It means knowing what motivates you and whether your motivations match up with your conscious decisions.

When you become clear you begin to awaken the higher faculty within. Consciousness is based on pure intellect, the intellect which is uncorrupted by the lower mind.

## CONSCIOUSNESS AND HUMAN INTELLECT

Consciousness is what sets us apart from animals. The human intellect encompasses the faculty of reasoning and freedom of choice. When we are faced with a dilemma, we can, with awareness, use our ability to reason and exercise choice and make a conscious decision. If you are using awareness, reasoning, and conscious choice, the decision will be rooted in the higher mind. If you are using your emotions to make the choice and you use our intellect to justify our emotions, your lower mind is controlling you.

- **Face the struggle between the lower and higher mind.** In the beginning, the struggle is inevitable. The heart and emotions say something, the intellect says something else, and then the two go into battle. But eventually, the opposing parts will thin out and awareness becomes apparent. Doubts will be cleared. Courage becomes strength, removes the fears, and Truth is revealed.
- **Being self-aware and intuitive means using the superconscious mind.** The second stage of the development of your mind would be from the conscious to the superconscious, from being discriminative to being intuitive. On the journey along the spiritual path, intuitive faculty will naturally become stronger and stronger. When intuition develops, struggle will lessen and a sense of effortless knowing will increase. You will no longer be a mass of contradictions. You will be able to just ride through—glide through, slide through—life.

There will be an ease to things. When the intuition is working well, there will be plenty of prana.

Prana is a sustaining energy but most of the time we lose prana because of our inner conflicts; we waste it all by running around, doing a hundred different things, most of them unnecessary. But when intuition comes into play, you will be able to live in harmony with yourself and others. Conflicts will fade away. You will be able to use your intuition to embrace others, to know them. That happens once self-knowledge dawns. You will only need to look at someone, turn your gaze inward, and then you will be able to see them from inside of yourself, as well as from outside. At that time, they are not separate from you. You will start to become one with all.

## CONTEMPLATING THE SELF WITH ANALOGIES IN VEDANTA

We are all waves in the same ocean; some are small, some are huge, but all are made of water. The waves are the same as the ocean. The universe and Brahman, absolute consciousness, are one. You are the infinite ocean of consciousness. See unity in diversity.

- We are clay becoming different, utilitarian pots and beautiful vases.
- We are gold turning into different shapes and forms of ornaments.
- We are spirit and consciousness in the guise of different varieties of people.

Under apparent differences, Nature is sacred and diverse, but it is the manifestation of one Consciousness. There are many types of fruits, flowers, insects, animals, beings, humans, races, and genders. Recognize unity in diversity. Spirit is one, and names and forms are many.

Consciousness is the essential nature of different minds, different people, different kinds of occupation or status. Consciousness is Real. Without consciousness, there would be no people, no objects. Without clay, there is no pot. Stop identifying yourself and others with outside appearances and occupations. See unity of consciousness at all times. We are one. I am you and you are me.

- **There is only one Self: The Sun is one, and the reflections are many.**

The Sun is compared to the *Atman*. It gives light to all indiscriminately. The *Atman* is That Consciousness that is common in all beings. It is One without a second. It is the Self in All, illuminating from within. It is independent, reflects brightly through the mirror, less through a wooden floor, and even less on a rock. The *Atman* is one reflecting through different minds and intelligence. The difference is the surface on which it shines. It is the same sun. The *Atman* is the source of Intelligence, therefore, no one is more intelligent than another. The same *Atman* is in an animal, a rock, a criminal, and a saint.

- When reflected through different containers of water, it looks like there are many suns. They are only reflections of the one sun. There is one *Atman*, but we think there are many individual souls.
- Remain unattached in the world of *maya*. Be like a lotus leaf growing in the water; drops of water roll off of it, but do not wet it. The *Atman* is untouched by good or bad.
- Be like the wind, carrying all odors, but untouched by ~~these~~ any. Same as the *Atman*, it remains untouched by any circumstance.

- Be like the crystal, reflecting any color it is placed against, but itself remaining pure, colorless, and unaffected.
- Be unattached in the world of *maya*, where all is relative—like the hardness of stone compared to the softness of mud. There is no absolute truth or value to anything in this world. The truth is to be found in the *Atman* alone.
- Cease to look for absolute happiness where it is not, like looking for the teeth of a crow or the baby of a virgin woman.
- Cease to look for the needle outside, when you have lost it inside.
- The mind is subjective; attachment makes things beautiful. What is poisonous and rejected by one, can be well sought by another. All is relative to the mindset only.
- The universe is endowed with consciousness, even though the nature of objects is quite different. In reality, the threads of a web are only part of the spider; the spider provides the energy and materials from his own body to create a web, something seemingly different from itself
- Do not try to change the illusions or the dreams. Work to change from within, you cannot change the outside, but change happens from within.
- Think properly; do not waste energy finding the logic in things. Find the essence and stay away from *maya*.

**The Self is all there is.**

- Love the Self in all. All is love (Bhakti Yoga)
- Serve the Self in others (Karma Yoga)
- Control the waves of the mind to see the underlying Self (Raja Yoga)
- Do Self-inquiry and reject false identification of your Self. (Jnana Yoga)

*This is the time for us to practice this meditation,*
*Wake up and learn what we can*
*To Remember ourselves.*
*Stay away from past and future,*
*Be in the moment, present.*
*See the essence and not the manifestations,*

*Respect the differences as it is in essence one.*
*Come back to unconditional love*
*Of Self and others*
*The Love and the Truth will set us free!*

## VEDANTIC MEDITATION: THE SELF AS SAT-CHIT-ANANDA

**The Self is Existence Absolute.**

- Birthless
- Deathless
- Eternal
- Distinct from the five sheaths
- Unlimited; has no beginning, no end
- All-pervading
- Unchanging reality
- Truth absolute
- Supreme Consciousness
- Witness of all phenomena
- Transcending appearance
- Undefinable
- Without name or form
- Unceasing
- Unbounded
- Undifferentiated
- Immeasurable
- Immutable
- Without parts
- Indivisible
- Transcendent
- Perfect freedom
- Neither inside nor outside

**The Self is Knowledge Absolute.**

- Consciousness absolute
- Unbroken awareness
- Giving intelligence to the mind
- Self-existent Light
- All-knowing, the knower
- Aware of mind and ego
- The source of all life
- Source of all knowledge
- Source of all creativity
- Source of all solutions to all situations
- The answer within
- Witness of three states: waking, dreaming, deep sleep
- Perfection, beyond action
- Beyond all mistakes
- Having no equal
- One without a second

**The Self is Bliss Absolute.**

- Infinite Joy, unending BLISS
- Inherent nature of the Self is Bliss
- Cannot be separated from Bliss
- If miserable, we have forgotten ourselves
- Love absolute
- Oneness
- Beyond all desires
- Fulfillment absolute
- Beyond all fears
- Beyond separation
- Gives light, love and beauty to the universe
- Residing in the pure heart

**"Knowledge of the Self is the only direct means to liberation (from suffering)" – Shankaracharya**

- In the story of ten friends swimming across a river and crying over a missing friend, we cry because we forget to count ourselves.
- We always look for happiness outside (wealth, fame, power), as in the story of the lady looking for her lost needle outside of the house.
- Happiness is our True Nature, as in the story of a dog chewing on a plastic bone. He enjoys blood coming from his own gums, thinking it is from the "bone."
- The musk deer looks for the smell that comes from his own sweat.

**Self-inquiry exercises:**

- Inquire into the story of your "I." What is the nature of your identity?
- Myself and My Body: What is your rapport with your body? What is your history with your body?
- Where does your fear come from? What do you do with it?
- What is your story of attachment? What attachments do you have?
- Look back to see the presence of the *Atman* in your life. How have you realized the presence of *Atman* in your life? What happens when it comes and goes?

## QUESTIONS

1. *Why do we practice self-inquiry?*
2. *How do we do self-inquiry?*
3. *What is Self-awareness?*
4. *What is self-surrender?*
5. *Give three Vedantic analogies.*

*INSPIRED STORY*

**Healing anxiety by awareness**

*I came back from a few months of traveling and pilgrimage in India and was not able to function. I was very fatigued and very spacey at that time and I had lymph node swelling. I learned afterwards, that it was a condition called vata imbalance, from too much traveling, too much feeling high and being ungrounded on pilgrimage, as well as an infection that made my gland swell.*

*When I went to the first medical doctor, seeing the lump in my gland, the doctor said, "Oh, it is cancer," then measured the lump and wanted me to come back for a biopsy. When I went to a second doctor, upon knowing I just came back from India, she said "Ah, it is tuberculosis!" In both encounters, I got very scared and my mind came up with all kinds of scenarios, swinging between diagnoses.*

*Then, I went to a Chinese doctor—an acupuncturist, an old man. He didn't say anything. He didn't say a big word, like the other two doctors. When I asked him, "What do I have?" he said, "Don't worry about this," and he treated me with acupuncture, which made me feel very good. During that time, I kept meditation every day and practiced asana and pranayama every day, despite my fatigue.*

*Then one day, I met with an Ayurvedic doctor, who gave me a dietary consultation and prescribed his blend of herbal rose tea, which I was supposed to drink when I did not feel well. I drank and drank... and realized that my mind was anxious. It was not the tea, per se, that healed me; it was the awareness that there was anxiety in my mind. This brought me back to a place of rest, poise, and strength, which healed the body and mind miraculously. Awareness removed the imaginative anxieties and brought me to the healthy, conscious and ever-present Self. The lymph node swelling, which came from a simple infection, disappeared without any effort. I'm fine—and learned a big lesson about trust in Mother Nature and in Self-awareness and not being scared of medical professionals with big words.*

**A journey from not-Self to Self**

*I grew up in a rough situation and developed self-destructive habits. I didn't even know I was being self-destructive. I was functioning in the world—I got an education, got married, and had children. From the outside, I seemed fine—but, inside, things were awful.*

*Suddenly, one day, my experience of being an addict and alcoholic for many years just brought me to my knees. I had always been critical of the Recovery program. But finally, I just stopped. I turned my life and my will over to the care of my sponsor and my teacher.*

*I begged her, "Tell me what to do." And she told me what to do. And I did everything she told me to do. And I still do that today. I go to 12-step meetings and have a community of people who I talk to. Getting sober is more than just stopping drinking and stopping using, it's about changing the way we live.*

*It is a work in progress. In Yoga philosophy, I had to grow in "discrimination," I had to relearn how to think. And now I ask the question, "What is real and unchanging and what is an illusion and changing?"*

*I think when I was young, I remembered myself, my true Self. I'm trying to tap back into that. The moments when I was in crisis were the moments that woke me up. I asked, "Is it important or not?" Death was so close—and real life was so close. I think we unconsciously distract ourselves from our search for the Truth.*

*There is so much similarity between the Recovery program and Yoga and Vedanta training. I have to learn about my passion via dispassion. I have to learn to recognize my emotions and know that they're not real. I know that feelings are not facts. I had to understand my cravings, my attachments, and my obsessive behaviors. This required a lot of humility. I had to ask for help all the time, every day, numerous times a day, and also to pray and ask for God's help.*

*My life is not perfect, but it's pretty good. I wake up every morning, sit outside on my back porch, and I just feel grateful. I had serious cravings for using and it was very hard to stop and to stay stopped. But I haven't used alcohol or my other vices for many years now. I have to keep my feet firmly planted on the ground. I'm no authority; I had to stop and accept the things I couldn't change. I had to learn that I don't need all the stuff that my mind comes up with. I had to realize that it was just triggering me to get back to the emotion. And it's not real. I learn to feel my feelings, as opposed to numbing them. It has been, and still is, hard for me. I had to accept my behavior and make amends for it, to forgive myself and ask for forgiveness from other people. If they didn't want to give me forgiveness, I was ready to accept that, too.*

*I have faith in God and I believe that in my recovery, on this Yoga path, I am blessed. The only thing I did was show up and something just kept drawing me to come back and come back. I have a busy life, but I keep my feet firmly planted in my Yoga and meditation routine. I keep open communications with my sponsors and teachers. I do service like teaching Yoga and recovery classes for my community. I feel stronger. I don't have cravings anymore. I have peace of mind—well, not completely with my emotions, I am still attached. I have old habits of self-pity and anxiety. I recognize them when they come up. I pray and call my sponsor and I meditate. I meditate every day. I have hope. I am conscious that I need to keep the peace of awareness, so calling somebody to talk about this helps me to be conscious. This is the path of awareness of that consciousness.*

*I love to be free from the suffering, from this unreality.*

*L., a Vedanta student*

**Awareness after death experience**

*After my health challenges and two near-death experiences, I am no longer attached to my role as bread-winner and provider for my extended family. I realized that life can cease at any moment. I was ready to become more detached.*

*In terms of self-inquiry, I remember the body that I had when I was growing up, playing with my brothers and sisters. It is not the same body now, but I still remember—but who is remembering? It is my inner coach, not the body that is changing. That realization shows me that progress can be made to continue the practice to realize my True Nature.*

*In terms of controlling the senses, I became a vegan, by choice, to control the tongue. I have not eaten Indian sweets for three years. Training myself has two purposes—one is saving energy, and the other, more importantly, is controlling my reactive tendency.*

*Detachment, detachment. I know very well that there is no guarantee that there will be a next moment. I surrender to the scriptures, to the teachers, and to the people who have traveled the path before. I learned that it requires devotion to follow the path of the Masters and to practice what they practiced.*

*I suffered a traumatic experience losing my parents when I was 12 and 17. I was always self-reliant, taking care of myself. That brought fear every step of the way.*

*I am no longer afraid, but began to feel anxious all the time, which created stomach issues—anxiety of the unknown, maybe anxiety of death. At that time, I did not quite understand that you don't die. We somehow subconsciously get attached to lies. We have anxiety about living projected in the future. I can't explain it. I have fun. I have no other responsibility besides living, but I still don't think I understand life. That is scary to me. I have faith in the scripture as a field that exists, and have faith in the wise because some of them already had the ultimate experience, but still it goes back to the mystery of the presence in the body, the life and death paradox.*

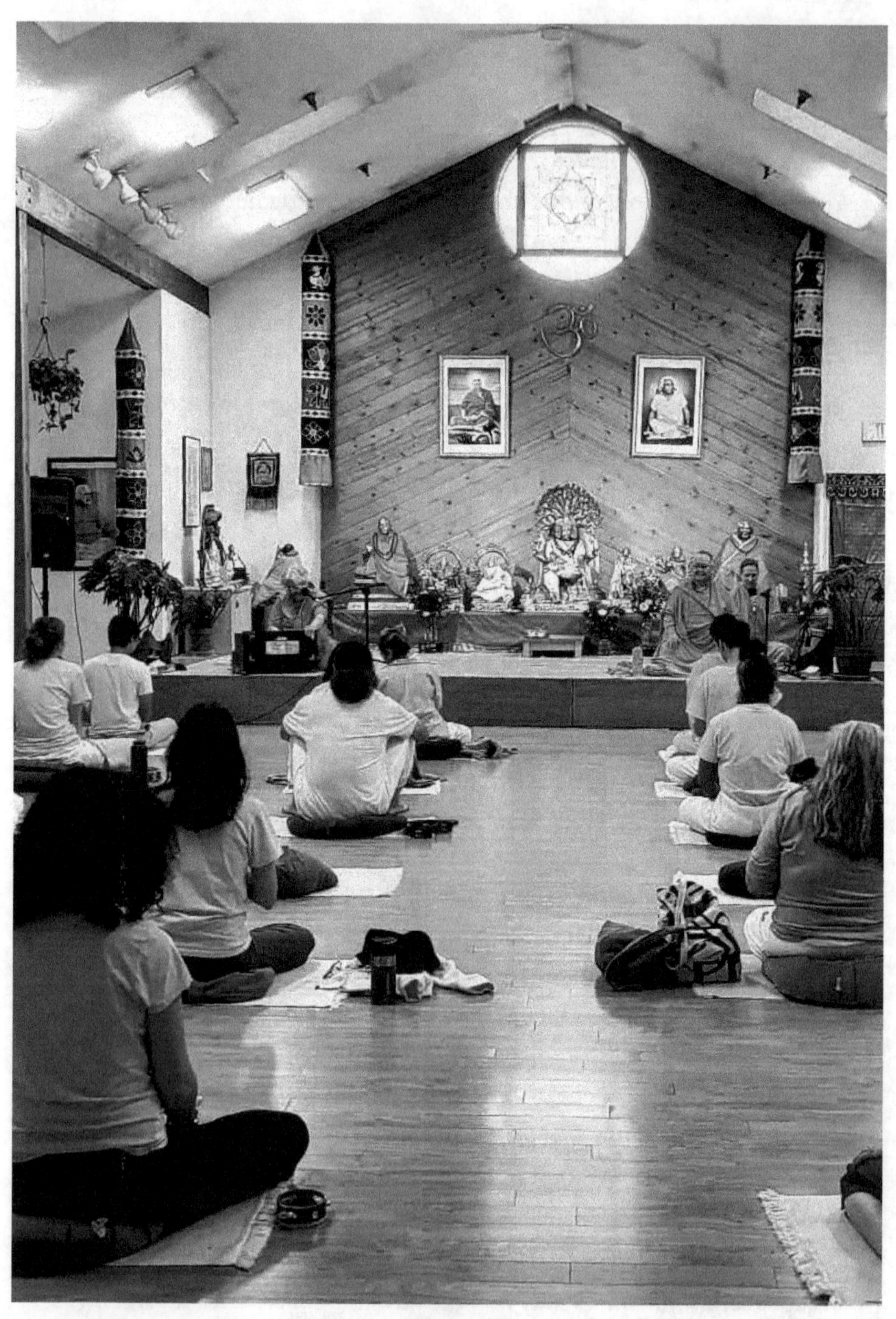

SATSANG IN YOGA FARM

## CHAPTER 18

# Nurturing Self-Awareness with Satsanga

***"One gets dispassion or vairagya by association with wise people. The state of freedom from moha (delusion) is induced by developing vairagya. Even a moment's company with wise people is quite sufficient to overhaul the old vicious samskaras of worldly-minded people. The magnetic aura, the spiritual vibrations, and the powerful thought currents of developed adepts produce a tremendous influence on the minds of worldlings. The personal contact of mahatmas is a blessing in reality for worldly persons. The service of saints purifies the minds of passionate persons rapidly. Satsanga elevates the mind to magnanimous heights."***

- SWAMI SIVANANDA in *Practice of Brahmacharya*

We need to connect and associate with positive people and those who have firm faith and clarity of purpose. When we do so, we feel much enthusiasm from them and our doubts and anxieties are automatically dispelled. The beginner on this spiritual journey of return, or journey of Self-healing, will need help. To light a candle, you need a burning candle; an illumined soul alone can enlighten or illumine another soul. Only a Guru or teacher can share this knowledge. A seeker on the path who is under the guidance of a master is safe from being led astray, from being lost along the way.

**Why is it so important to have a spiritual mentor, teacher, guide, or guru?** The nature of egoism is such that we will not be able to discover our defects. There will be some blind spots. You can turn your head as much as you want, but you will not be able to see your own neck. In a similar way, the ego is obstructing our view. Our identification with the body and mind—and especially the ego, identification with something that we are not—prevents us from seeing things correctly. We will be unable to see our defects and will need the help of someone who has been there, who knows the pitfalls and difficulties to be encountered, and who can point them out to us. That person can help us move from where we are, toward where we want to be.

## PITFALLS OF THE BEGINNER

*Satsanga* and association with the guru is an armor and fortress to guard against all temptations and unfavorable forces of the material world. We constantly feel the pull of those forces and we need help to pull us up and guide us inward. The mind has absorption power; we are easily influenced by the company we keep, including our loved ones. We can easily feel pressured to conform to peer pressure or societal norms, or at least to doubt our path and our endeavor.

Swami Sivananda said, *"A new person or beginner on the path must have personal help, a personal teacher, mentor, or Guru first. He cannot have God as a guru, to begin with; he must have a pure mind first."*

## WHAT DO WE MEAN BY THE WORD GURU?

*Guru* means "the one who dispels darkness." To be a guru, one must have a command from God, meaning that a person has to attain a certain level of purity. Then the voice of intuition, a higher voice, can give a command to the guru, *"You need to go and teach this."*

In Swami Sivananda's words, *"The Guru is a being who has raised himself or herself from this domain of the material consciousness to that which is supreme consciousness and thus has free access to both realms."*

It is like a person standing with half their body in water and half out in the air and bending down to lift other people out of the water. The guru can do this, because they have experience of both worlds. When the beginner lives in the company of the guru, it is spiritual education. The Sivananda ashrams and centers, founded by Swami Vishnudevanandaji in the lineage of Swami Sivananda, run like *gurukulas*. The teachers are called *acharya*, which means "a spiritual teacher, holder of lineage," and they teach from scriptures. The swamis and the *acharyas*, or the senior teachers, are disciples of the lineage.

A special feature is that the teachers are themselves immersed in the Yoga life. It's not like an academic setting, where the teacher can educate a student's intellect and then go home, and there is no personal connection between student and teacher. In the ashram, we live together day in and day out. It's not a question of one or two months, or even one or two years—it's a long time. When students live in a spiritual community, in company with each other, they also learn from each other, their brothers and sisters of the same spiritual family. These are helpful connections to be cherished for a long time on the Self-healing journey.

## GURUKULA AND THE TRADITION OF LINEAGE

The *gurukula* is a traditional system of learning where the student lives with the teacher. *Gurukula* literally means "the guru's home." The student prepares for Self-knowledge and the teacher has time to understand the student's readiness to receive this knowledge. For young students, sometimes it takes more than ten years. In ancient times, the youngest student could be sent at the age of six to live with the guru and stay ten to twelve years, during which the teacher would guide them like a parent. The teacher would then indicate the path for the student to follow. For some students, the teacher would say, "Go and lead a good life as a householder," and for other students, "Stay in the ashram and continue your spiritual journey here."

## THE TEACHER'S TRADITION

This system of transmission of spiritual knowledge is based on the direct guru-disciple relationship. It is a spiritual relationship, based on the need of the disciple to be guided out of their spiritual ignorance. The main theme of the teaching is always: how to be free from ignorance and how to come closer to the Atman. The relationship is based on the student's quest for knowledge and the teacher's compassion and desire to uplift the student.

Self-knowledge is revealed directly to the seeker of truth after a period of preparation, after the students have undergone a period of scriptural studies, training in renunciation of selfishness and development of wisdom.. It doesn't come merely because we desire it. We have to do the practice of purification, study, and learn to renounce the ego. The practice of Karma Yoga helps to renounce the ego. We avoid saying, *"Oh, I like to do this and I don't like to do that,"* or *"Why is this person doing this, and I have to do that."* We don't say, *"I don't like to study with a certain person, because they don't know much; I like the other person, because they are smarter."* All of these thoughts come from the ego.

The teacher is the classical instrument of spiritual realization for the student; the teacher is important. The student should remember that they, too, will one day become a teacher. The teacher/student relationship is a karmic one, fulfilling the desire for knowledge of the student and the willingness and compassion of the teacher to share knowledge.

### Guru Parampara

**The lineage of Self-knowledge,** called *Guru Parampara,* is alive. It is the lineage of passing spiritual knowledge from teacher to student in an unbroken chain.

In Sivananda Yoga Vedanta Centers, we display pictures of Swami Sivananda and Swami Vishnudevananda, together representing the Self-knowledge lineage, which can be traced back to the founder of the lineage, Adi Shankaracharya in the eighth century AD.

The purpose of the lineage traditionally is to preserve, store in memory, and transmit the knowledge that leads to self-realization. In this system of education, you learn with your entire being, body, mind, and spirit in daily life; it's not merely academic or intellectual. You receive something important, something that becomes your way of life, and you pass it on naturally to the next generation of students, who will one day become teachers. But it cannot be passed on by ego; it's passed on by realization. And if you follow a lineage, it will increase the preciousness and the value of the teaching, as it passes through the memory of the ages. This is the gift, the value of the lineage.

## PROCESS OF SELF-KNOWLEDGE ACCORDING TO VEDANTA

Vedanta proposes a rational understanding of the self as a prelude to an intuition of the Self. There are many steps to go through in this process. They are the four classical paths of Yoga: Karma Yoga, Hatha Yoga/Raja Yoga, Bhakti Yoga, and Jnana Yoga. Practice the four paths in daily life, plus meditation and Vedanta philosophy and Self-knowledge will deepen.

The Vedantic process for Self-knowledge is: 1) being exposed to knowledge through teachings and scriptures, 2) contemplation and self-inquiry on the truth of the teachings, and 3) long meditation on the truth of the teachings until Self-realization through intuition. The guru is involved in this process throughout: 1) by educating the intellect of the student about the truth of the scriptures, 2) by helping the student to purify and to do self-inquiry in daily life, thus developing the qualifications of discrimination (*viveka*) and detachment (*vairagya*), and 3) by being a lifelong living example of the state of being in the world and simultaneously being out of the world—established in the Truth of oneness of the Self.

Initiation into a tradition activates the memory of the past and awakens the traditional knowledge, the classical Yoga, that stands the test of time and has been passed down silently over a long period of time. It has the value of Truth. The practice is lifelong, bringing into memory the intuition and the consciousness of past teachers.

Through this connection to the lineage, one taps into the eternal knowledge of Truth. Meeting the guru is meeting your *Atman* or Self. When we meet the guru, we can see ourselves through the eyes of self-awareness, through the eyes of the guru. Normally, we only see ourselves through the eyes of other people, society, family, books, and secular teachers. We might have many teachers, but the teacher of Self-knowledge is the only true guru, the only real teacher of the Truth.

## THE PROCESS OF SELF-KNOWLEDGE IN THE GURUKULA

Gaining Self-knowledge and self-awareness is a slow process. Each person is unique. The teacher must uncover the veils over our eyes; this process can take a long time. Each student has their unique relationship with the teacher; it's not one size fits all. Some teachers will have a few students, but other teachers will have many students. Swami Sivananda and Swami Vishnudevananda taught the masses—they had a lot of students—but they had only a few disciples or fully-committed students. We cannot compare teachers. Nor can we compare ourselves with our classmates—out of jealousy, or even for the sake of comparison—because most of the time, in this journey of Self-knowledge, through the guru-disciple relationship, we are unique and it is our behavior that will qualify us as an *adhikari* (a ready student) or not.

Most of the time, we will struggle when trying to acquire the qualifications of a ready *sadhaka*, but this is mostly a struggle within ourselves. There is also a struggle with the teacher; often, we blame the teacher for our miseries. Our ego expects a teacher to behave a certain way, we expect that the teacher is there to love us, please us and praise us. We think that our ego is correct all the time. But often, it's the opposite; the teacher might be stern towards you and not acknowledge you.

### Testimony of Swami Sitaramananda

*When I was initially serving Swami Vishnudevanandaji as his correspondence secretary, or sometimes as his driver, and he said thanks to me for whatever I had done, it felt like pinpricks, because if I am serving him, and I am him, it doesn't make sense for him to thank me.*

*So I thought, "Oh my God, what did I do wrong?" It's like every day you talk to your hand saying, "Hand, thank you for doing the job for me." It doesn't make sense. We are part of one whole, the same, but our ego expects and projects this separation. So we like praise and we like to be praised.*

Life in an ashram, in company of the ashramites, is amazingly rich and intense. It is a life of Yogic purification. We learn to see the Self in all, experiencing multitudes of circumstances and people. We learn detachment from our mental patterns. We learn tolerance, selflessness and flexibility in daily life.

## THE HIDDEN MYSTICAL SCIENCE OF GURUPARAMPARA

During the journey of self-qualification, when the intuitive knowledge is not yet accessible, according to Swami Sivananda, one positive thing we can remind ourselves of is that this transmission of spiritual knowledge is real; the transmission through the ages, the *Guru Parampara,* is real.

Swami Sivananda said, *"Just as you can give an orange to a person, so this spiritual power, spiritual knowledge, can be transmitted from one person to another. This is a hidden mystical science."*

Thus to receive the teacher's guidance, to access this hidden mystical science, service to teachers is necessary. The student must do a lot of hard inner work. The grace of the guru is necessary, however, the whole work must be done by the student. The most important person in the guru-disciple relationship is the student. The student is the one who wants Self-knowledge. The student is the one who is coming closer to the Truth; the majority of the work is done by the student, not the teacher. The hungry man has to eat for himself; the thirsty person has to drink for himself. At the same time, guru's grace is important and *satsanga* is important. As much as possible, try to keep the company of teachers.

### Testimony of Swami Sitaramananda

> *"I did not know that I was suffering from a condition quite common to many, a state of fragmentation, stress, and disharmony that comes from being disconnected from the divine spirit or being unable to see your Self. I did not know that I was a prisoner of my mind and my moods. The radiance emanating from Swamiji was overwhelming and impressive. I felt an unconditional love, that was like a fresh breeze in the desert land of normal human relationships. Swamiji was warm, direct, happy, and simple. No place for nonsense and complications.*
>
> *At 28, I already knew that my academic learning and professional achievements had not given me the formula to understand myself and life, how to be happy, and how*

*everything fit together. I did not understand that true learning involved embracing the idea, "I know that I don't know," then learning, "I don't know that I know," and finally asserting, "I know that I know." This is all about ego and non-ego, how to manage the ego and the mind for true knowledge to happen."*

## HOW TO CHOOSE YOUR GURU

Swami Sivananda gave some guidelines on how to choose your guru. *"If you find peace in the presence of a Mahatma (*Atman *means "soul" and* maha *means "great," so "a great soul"), if you are inspired by his or her speeches, if he or she can clear your doubts, if he or she is free from greed, anger, and lust, if he or she is selfless, loving, and I-less, you can take him or her as your guru. Once you choose your guru, implicitly follow him or her."*

**If you're not able to find your guru,** for a sincere *sadhaka*, or seeker, who is on the path of purification, help comes mysteriously. When the time is right, guru and disciple are brought together by the law of karma in an mysterious way.

### Testimony of Swami Sitaramananda

*"My meeting with Swami Vishnudevananda and the Sivananda Yoga Vedanta Center was like a miracle. I used to go to work passing in front of the Yoga Center, but I never noticed it. It took a burnout crisis due to overwork (I used to be a social worker) to slow me down. I took a leave of absence and was, for the first time, awakened to a humble, non-action, contemplative attitude and a new reverence for life. I recognized that I needed to work on myself before trying to save the world. I found out that the books and teachers around me did not have the answers to the questions I had in mind about life; I was craving for answers. The answers came in the form of Swami Vishnudevananda's lectures and company, Swami Sivananda's books and the teachings of the Vedantic lineage they belong to."*

## STICK TO ONE GURU

Swami Sivananda advised to *"stick to one guru," because, "the truth is one, but the paths are many." Swami Sivananda's advice in learning is to "listen to all, but follow one; gather knowledge from all, but adopt the teachings of one master. Dig deeply in one place and you are sure to find water."*

Beware of the temptation to compare or mix different teachings and teachers. Why? Because Sivananda said, it's like following different doctors. When you don't feel well, you go to multiple doctors, and you mix their advice. He said, *"From one doctor you get a prescription, from two doctors you get a consultation, and from three doctors you get your cremation."*

If we have many gurus, we'll be bewildered and lost as to what to do. We must beware of our egoistic tendency to question the teacher and not surrender. When we do so, we put the knowledge relationship in jeopardy, because the teacher has to have empathy for the student to transmit energy and teach them. On the contrary, the student must have openness, love, respect, and devotion to receive the knowledge. But, if something does not please the student, and they question and fight, the knowledge relationship is in trouble. Then we may return to the old, individualistic self from the beginning of our journey!

## SATSANGA IN DIFFERENT FORMS

If we don't have the presence of a teacher in our life, we can have *satsanga* through books and the writings of a master.

> **Story of Swami Sitaramananda**
>
> *"The powerful words of Swami Sivananda in his books paved my way to knowledge and practice. No aspect of life is not covered by him. His books gave me the answers I had been seeking for so long. Swami Vishnudevananda's lectures and practical teaching in the ashrams and centers bridged the teaching of theory and practice and transformed my life."*

We want everything to come easily. We want the teacher to come to us. We don't want to go to the teacher. But, if we cannot find the live *satsanga* of a master, we can resort to reading their books. Swami Sivananda wrote over 200 books; we can read these or listen to his *satsanga*. Nowadays, we can find *satsanga* online. Swami Vishnudevananda did not write many books, but he made thousands of audio recordings. His disciples continue the teaching of the lineage through many different courses containing the teaching of the masters. For example, the Yoga Teachers Training Courses come directly from the lineage.

## INCREASE SATSANGA, DECREASE KUSANGA

In order to increase and protect our practice, we need to increase our *satsanga*, our wise company, association with like-minded individuals who support our spiritual journey. We need to engage in activities that uplift and inspire our devotional attitude.

At the same time, decrease our *kusanga*, time spent in negative company or association with individuals or activities that are considered unfavorable or detrimental to our spiritual growth and well-being. This can include associating with individuals who have negative attitudes, engaging in harmful behavior, or indulging in materialistic and ego-driven activities. *Kusanga* is believed to have a negative influence on our consciousness and can lead to distraction, attachment to worldly desires, and a decrease in devotion and connection to the Divine.

Usually, it is not helpful to keep negative company—based on material connections, familial connections, convenience and alliances, personal friendships—devoid of a common endeavor to search for truth and self-realization. Eventually, try to spiritualize all relationships.

People who are seekers on the path after truth can become spiritual brothers and sisters. Keep *satsanga*, always being in the company of those who are also seeking to know the truth, as it will protect emerging spiritual aspirations. Of course, when we are strong, we can have such *satsanga* with everybody; we can see the Divine in everyone and learn lessons from them. However, at the beginning of our journey, when we are not strong and established in sadhana, it is better to detach from *kusanga*.

**Daily Satsanga format and schedule** in the Sivananda Yoga Vedanta Organization

- **6:00–7:30am,** guided group silent meditation, group call-and-response kirtan, and a lecture from a teacher of the lineage or readings from books and materials from the gurus. (Not material from Google the guru! We speak from books and material from the gurus, because the words used by the gurus have power in themselves.) The *satsanga* format also includes closing prayers, peace prayers, closing *arati*, or the ceremony of light.
- **7:30–9:00pm,** to end the day, the same session is repeated.

**Satsanga is forever.** In the *Bhagavad Gita*, Shri Krishna said, *"Neither in this world, not in the next, is there destruction for him that follows the teaching. Verily, none who does good ever comes to grief. Having attained to the world of the righteous and having dwelt there for everlasting years, he who fell from Yoga is reborn in the house of the pure and wealthy, or he is born in a family of the wise Yogis"* [VI:40–42].

Spiritual connections and spiritual support on the path of Self-healing might take a lifetime, or many lifetimes; they are eternal or timeless connections.

A disciple will find their guru from lifetime to lifetime, as we continue from where we left off. No spiritual learning goes to waste.

### Story of a six-year-old Yogi

*During our annual Yoga Children's Camp, there was a little boy, six years old, born in a family of Yogis. He was the youngest of all the students, but he was the most mature. Other children, older than him, just wanted to play and go on outings like water sliding, etc. But this young boy came up to me and asked, "Is this a Yoga camp or an outing camp?"*

### Testimony of Swami Sitaramananda

*When I had initiation with my teacher, Swami Vishnudevanandaji, I felt a very, very old connection, as if I had known him for a long, long time. I come back, time and time again, to visit this memory, which has guided me all these 40 years.*

*Does this mean I met the same Swami Vishnudevanandaji in a past lifetime? No. It just means that I have been practicing over many, many lifetimes and the desire for knowledge was very strong. According to the karmic law of the universe, a teacher will manifest and teach exactly what you need in this lifetime.*

*In this lifetime, I was born in Vietnam and had to battle for many years with the question of war and peace. I was sent to snowy Quebec, by accident, to study. There I met a particular Yogi, Swami Vishnudevananda, who came from India and from the Yogic lineage of Swami Sivananda and who was dedicated to world peace. This is how the universe gave me what I needed.*

## IMPORTANCE OF A SPIRITUAL DIARY

Our last point on satsanga and how to protect our self-awareness is the importance of keeping a spiritual diary, as a method of satsanga. Let's say that a student is not in company with the teacher. Perhaps the student has already studied from spiritual books and, periodically, takes some courses. It is good, at that time, that the student keeps a spiritual diary, recording the sadhana, but also speaking with his higher mind that is close to the Self, the *Atman*. The student will be following their own progress by objectively recording sadhana practice daily and facing their lower mind.

It is important to keep a daily routine, and the spiritual diary is the record of our practice. It keeps us honest—our own soul is watching. The spiritual diary is essential in establishing the practice, and not falling victim to short-term enthusiasm, or the illusions of the mind.

## CONCLUSION

To understand the teacher/guru tradition and this unique system of transmission of spiritual knowledge, we need to tune deep within and tap to the source of our own inner voice seeking for perfection and for release from suffering. Many misconceptions of the sacred teacher/student relationship are circulating in the world today.

We are blessed to be exposed to this ancient system and we pray that more can have access to it in this modern technological, egalitarian, utilitarian, separated and individualistic era, where there is confusion between wisdom and information and where it is still debated whether AI (artificial intelligence) is sentient or not.

Being highly intellectual, added to being highly emotional, will not equal being devotional.

Devotion is, in itself, wisdom. It is entirely different than being emotional.

May we all become wise through devotion and *satsanga.*

*Loka samastha sukhino bhavantu*
May the whole world attain peace and harmony.

*Asato Ma Sat Gamaya*
*Tamaso Ma Jyotir Gamaya*
*Mrityor Ma Amritam Gamaya*
Lead me from the unreal to the real

From darkness to light
From mortality to Immortality

*Om Purnamadah Purnamidam*
*Purnat Purnamudachyate*
*Purnasya Purnamadaya*
*Purnameva Vashishyate*
Om. That is whole. This is whole.
From the whole, the whole becomes manifest.
From the whole, when the whole is negated,
What remains is again the whole.

*Om Shanti Shanti Shantihi*
Om Peace Peace Peace

# Sample Spiritual Diary

| | MONDAY | TUESDAY | WEDNESDAY | THURSDAY | FRIDAY | SATURDAY | SUNDAY | TOTAL |
|---|---|---|---|---|---|---|---|---|
| What time did you get up? | | | | | | | | |
| How many hours did you sleep? | | | | | | | | |
| How long did you meditate? | | | | | | | | |
| How long did you do Kirtan? | | | | | | | | |
| How long did you do Pranayama? | | | | | | | | |
| How long did you do Asanas? | | | | | | | | |
| How long studying spiritual books? | | | | | | | | |
| How long in Karma Yoga? | | | | | | | | |
| How long in mouna? | | | | | | | | |
| How much charity given? | | | | | | | | |
| How many lies told? | | | | | | | | |
| How long and how often angry? | | | | | | | | |
| What virtue are you developing? | | | | | | | | |
| What vice are you eradicating? | | | | | | | | |
| What time did you go to bed? | | | | | | | | |

## *INSPIRED STORY*

### "I am not this body"

*Swami Vishnudevanandaji was in a very bad car accident in Canada. It was a front-end collision. Not wearing a seat belt, Swamiji had a concussion, broken ribs, and punctured lungs. He was put on a waterbed, because he could not move without significant pain. Upon hearing the news, I felt for his injured body and thought to myself, "Oh, poor Swamiji!" I flew in to visit him from California.*

*When I entered his hospital room, with one glance at him, the thought came, "Poor me! I am the one who is young and with a strong body; his body is completely smashed. And yet, it is clear that he is not his body; he was radiating peace, strength, wisdom, and prana while in this physical state." I was in a completely different state of mind and consciousness. The only thing that moved in his body were two of his fingers, holding the mala beads and doing japa.*

*All the nurses in the hospital liked to come and serve this special patient!*

### QUESTIONS

1. *Explain the beneficial relationship of a beginner on the spiritual path with the cultivation of satsanga. Why is it important to have a teacher, guide, guru?*
2. *Describe the connection between the ancient teacher/student tradition, the notion of lineage of Self-knowledge and the process of Self-knowledge according to Vedanta.*
3. *Why is it advisable to stick to one guru/lineage?*
4. *What is kusanga? Give some examples.*
5. *How can the practice of keeping a spiritual diary be compared with the practice of satsanga?*

# Glossary

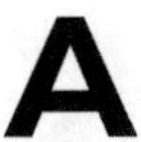

**Abhinivesha** ............................ Will to live; fear of death or attachment to life

**Abhishekam** ............................ In puja, bathing the deity with water

**Abhyanga** ............................... Ayurvedic warm oil massage

**Abhyasa** .................................. Consistent practice

**Acharya** .................................. Spiritual teacher; holder of a lineage; one who teaches from the scriptures

**Adhibhautika** ........................ The afflictions caused by beings around you

**Adhidaivika** ........................... Suffering caused by Divine forces or the forces of heaven, including natural disasters

**Adhyatmika** ........................... The afflictions or problems caused by one's own body

**Adi Shankaracharya** ................ 8th century Indian Vedantic scholar and teacher, who teaches advaita vedanta and who found 10 classical monk orders in India.

**Adikhari** ................................. A prepared, ready student

**Advaita** .................................... Non dual

**Agami karma** .......................... Future karma that you create in this lifetime

**Agni** ........................................ Fire; the cosmic fire; fire of digestion

**Agnihotra** ............................... Vedic fire offering; homa

**Aham** ....................................... "I"; the root of ahamkara

**Aham Bhahman Asmi** .......... "I am Brahman"

**Ahamkara** ............................... Ego; egoism; process of individuation or identifying ourselves with the body and mind in opposition to everything else in the world

**Ahimsa** .................................... Principle and practice of non-violence and non-injury toward all living beings; respect for life

**Aim** .......................................... Bija mantra of Saraswati

**Ajna chakra** ............................ Third eye chakra; energy center located between the eyebrows

**Akhanda** .................................. Continuous

**Akhanda kirtan** ...................... Continuous kirtan

**Alabdhabhumikatva** .............. Doubting progress, lacking optimism, doubting potential for further progress

**Alayasa** ................................... Burnout, laziness in body and mind

**Ama**........................................ Toxins that come from undigested food
**Ambika Devi**.......................... The name of the strong form of the power of the universe that removes all nonsense
**Anahata chakra**..................... Heart chakra; energy center located in the heart center
**Ananda** ....................................Bliss absolute
**Anandamaya kosha** ............ Bliss sheath; corresponds to causal body; the seed of karma
**Anavasthitatva** ...................... Inability to maintain stability, inability to maintain progress or gains, tendency to slide backwards
**Annamaya kosha** ................. Food sheath; physical layer of the body
**Antah** .................................... Inner
**Antahkarana**.......................... The totality of the mind; the instrument of seeing
**Anuloma viloma**.................. Alternate nostril breathing
**Anuvasana** ............................ Enema using medicated oil - oil enema helps lubricate the system and remove all the lipid soluble waste; one of five actions of Ayurvedic Pancha Karma
**Apana vayu** ........................... Downward moving air; subdosha of vata that governs elimination of negative thoughts
**Aparigraha**............................ Non-grasping; non-accumulation; not taking more than one needs in life
**Arati** ...................................... Light ritual when light is waived and offred to deities along with mantras and songs
**Archana**.................................. Worship, such as puja
**Arjuna**.................................... One of Pandava prince, main character in Bhagavad Gita
**Artha** .......................................Prosperity; economic values, material gain; ability to earn income and take care of oneself and one's family; accumulation of wealth; desire for wealth; one of the four goals of life
**Asana** ...................................... Yoga posture; steady pose; yogic exercise; in puja, giving the deity a seat
**Ashram** ................................... Yogic spiritual center or monastery
**Ashramas**................................ Four phases of human life according to physical age and psychological maturity, asociated with these stages in life are corresponding duties and responsibilities.

**Ashtanga yoga**........................ 8 limbs yoga, Raja Yoga
**Asmita**.................................... Egoism or I-ness, sometimes also describes as ahamkara, the individuation or development of ego
**Asteya**.................................... Non-stealing; non-covetousness; not desiring something that is not yours
**Astral body** ............................ Subttle body
**Atma-nivedanam** ....................Complete self-surrender to the Divine
**Atmakaraka** ........................... Indicator of the purpose or mission in life of the soul
**Atman** .................................... Soul; immortal Self
**Aum** ....................................... A-U-M; the mantra Om written to indicate the three syllables of the word though it is pronounced as one syllable
**Avidya** .................................... Spiritual ignorance; forgetting one's true nature as Spirit; lack of awareness of the real truth of existence
**Avirati** .................................... Desires, cravings, self-indulgence, non-dispassion
**Ayurveda**................................ Ancient system of medicine of India

# B

**Bandha** ....................................Lock; energetic lock
**Bhagavad Gita** .........................Ancient hindu scripture, scripture on Yoga
**Bhagavate**............................... Divine
**Bhakta**..................................... Devotee
**Bhakti**...................................... Devotion
**Bhakti Yoga**............................ The yoga of devotion; the practice of sublimation of desire and relationships; one of the four paths of yoga
**Bhrantidarsana**...................... False perceptions, delusion, misunderstanding
**Bija mantra** ............................ The mono syllable seed sound that is hidden in all the formula mantra
**Brahmachari**........................... One whose whole life is focused and moving inward and upward towards Brahman
**Brahmacharya**........................ Sensory and sexual restraint; control or one's passions and desires; control or sublimation of sexual energy and sensual desires; practice of restraining the tendency to seek sensual pleasure as the goal of life; sexual continence or complete abstinence

**Brahmacharya Ashrama** ...... Student phase of life 6-25 years of age, focused on learning, self-development and control

**Brahmacharya Life** ............. A celibate life dedicating to realizing Brahman; a life of self-restraint and sublimation of sexual energy, of all energy, into ojas shakti

**Brahmamuhurta**.................. Time between 4 a.m.-6 a.m.; sunrise; auspicious time in morning for spiritual practices

**Brahman** .............................. Pure consciousness; the ultimate reality underlying and pervading everything

**Brahmin**............................... The highest category or varna of the four types of humans in which sattvic qualities dominate characterized by purity, knowledge and wisdom; represented by teachers, scholars and priests

**Bramasthan** ......................... In traditional Indian architecture, the most powerful and holy spot of any property or house; the space at the middle of the house

**Buddhi** ................................. Intellect; intelligence; the higher mind

# C

**Chaitanya**............................. Spiritual consciousness or the knowledge of the Divine

**Chakra** ................................. Energy center

**Chamunda** ........................... The demon

**Charya** ................................. Occupation with, engaging, or following; connected to the idea of acharya or teacher

**Chit** ...................................... Knowledge absolute

**Chitta** ................................... Total mind

# D

**Dama**.................................... Control over the senses; the ability to control the senses and, therefore, reactions to external stimuli

**Dasha** ................................... In Vedic Astrology, a period of life

**Dasya**.................................... Cultivate feelings of being servant of God

**Deepa** ................................... In puja, waving a lamp or offering the fire to illuminate the freshly decorated deity

**Deva** ..................................... God

**Devanagari**........................... Sanskrit; the language of the Gods

**Devata** .................................. Deity

**Devi**....................................... The Goddess

**Dharana** ................................ Concentration of the mind

**Dharma** ................................ Purpose, duty, truth; righteousness; morality; duties, rights, laws, conduct and virtues and the right way of living; the desire to grow, to understand, to be in line with the rules of life; desire to do good and be good; one of the four goals of life

**Dhoopa** ................................ In puja, spreading incense smoke throughout the altar

**Dhyana** ................................ Meditation, 7th rung in Raja Yoga scripture

**Dhyana Slokas** ...................... Sacred prayers; special mantras recited before you start any kind of spiritual endeavor or spiritual learning class

**Diksha1** ................................ Initiation

**Doctrine of Karma** ............... Doctrine comprised of the Law of Action and Reaction, the Law of Compensation and the Law of Retribution

**Dosha** ................................... Ayurvedic constitution

**Dukkha** ................................ Suffering

**Durga** ................................... Divine mother, represents inner strength, divine protection

**Dvesa** ................................... Repulsion; tendency of the mind to move away from things it dislikes; together with raga refers to the swinging of the mind between likes and dislikes, love and hate

# E

**Ekagrata** ............................... The one-pointed state of mind; deeply concentrated state of mind

**Existential** ............................ Relating to our own existence as human beings

# G

**Govinda** ............................... Name of Krishna

**Grihastha Ashrama** ............. "Householder stage of life 25-50 years of age, focused on raising a family, fulfilling societal and family responsibilities and accumulating wealth and material possessions"

**Guna** .................................... Temperment; attribute or quality of nature, of which there are three - sattva, rajas and tamas

**Guru** ..................................... Spiritual teacher; guide; one who dispels darkness;

**Gurukula** ............................. The guru's home; the place where the teachers and students live together; the traditional yogic system of the the student living with the teacher

**Guruparampara**.................... The lineage of spiritual knowledge passed on from teacher to student, from one generation to the next

## H

**Ha**......................................... Solar energy

**Hanuman**.............................. The monkey God; the God of wind; the power of devotion and selfless service

**Hara** ...................................... Name of Siva

**Hari**....................................... Name of Vishnu

**Hatha Yoga**........................... Yoga method focusing on balancing Ha and Tha - sun and moon energy

**Hatha Yoga Pradipika** .......... scripture on Hatha Yoga

**Homa** .................................... Vedic fire offering; agnihotra

**Hridaya** ................................. Spiritual heart

## I

**Ida nadi**................................. Lunar energy channel of the body; corresponds to left nostril

**Indra** ..................................... King of the Gods

**Indriyas**................................. The organs of perception and the organs of action

**Ishanya**.................................. In traditional Indian architecture, northeast corner of the house which is considered the most auspicious corner of the house and the location where God resides

**Ishta Devata**.......................... One's personal, chosen deity of worship

**Ishwara** ..................................God, highest ideal on world of Maya

**Isvarapranidhana** ................. Self-surrender; surrender to a higher power or committing oneself completely to Brahman

## J

**Japa** ....................................... Mantra repetition

**Japa mala** .............................Strand of prayer beads

**Japa yoga**.............................. A method of meditation using the sound vibration of mantra

**Jaya**........................................ Victory

**Jiva** ........................................ Individual soul, Atman identifying with body and mind

| | |
|---|---|
| **Jnana Yoga** | The yoga of knowledge; path of yoga that focuses on discrimination and vairagya or dispassion through self inquiry; one of the four paths of yoga |
| **Jyotish** | Vedic astrology; "science of light" |

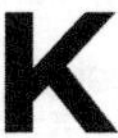

| | |
|---|---|
| **Kailasa** | Holy abode of Siva |
| **Kama** | Sensual pleasures; love; seeking of pleasure and the enjoyment of the senses; one of the four goals of life |
| **Kapalabhati** | Strong, quick inhalation/exhalation breathing technique; "shining skull" breat" |
| **Kapha dosha** | Constitution made up of earth and water elements; energy of construction, lubrication and nourishment |
| **Karakas** | Planet significators that determine on which person or thing a planet has influence |
| **Karana** | Instrument |
| **Karma** | The universal law of cause and effect; action and the result of action |
| **Karma indriya** | Organs of action |
| **Karma Yoga** | Purification through selfless service; sublimation of your actions, the desires for the results, the desire to be somebody; resolving all the karmic debts that are the results of past thoughts, desires and actions by not continuing to desire, expect and act out of ignorance; detachment to your actions and the results of your actions; one of the four classical paths of yoga |
| **Kartikeya** | Also called Subramanya; Lord of War; son of Lord Shiva and Parvathi; brother of Lord Ganesh |
| **Ketu** | Considered like a planet in Vedic Astrology, it is the south intersection point of the path of the sun and the moon |
| **Kirt** | To praise |
| **Kirtan** | Singing God's glory; singing of Divine names; glorification of the Divine through singing |

**Klesha** .................................... "Poison," or mental state; there are five kleshas in the yogic tradition, considered to be the causes of suffering or impediments to spiritual growth

**Kosha** .................................... Veil; layer; sheath

**Krishna** .................................... A major deity in Hinduism, worshiped as the eighth avatar of Lord Vishnu and as a Supreme God in his own right; the god of protection, compassion, tenderness and love; the aspect of the Divine that brings peace, sustenance and harmony; representation of Divine Love

**Kriya** .................................... Action, deed, effort; a "completed action;"; a technique or practice within a yoga discipline meant to achieve a specific result

**Kshatriya**.................................... The second highest category or varna of the four types of humans in which the qualities of rajas mixed with sattva predominate characterized by passion, energy and action; represented by the warrior or ruling class

**Kundalini** ....................................High spiritual energy or force; the serpent power

**Kusanga** .................................... Negative company or association with individuals or activities that are considered unfavorable or detrimental to one's spiritual growth and well-being

## L

**Lagna**....................................Ascendant sign in Vedic Astrology

**Lagnesh**.................................... In Vedic Astrology, planet ruler which represents your overall life

**Lakshmi** .................................... One of the principal goddesses in Hinduism; the goddess of prosperity, wealth and spiritual progress

**Likhita Japa**.................................... The practice of continuous writing of a mantra

**Lokah Samasta**.................................... chant Prayer for the world: "May the whole world attain peace and harmony"; Loka samastha sukhino bhavantu

# M

**Madhyama** ............................ An inner, subtle, more eternal state of sound; it's inaudible to the physical ear but higher in wavelength and is more powerful

**Maha** .................................... Great

**Maha Myritunjaya mantra** .................................. Also known as Om Tryambakam mantra; mantra for protection that can be used for many different occasions

**Mahadeva** .............................. Siva

**Mahamrityunjaya mantra** .................................. Om Tryambakam mantra; mantra used for daily protection

**Mahatma** ................................ A person revered for high-mindedness, wisdom and selflessness

**Mala bead** .............................. Rosary, prayer bead

**Mananam** .............................. Reflection, thinking; referring to reflecting on and thinking about the teachings

**Manas** .................................... The sensory mind; outer mind

**Manipura chakra** ................. Navel chakra; energy center located at the navel center

**Manomaya kosha** ................. Mental sheath; layers of the mind; the mind, emotions and senses

**Mantra Sanskrit** ................... invocation of the Supreme Being

**Mantra diksha** ...................... Mantra initiation

**Meru bead** .............................. Central bead in a mala beard, not to cross over while doing japa

**Mitahara** ............................... Eat half or half full

**Moha** ..................................... Delusion

**Moksha** .................................. Liberation; the soul's emancipation from the cycle of death and rebirth; the desire to be free from spiritual ignorance, which is the cause of suffering; the highest of the four goals of life

**Mudra** .................................... Seal; energetic seal

**Muhurta** ................................. In Vedic Astrology, the timing of events

**Muladhara chakra** ............... Root chakra; energy center at the base of the spinal column

**Mumukshutva** ....................... Desire for liberation

**Murti** ...................................... A statue or symbol of the Divine

**N**

**Nadi** .................................... Subtle energy channel
**Namaskara** ............................ Respecful greeting or parting salutation in Hindu and yogic traditions
**Namo**.................................... salutations and prostrations, to bow
**Narayan**................................. Lord Vishnu
**Nasya oil**............................... Medicated herbal oil
**Nasyam** ................................. Oiling of the nostrils or nasal instillation of medicated substances helps clear the respiratory tract and sinuses and helps eliminates high kapha; one of the five actions of Ayurvedic Pancha Karma
**Nauli** ..................................... One of kriya cleansing exercise
**Neti pot** ................................ Special pot for dispensing salt water for nasal irrigation
**Neti-neti** ............................... "Not this, not that"; the Vedantic refutation or negation method that brings one to their true nature
**Nididhyasan**........................... Meditation
**Nirguna Mantra**.................... Mantra without form
**Niyamas** ................................ The five yogic inner observances

**O**

**Ojas** ....................................... Energy of contentment, endurance and sustenance; immunity; the subtle energy that sustains health and life
**Ojas shakti** ............................ The power and sustenance of life that gives you contentment, endurance or perseverance and happiness in living this life
**Om** ......................................... The universal mantra
**Om Namah Sivaya** ................ Mantra of Lord Siva
**Om Namo Narayanaya**...........Mantra of Lord Vishnu
**Om Tryambakam mantra** .................................. Mahamrityunjaya mantra; mantra for protection that can be used for many different occasions

**P**

**Panchanga**.............................. Five qualities of light at the moment of birth; how the Sun and Moon relate to each on a daily basis and in particular on your day of birth
**Pada-sevana** ........................... Service with humility, or literally 'service at the feet

of the lord'

**Pancha Karma** ...................... Ayurvedic detoxification and rejuvenation therapy

**Pancha koshas**........................ The five veils of consciousness; the five layers or sheaths of the body

**Para Brahman**........................ Supreme reality; supreme consciousness

**Para Shakti**............................ Universal, high feminine Divine energy; the Divine creative force

**Para state of sound** ............... A potential state of sound, undifferentiated; sound that is not expressed

**Parvati**.................................... Wife of Lord Shiva

**Pashyanti**................................ A very high and powerful wavelength of sound; sound at a telepathic or universal level

**Patanjali Maharishi**................ Great sage and teacher of yoga, compiler of yoga sutras

**Pingala nadi** ............................ Solar energy channel of the body; corresponds to right nostril

**Pitta dosha** ............................. Constitution made up of fire and water (oil) elements; energy of transformation

**Pradakshina**........................... In puja, circumambulating the altar and bidding farewell to the deity

**Prakriti** ................................. The manifest world; nature

**Prakruti** ................................. Original constitution at conception

**Pramada**................................. Distraction, negligence, impatience, haste

**Prana**...................................... Vital energy; universal energy or life force

**Prana vayu** ............................. Inward moving air of the body; subdosha of vata that governs receptivity and vitalizes mind

**Pranamaya kosha**.................. Prana sheath; breath sheath; vital energy layer

**Pranayama** ............................ Yogic breathing practices; the control of prana

**Prarabdha karma**.................. Karma of the present life; the result of past actions that manifest in the present in this life

**Pratyahara** ............................ Withdrawal of the senses; control of the senses as a practice to purify the senses

**Pranava mantra** ..................... Repetition of the "OM" mantra

**Prema** ..................................... Love of God; Divine or unconditional love, devotional love; pure love

**Puja** ......................................... A ritual or ceremony through which you express Divine love

**Punya** ...................................... Merit

**Purushartha**........................... Self-effort; inner motivation; (four kinds of)

desires or motivations we are born with

**Pushpa** ................................ In puja, offering fresh flowers while chanting the deity's names

# R

**Radha** ................................ Lord Krishna's favorite devotee

**Raga** ................................ Attachment; tendency of the mind to gravitate toward things it likes; together with dvesa refers to the swinging of the mind between likes and dislikes, love and hate

**Rahu** ................................ Considered like a planet in Vedic Astrology, it is the north intersection point of the path of the sun and the moon

**Raja Yoga** ................................ Kingly Yoga, classical 8 limbs Yoga

**Rajas** ................................ Quality of action, passion, egoism

**Raktamokshana** ................................ Blood-letting, this is not commonly used in modern times; one of the five actions of Ayurvedic Pancha Karma

**Rama** ................................ Incarnation of Vishnu

**Rasa** ................................ Essence

**Rishi** ................................ Sage or seer of ancient times

**Rudraksha mala** ................................ Mala made of the sacred rudraksha bead, also known as Shiva's tears; mala to Lord Shiva

# S

**Sadashiva** ................................ Name of Siva

**Sadguru** ................................ True guru

**Sadhaka** ................................ Spiritual aspirant; spiritual student

**Sadhana** ................................ Conscious spiritual practice; ; conscious training of the mind, body, heart and spirit; daily yogic routines of asana, pranayama and meditation

**Sadhu** ................................ A holy man, sage or religious ascetic that has renounced the worldly life; often one who travels from place to place living off food given to them

**Saguna mantra** ................................ Mantra with the form of the deity

**Sahasrara chakra** ................................ Crown chakra; energy center located at the crown of the head; corresponds to the pineal gland

**Sakhya** ................................ Cultivate feelings of friendship with God

**Sakshi** ................................ Silent witness

**Sama**........................................ Serenity, calmness, tranquility; maintaining a state of equanimity

**Samadana**................................ Balance with attention; when the mind no longer gets distracted and no longer loses balance and is always focused on the goal; one-pointedness of mind or total concentration and focus

**Samadhi**................................... Deep meditative state; experience of complete meditation; the superconscious state

**Samana vayu**............................ Assimilating air of the body; subdosha of vata that helps mental digestion and gives contentment to mind

**Samsara**.................................... The cycle of death and rebirth

**Samsaya**.................................... Self-doubt, lack of self-worth, low self-esteem

**Samskara**................................... Impressions in the mind; deep pattern of thinking or behavior

**Sanchita karma**........................ The accumulation of all of the actions that you have done through all past lifetimes

**Sankalpa**.................................... Intention

**Sankara**...................................... Name of Siva

**Sannyasa**.................................... Renunciation stage of life

**Sannyasa Ashrama**.................. Final stage of life 75 - end of life focused on attaining God-realization and Moksha, liberation from the cycle of birth and death

**Santosha**..................................... Contentment; without desires or expectations

**Sanyasin**..................................... Renunciate

**Sara adhija vyadhji**.................. Causation of disease

**Saraswati**.................................... Goddess of knowledge, wisdom and creativity

**Sarvangasana**........................... Shoulderstand

**Sat**................................................ Truth consciousness

**Sat Sampat**................................ The six-fold virtues that must be acquired to become a sadhaka or practitioner of yoga

**Satchitananda**........................... Truth-consciousness-bliss

**Satsampat**.................................. Six virtues of the mind to cultivate to make the mind stronger and realize the truth

**Satsanga**.................................... Association with wise, good, uplifting people; like-minded individuals who support your spiritual journey

**Sattvic**......................................... Characterized by purity, clarity, light, balance

**Sattva** .................................... Quality of purity, knowledge, balance

**Satya** .................................... Truth; the virtue of truthfulness; the practice of sincerity and honesty; honest living

**Saucha** .................................... Cleanliness; the practice of both internal and external purity;

**Savasana** .................................... Corpse pose; resting pose; proper relaxation; conscious relaxation

**Shakti** .................................... Cosmic energy; universal, high feminine Divine energy; the Divine creative force; power

**Shambo** .................................... The quiet, auspicious form of Lord Shiva

**Shankaracharya** .................................... Adi Shankaracharya; 8th century Indian Vedantic scholar and teacher of advaita vedanta

**Shanti** .................................... Peace

**Shanti mantra** .................................... A Vedic chant with a certain specific way of chanting it

**Shinrin-yuoku** .................................... Forest bathing; being in nature in a conscious and mindful way

**Shiva** .................................... The supreme lord of yoga; the third god of the Hindu triad and he is the God of Destruction

**Shradha** .................................... Faith; trusting in the path of Jnana Yoga

**Shravanan** .................................... Listening, particularly listening to stories of the Divine

**Shudra** .................................... The lowest category or varna of the four types of humans in which tamasic qualities dominate characterized by ignorance and inaction; represented by the service providers or laborers

**Siddhasana** .................................... Accomplished pose of meditation

**Siddhi** .................................... Spiritual power

**Sirsasana** .................................... Headstand

**Sita** .................................... Wife of Rama

**Siva** .................................... The supreme God in Hinduism; supreme consciousness

**Smaranam** .................................... Remembrance, with regard to the teachings; remembrance of God's name and presence in prayers

**Snaana** .................................... In puja, bathing the deity with various auspicious items

**Soma** .................................... Divine nectar

**Sraddha** .................................... Faith

**Sri** ........................................ Title of respect
**Styana** ........................................ Mental torpor, apathy, lack of motivation, disinclination
**Sublimation** ........................................ Channel the energy of lower desires and pursuits into higher spiritual pursuits
**Subrahmanya** ........................................ Also called Kartikeya; son of Siva and Parvati; brother of Lord Ganesh, chief general of army of Gods
**Sukha sthanam** ........................................ Well-being of body-mind-spirit
**Surya** ........................................ The sun god
**Sushumna nadi** ........................................ Central energy channel of the body
**Svadharma** ........................................ Personal dharma; the basic dharma is towards one's own body; practicing dharma that includes our specific, unique duties, responsibilities and righteousness
**Svadyaya** ........................................ Self-study; long, deep contemplation about the truth and your true nature; introspection based on the study of the Vedantic scriptures
**Swa** ........................................ Self
**Swadhisthana chakra** ........................................ Sex chakra; energy center located at the genital area
**Swami** ........................................ "One who is one with himself"; A Hindu ascetic or religious teacher; specifically a senior member of a monastic religious order

## T

**Tamas** ........................................ Quality of inertia, darkness, ignorance
**Tantra** ........................................ The classical tradition that teaches us about gods and goddesses around us and teaches us how to communicate with them through sacred worship
**Tapas** ........................................ Austerity or self-discipline
**Tat Twam Asi** ........................................ "That you are"
**Tejas** ........................................ Subtle fire energy of pitta; gives one courage, fearlessness, insight to spiritual path
**Tha** ........................................ Lunar energy
**Titiksha** ........................................ Endurance, strength of mind to keep you going on the spiritualpath through the long, slow journey of purification; endurance or perseverance through suffering

**Tra** ........................................ To protect, our to free
**Twameva song** ..................... Dedication song; daily song offering dedication of all of your actions

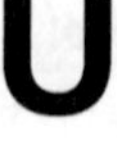

**Udana vayu** ........................... Upward moving air of the body; subdosha of vata that provides mental energy, will and strength
**Uddiyana bandha** ................ one of Hatha yoga lock of energy
**Upadhi** .................................. Separating or limiting factor; limiting adjunct; often used in referring to the mind and physical body
**Upanishads** ........................... Vedantic scripture
**Uparati** ................................. Satiation; meaning having had enough of external pleasures, the mind is ready to turn inward, away from the allurements of the senses; renouncing anything that doesn't fit your dharma (duty)

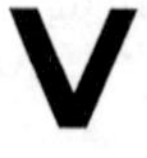

**Vandana** ................................ Worship
**Vaidya** .................................. Ayurvedic practitioner
**Vaikhari** ................................ A gross audible sound; dense audible sound, sound in its maximum differentiation
**Vairagya** ............................... Detachment; dispassion; detachment from the unreal or from what by nature is changing and is not true
**Vaishya** ................................. The second lowest category or varna of the four types of humans in which rajas and tamas predominate characterized by passion, egoism and lethargy; represented by business people, trades people, merchants
**Vamanam** ............................. Therapeutic emesis, induced vomiting helps clear the upper gastro till the duodenum (end of stomach); one of the actions of the five Ayurvedic Pancha Karma
**Vanaprastha** ......................... Retirement stage of life 50-75 years of age focused on focus on spiritual pursuits such as meditation, the study of scriptures, and reflection and preparing for the final stage of life

**Varnas** ........................................ Four categories of humans based on their gunas or innate qualities

**Vasana** ........................................ Deeply rooted thoughts; thoughts and mental tendencies of the mind; mental thought waves which are considered to be the primary cause of disease; desire

**Vastu** ........................................ Vedic science of space; the study of how to live according to natural law, according the cosmic energy, and it is the natural basis for architecture

**Vastu Shastra** ........................ The traditional system of Indian architecture based on Vedic science of space

**Vasudeva** ................................ Lord Krishna

**Vata dosha** .............................. Constitution made up of air and wind elements; energy of action and movement

**Vayu:** ........................................ Wind; wind of the body

**Vedanta** ..................................... A Hindu philosophy based on the doctrine of the Upanishads, especially in its monistic form; the teaching of oneness or unity consciousness

**Vedantic mantra** ...................... Repetition of the Mahavakyas

**Vedantin** .................................. One who practices the philosophy of Vedanta

**Vedas** ........................................ Books of knowledge, ancient scriptures

**Vedic Sciences** ......................... The Vedic sciences include Jyotish (vedic astrology, science of time), Ayurveda (the science of healing), Tantra (the knowledge of universal patterns of energies underlying visible and invisible worlds, includes science of mantras, yantra, and sacred myths) and Vastu (science of space and placement) and last but not least, the science of Yoga and Vedanta philosophy.

**Vichara** ..................................... Self-inquiry

**Vidya** ........................................ True knowledge

**Vijnanamaya kosha** ................. Intellectual sheath;

**Vikruti** ...................................... Present constitution that is changed or imbalanced

**Virechanam** ............................. Purgation - induced purgation clears the intestines evacuating the bowels and eliminates high pitta; one of the five actions of Ayurvedic Pancha Karma

**Visuddha chakra** ........ Throat chakra; energy center located at the base of the throat

**Viveka** ........ Discrimination, particularly between the real and unreal; discriminative intelligence

**Vritti** ........ A modification of the mind; thought; thought energy force

**Vyadhi** ........ illness or disease

**Vyana vayu** ........ Circulating air of the body; subdosha of vata that helps free flow of ideas and independence in the mind

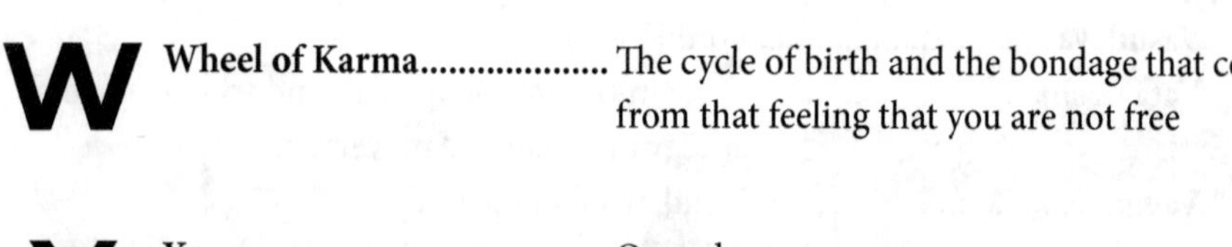

## W

**Wheel of Karma** ........ The cycle of birth and the bondage that come from that feeling that you are not free

## Y

**Ya** ........ One who goes or moves

**Yamas** ........ The five yogic restraints or moral codes

**Yantra** ........ A sacred geometrical figure, used for meditation

**Yoga** ........ Union, completeness, wholeness; balanced state of mind

**Yoga asana** ........ Yogic exercise, yoga póture

**Yoga chikitsa** ........ Yoga therapy

**Yoga chitta vritti nirodhah** ........ This verse is most important verse in Raja Yoga sutras, referring to yoga is the control of all mental modifications

**Yoga nidra** ........ Yogic sleep; deep relaxation

**Yoga Sutras** ........ Raja yoga scripture from Patanjali. A sutra is a condensed string of words

**Yoga Vasishta** ........ Jnana Yoga scripture

**Yogi** ........ A person who practice yoga

**Yuga** ........ A period of time

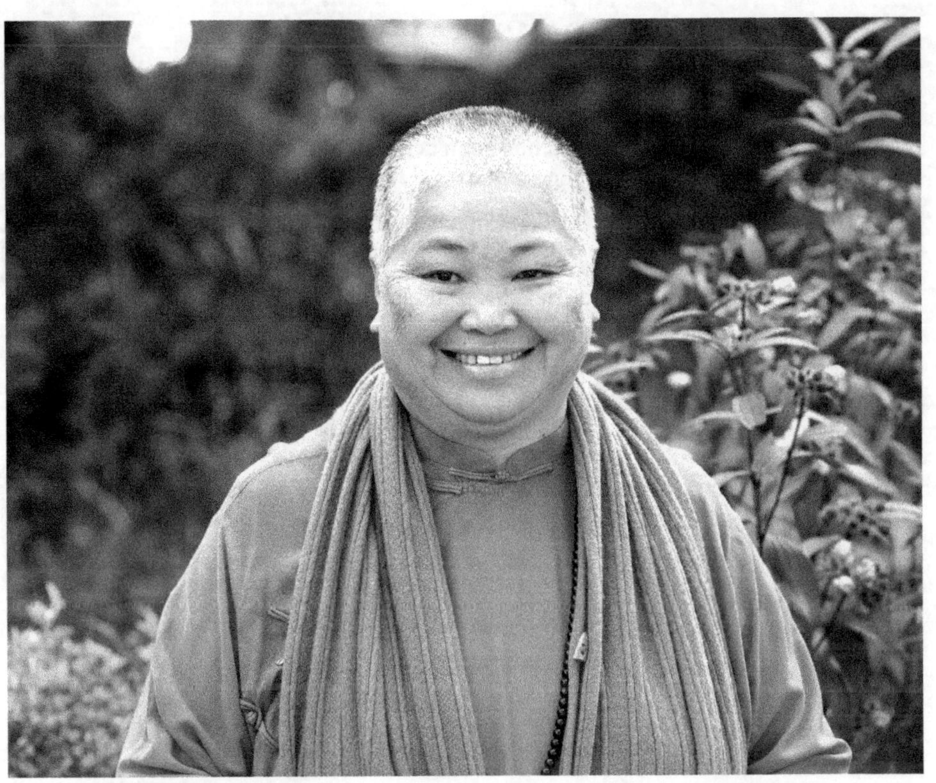

**Swami Sitaramananda** is the acharya of SYVC and direct disciple of Swami Vishnudevananda scince 1982. She is spiritual director of the Sivananda Ashram Yoga Farm in Grass Valley, CA, USA and the Sivananda Yoga Resort and Training Center in Dalat, Vietnam.

She is author of many books: Essentials of Yoga Practice and Philosophy (translated into Chinese, Japanese and Vietnamese), Positive Thinking Manual, 108 Yoga Health Tips, Guru's Grace, The Answers lie within, Learning Selfless Love.

Swami Sita's Blogs
https://sivanandayogafarm.org/blog/

Swami Sita's Podcast
https://sivanandayogafarm.org/podcast/

## ABOUT THE SIVANANDA ASHRAM YOGA FARM

The Sivananda Ashram Yoga Farm was founded by Swami Vishnudevananda in 1971, on 80 acres in the beautiful Sierra-Nevada foothills, three hours north of San Francisco. Swami Sitaramananda has been acharya of the Ashram for last 30 years.

One of the oldest classical ashrams in North America, the Yoga Farm has become a recognized center of classical Yoga training on the West coast, and has been renovated and expanded over the years. The concepts and teachings detailed in this book are put into daily practice in ashram life, through various programs, courses, workshops, asana classes, and community meals.

### Contact Information

To register for programs, courses, or retreats, or to register as a volunteer Karma Yogi or work-study, please contact us:

**Yoga Farm Sivananda Ashram**

*14651 Ballantree Lane*

*Grass Valley, CA 95949*

*Tel: 532 272 9322*

*Web: sivanandayogafarm.org*

*Email: yogafarm@sivananda.org*

The Sivananda Yoga Resort and Training Center was founded in Dalat Vietnam in 2017 by acharya Swami Sitaramananda. Like Sivananda Ashram Yoga Farm, the Ashram offers classes, retreats, and courses outlined in this book.

**Sivananda Yoga Resort and Training center**

*K'Lan Resort, Hoa Hong Str., Ward. 4, Tuyen Lam Lake,*

*Dalat City, Vietnam*

*Tel: (+84) 263 6501100*

*Web: sivanandayogavietnam.org*

*Email: vietnamyogaresort@sivananda.org*

# Acknowledgments

We would like to give thanks to Sivananda Ashram Yoga Farm Grass Valley CA and Sivananda Yoga Resort and Training center Dalat, Vietnam staff, for their dedication and assistance in gathering materials, in transcribing and in editing and particularly to Swami Jnaneswariananda, Swami Pranavananda, Swami Sivasankariananda, Shakti Chaitanya, Sivakami Chaitanya. We would also like to thank the graphic design work of Sivashakti Chaitanya.

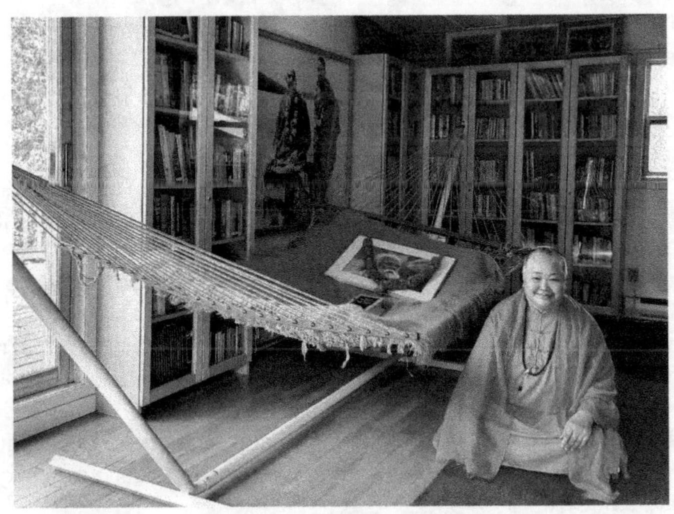

## INTERNATIONAL SIVANANDA YOGA VENDANTA ASHRAM AND CENTERS

Founded in 1957 by Swami Vishnu-devananda

### ASHRAMS

**Sivananda Ashram Yoga Camp**
673 8th Avenue, Val Morin
Québec, J0T 2R0, CANADA
+1 819 322 3226
www.sivananda.org/camp
yogacamp@sivananda.org

**Sivananda Ashram Yoga Retreat**
P.O. Box N 7550
Paradise Island, Nassau, BAHAMAS
+1 416 479 0199
www.sivananda.org/bahamas
nassau@sivananda.org

**Sivananda Ashram Yoga Ranch**
P.O. Box 195, 500 Budd Road
Woodbourne, NY 12788, U.S.A.
+1 845 436 6492
www.sivananda.org/ranch
yogaranch@sivananda.org

**Sivananda Ashram Yoga Farm**
14651 Ballantree Lane, Comp. 8
Grass Valley, California 95949, U.S.A.
+1 530 272 9322 | +1 800 469 9642 (USA)
www.sivananda.org/farm
yogafarm@sivananda.org

**Ashram de Yoga Sivananda**
26 impasse du Bignon,
45170 Neuville aux bois, FRANCE
+33 2 38 91 88 82
www.sivananda.org/orleans
orleans@sivananda.net

**Sivananda Yoga Retreat House**
6370, Reith near Kitzbühel, AUSTRIA
+43 53 56 67 404
www.sivananda.org/tyrol
tyrol@sivananda.net

**Sivananda Yoga Vietnam Resort and Training Center**
K'lan Resort, Hoa Hong Street
Ward 4, Tuyen Lam Lake
Dal Lat City, Lam Dong Province, VIETNAM
+84 263 650 1100
www.sivananda.org/vietnam
vietnamyogaresort@sivananda.org

**Sivananda Yoga Vedanta Dhanwantari Ashram**
P.O. Neyyar Dam, Dt. Thiruvananthapuram Kerala 695 572, INDIA
+91 94 9563 0951
www.sivananda.org/neyyardam
guestindia@sivananda.org

**Sivananda Kutir**
P.O. Netala, Uttara Kashi District
Uttaranchal, Himalayas 249193, INDIA
+91 90 12 78 94 28 | +91 99 27 09 97 26
www.sivananda.org/netala
Himalayas@sivananda.org

**Sivananda Yoga Meenakshi**
New Natham Road, Saramthangi
Village Vellayampatti P.O. Madurai
Dt. 625 503, Tamil Nadu, INDIA
+91 98 6565 5336, +91 98 6515 5335
www.sivananda.org/madurai
madurai@sivananda.org

**Sivananda Yoga Tapaswini**
Guthavaripalem, Kadivedu P.O.,
Chilakur Mandalam – 524410, Gudur
Nellore DT., Andhra Pradesh, INDIA
+91.89850 45125 | +91 89850 45251
www.sivananda.org/gudur
gudur@sivananda.org

## SYVC CENTERS
## SOUTH AMERICA

**Asociación de Yoga Sivananda**
Acevedo Diaz 1523
Montevideo 11200, Uruguay
Tel: +598 2401 0929/6685
Mobile: +598 98 200 070
montevideo@sivananda.org
www.sivananda.org/montevideo

## ISRAEL

**Sivananda Yoga Vedanta Centre**
6 Lateris Street, Tel Aviv 64166, Israel
Tel: +972 3 6916793
telaviv@sivananda.org
www.sivananda.org/telaviv

## NORTH AMERICA

**Sivananda Yoga Vedanta Center**

243 West 24th Street
New York, NY 10011, U.S.A.
Tel: +1 212 255 4560
newyork@sivananda.org
www.sivananda.org/newyork

**Sivananda Yoga Vedanta Center**
1246 West Bryn Mawr
Chicago, Illinois 60660, U.S.A
Tel: + 1 773 878 7771
chicago@sivananda.org
www.sivananda.org/chicago

**Sivananda Yoga Vedanta Center**
3741 West 27th Street
Los Angeles, California 90018
Tel: + 1 310 822 9642
losangeles@sivananda.org
www.sivananda.org/la

**Sivananda Yoga Vedanta Centre**
5178 Saint Laurent Boulevard
Montreal, Quebec, H2T 1R8, Canan-
da
Tel: +1 514 279 3545
montreal@sivananda.org
www.sivananda.org/montreal

**Sivananda Yoga Vedanta Centre**
77 Harbord Street
Toronto, Ontario, M5S 1G4, Canada
Tel: +1 416 966 9642
toronto@sivananda.org
www.sivananda.org/toronto

## SYVC CENTERS
### EUROPE

**Sivananda Yoga Vedanta Centre**
45 – 51 Felsham Road
London SW15 1AZ, UK
Tel: +44 20 8780 0160
london@sivananda.net
www.sivananda.org/london

**Sivananda Yoga Vedanta Zentrum**
Luisenstraße 45,
80333 München, Germany
Tel: +49 89 700 9669 0
munich@sivananda.net
www.sivananda.org/munich

**Sivananda Yoga Vedanta Zentrum**
Schmiljanstrasse 24
D-12161 Berlin, Germany
Tel: +49 30 85 99 97 98
berlin@sivananda.net
www.sivananda.org/berlin

**Sivananda Yoga Vedanta Zentrum**
Prinz Eugen Straße 18
Vienna 1040, Austria
Tel: +43 1 586 34 53
vienna@sivananda.net
www.sivananda.org/vienna

**Centre Sivananda de Yoga Vedanta**
1 rue des Minoteries
Geneva 1205, Switzerland
Tel: +41 22 328 03 28
geneva@sivananda.net
www.sivananda.org/geneva

**Centre Sivananda de Yoga Vedanta**
140 rue du Faubourg Saint-Martin
75010 Paris, France
Tel: +33 1 40 26 77 49
paris@sivananda.net
www.sivananda.org/paris

**Centro de Yoga Sivananda Vedanta**
Calle Eraso 4
Madrid 28028, Spain
Tel: +34 91 361 51 50
madrid@sivananda.net
www.sivananda.org/madrid

**Sivananda Jogos Vedantos Centras**
M.K. Ciurlionio g. 66
Vilnius 03100, Lithuania
Tel: +370 8 64 87 28 64
vilnius@sivananda.ne
www.sivananda.org/vilnius

## INDIA

**Sivananda Yoga Vedanta Centre**
TC 37/1927 (5), Airport Road West Fort P.O.
695 023 Thiruvananthapuram, Kerala, India
Tel: +91 471 245 0942, mobile: +91 9497008432
trivandrum@sivananda.org
www.sivananda.org/trivandrum

**Sivananda Yoga Vedanta**
**Nataraja Centre**
A-41 Kailash Colony, New Delhi 110 048, India
Tel: +91 11 4059 1221, +91 11 2924 0869
mobile: +91 88 60 95 44 55
delhi@sivananda.org
www.sivananda.org/delhi

**Sivananda Yoga Vedanta**
**Dwarka Centre**
PSP Pocket, Sector – 6
(near DAV school, next to Kamakshi Apts)
Swami Sivananda Marg
Dwarka, New Delhi 110 075, India
Tel: +91 11 64 56 85 26, +91 11 45 56 6015/6
dwarka@sivananda.org
www.sivananda.org/dwarka

**Sivananda Yoga Vedanta Centre**
3/655 (Plot No. 131) Kaveri Nagar Kuppam Road
Kottivakkam, Chennai 600 041, India
Tel: +91 44 2451 1626, +91 44 2451 2546
chennai@sivananda.org
www.sivananda.org/chennai

**Sivananda Yoga Vedanta Centre**
444, K.K. Nagar, East 9th Street
625 020 Madurai, Tamil Nadu, India
Tel: +91 0452 2581170, +91 0452 4393445
Mobile: +91 9092240702
maduraicentre@sivananda.org
www.sivananda.org/maduraicentre

## SYVC CENTERS
### ASIA

**Sivananda Shojiko Retreat**
789 Shoji, Fujikawaguchiko-Machi, Minamitsuru-Gun,
Yamanashi-Ken, Japan 401-0336
Tel: +81 555 87 2250
shojikoretreat@sivananda.jp
www.sivananda.jp/eng/shojiko-retreat/

**Tokyo center**
Funabashi4-21-3, Setagaya-ku, Tokyo, Japan
156-0055
Tokyo@sivananda.org
https://sivanandajp.org/

**Sivananda Yoga Vedanta Centre Hochiminh**
147/8 Nguyen Dinh Chinh, Ward 11, Phu Nhuan Dist., HCM City, Vietnam
Ho Chi Minh City, Vietnam
Tel: +84 6680 5427, +84 6680 5428
hochiminh@sivananda.org
www.sivananda.org/hochiminh

**Sivananda Yoga Vedanta Centre Dalat**
B2-11 Golf Valley, Ward 2, Dalat city, Lam Dong, Vietnam
Tel.: +84 263 650 1900
dalat@sivananda.org
www.sivananda.org/dalat

**Sivananda Yoga Vedanta Centre Hanoi**
68, Alley 12, Dang Thai Mai str., Quang An Ward, Tay Ho, Hanoi, Vietnam
Tel.: +84 243 996 3339
hanoi@sivananda.org
www.sivanandayogavietnam.org

# Index

SWAMI SIVANANDA, renowned sage and yogi of Rishikesh, Himalayas, foresaw, the need for Yoga in the modern world and sent his disciple SWAMI VISHNUDEVANANDA to the West in 1957.

Swami Vishnudevananda took the core of yogic teachings and broke it down for the Western mind, eventually creating the International Sivananda Yoga Vedanta Centres to educate and train yogis in both the East and West.

In this stressful world, Yoga transcends all differences and helps millions of people worldwide to reconnect with their inner life, to find peace of mind in a world of conflict and distractions, and to recognize their inner joy, power and health.

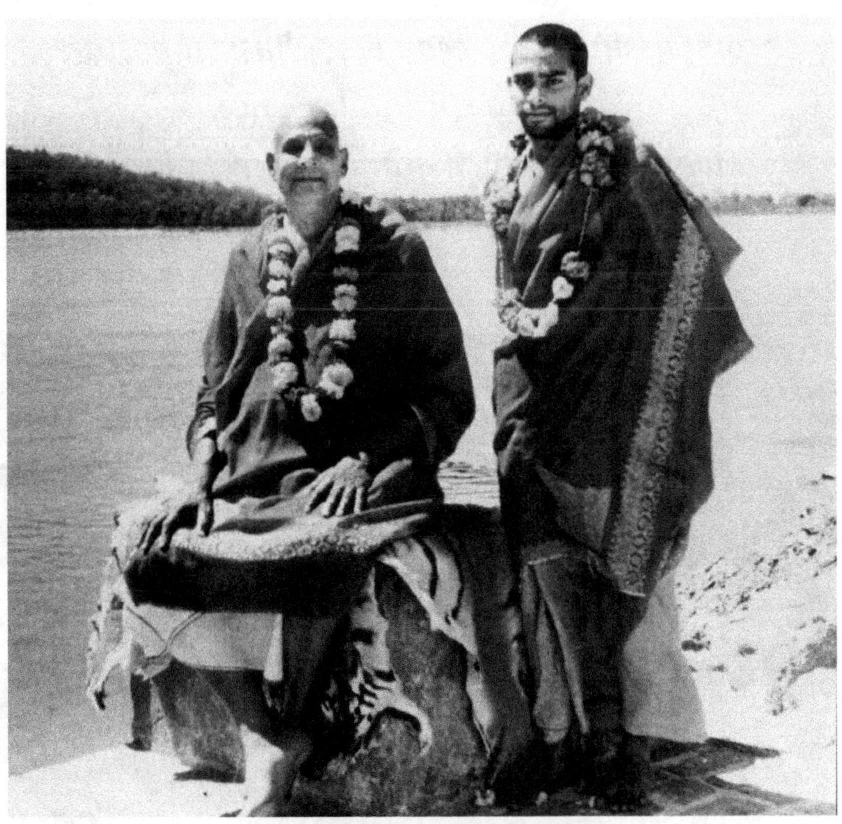

*Encompassing more than just physical postures,*
*Yoga is a spiritual science,*
*a way of life which grants peace, balance,*
*and freedom from suffering.*

# *Endorsements for*
# *Yoga Sadhana for Self-Healing*

"*Yoga Sadhana for Self-Healing* is an insightful, in-depth and many-sided explication of the profound powers and practices of Yoga, Ayurveda and Vedanta to heal body and mind, and to guide us to the highest Self-awareness and harmony with the whole of life. Swami Sitaramananda shares her many years of study, practice and teaching to make these yogic secrets accessible today. Natural Healing and experiential spirituality should go together as part of a deeper path to Self-Realization such as she explains.

**David Frawley,**
American Institute of Vedic Studies

"This book is a much-needed and comprehensive primer for emotional maturity and spiritual awakening. It offers a safe blueprint for liberation from samsāra, a life of constant complaints and discontent. The magnum opus of Sri Swami Sitaramamanandaji, *Yoga Sadhana for Self Healing* is a compilation of a life-time of expertise and experience written in a language that is easy to read and retain. Sri Swami Sitaramamanandaji's pragmatism, incisive clarity, and compassion are evident in her in-depth discussion of all matters pertaining to yoga as a way of life that helps one to eventually discover the Vedantic vision of oneness with everything and everyone. Through this book— a priceless offering to the world— Swamiji has demystified the spiritual path, laying bare the inner work that one has to do to regain physical and emotional equilibrium, and discover a sense of connection and purpose in one's life.

**Swamini Swatmavidyananda,**
Arsha Vijnana Gurukulum

"In this time of transition and uncertainty, when many are grappling with stress-related physical, emotional, mental, and spiritual challenges, Swami Sitaramananda's book emerges as a beacon of light. It delves deeply into holistic health, self-knowledge, purification, resilience, stress management, and the integration of Yoga and Ayurveda into daily life.

*Yoga Sadhana for Self-Healing* offers profound insights into increasing vitality, understanding karma and the causes of suffering, and the transformative power of sadhana (spiritual practice).

Swami Sitaramananda's vast experience and compassionate teaching shine through every page, making complex and ancient wisdom accessible to all readers. This book is not only practical but also deeply rooted in ancient traditions, bringing profound knowledge in an easily comprehensible manner.

It is an invaluable resource for personal growth and spiritual awakening."

**Swami Swaroopananda,**
acharya of Sivananda Yoga Vedanta Centers